Toxicity and Human Health Assessment of Air Pollutants

Toxicity and Human Health Assessment of Air Pollutants

Guest Editors

Ting Wang
Tingting Ku
Jia Xu

MDPI

Basel • Beijing • Wuhan • Barcelona • Belgrade • Novi Sad • Cluj • Manchester

Guest Editors
Ting Wang
College of Environmental Science and Engineering
Nankai University
Tianjin
China

Tingting Ku
College of Environment and Resource Sciences
Shanxi University
Taiyuan
China

Jia Xu
State Key Laboratory of Environmental Criteria and Risk Assessment
Chinese Research Academy of Environmental Sciences
Beijing
China

Editorial Office
MDPI AG
Grosspeteranlage 5
4052 Basel, Switzerland

This is a reprint of the Special Issue, published open access by the journal *Toxics* (ISSN 2305-6304), freely accessible at: https://www.mdpi.com/journal/toxics/special_issues/LZOA06Q27O.

For citation purposes, cite each article independently as indicated on the article page online and as indicated below:

Lastname, A.A.; Lastname, B.B. Article Title. *Journal Name* **Year**, *Volume Number*, Page Range.

ISBN 978-3-7258-5677-0 (Hbk)
ISBN 978-3-7258-5678-7 (PDF)
https://doi.org/10.3390/books978-3-7258-5678-7

Contents

About the Editors

Ting Wang

Ting Wang is an associate researcher of the College of Environmental Science and Engineering, Nankai University. Her research field focuses on the health impacts of air pollution and related mechanisms, including clarifying the characteristics of key source pollution, providing data support for precise source tracing and targeted governance of atmospheric pollution, revealing the key mechanisms of health hazards, providing a scientific basis for the assessment of health effects and early prevention of pollution exposure, and quantitatively evaluating the effects of emission reduction policies. She has published over 50 SCI-indexed papers in prestigious international journals such as *Adv Mater*, *JGR–Atmos* et al. She obtained four authorized inventions, two utility models, and authored a monograph. She has led numerous national, provincial, and ministerial-level scientific research projects. She has been selected into the Tianjin Innovation Talent Program, the first batch of young scientific and technological talents in the ecological environment field of Tianjin, and outstanding young scientific and technological workers of the Tianjin Youth Scientific and Technological Workers Association and holds various social positions. She was awarded the First Prize of Tianjin Science and Technology Progress.

Tingting Ku

Tingting Ku is a professor at the College of Environmental and Resource Sciences, Shanxi University. Her research focuses on the health effects of air pollution and its toxicological mechanisms, including elucidating the key molecular initiating events and adverse outcome pathways underlying its toxicity, providing a scientific basis for accurate health risk assessment, identifying critical toxic components, and quantitatively evaluating the effectiveness of regulatory measures and green alternative chemicals. Dr. Ku has led several important research projects, including two funded by the National Natural Science Foundation of China. In addition, she has contributed to key research initiatives under the National Key Research and Development Program of China. Dr. Ku has also led one General Program funded by the China Postdoctoral Science Foundation and one youth project supported by the Shanxi Provincial Foundation. She has published over 20 high-impact SCI papers in leading journals in environmental science and toxicology, including *Proceedings of the National Academy of Sciences*, *Environmental Science & Technology*, *Environmental International*, *Particle and Fibre Toxicology*, and *Journal of Hazardous Materials*. She has been recognized as an Outstanding Young Talent of the Three Jin Talents Program, Shanxi Province, and as a Wenying Scholar at Shanxi University. Additionally, she is an active young member of the Chinese Society of Toxicology in the field of analytical toxicology.

Jia Xu

Jia Xu is an Associate Research Fellow at the State Key Laboratory of Environmental Criteria and Risk Assessment, Chinese Research Academy of Environmental Sciences (CRAES). She earned her Ph.D. in Environmental Science from Nankai University in 2014 and completed postdoctoral training at the University of Washington, USA, from 2016 to 2019. She joined CRAES in August 2020 and was promoted to Associate Research Fellow in the same year. Her research primarily focuses on air pollutant exposure modeling and health risk assessment, source apportionment and oxidative toxicity of atmospheric particulate matter, and the mechanistic links between air pollution and adverse health effects. She has led multiple research projects, including the National Natural Science

Foundation of China (Youth Program), and subprojects under the National Key R&D Program. To date, she has published 12 SCI papers as the first or corresponding author in high-impact journals such as *Environmental Science & Technology*, *Science of the Total Environment*, *Environmental Pollution*, and *Environmental Research*. She also serves as a reviewer for several leading journals in environmental science.

toxics

MDPI

Editorial

Toxicity and Human Health Assessment of Air Pollutants

Ting Wang [1,*], Tingting Ku [2] and Jia Xu [3]

[1] Tianjin Key Laboratory of Urban Transport Emission Research, College of Environmental Science and Engineering, Nankai University, Tianjin 300071, China

[2] Shanxi Key Laboratory of Coal-based Emerging Pollutant Identification and Risk Control, Research Center of Environment and Health, College of Environment and Resource Sciences, Shanxi University, Taiyuan 030006, China; kutingting@sxu.edu.cn

[3] State Key Laboratory of Environmental Criteria and Risk Assessment, Chinese Research Academy of Environmental Sciences, Beijing 100012, China; xu.jia@craes.org.cn

* Correspondence: wangting@nankai.edu.cn

1. Introduction

Air pollution has been shown to be responsible for the morbidity and mortality of a variety of major diseases [1–3]. The World Health Organization (WHO) estimates that almost all of the global population breathes air that exceeds the WHO's guidelines and contains high levels of pollutants [4,5]. To date, however, the key constituents of air pollution that impact health and the potential mechanisms remain largely unstudied [6]. In addition, comprehensive assessments of evidence from in vitro and in vivo studies, high-quality cohort studies, and high-resolution model simulations of health impacts are still substantially sparse [7].

This Special Issue, entitled "Toxicity and Human Health Assessment of Air Pollutants", aims to understand the mechanisms of the health effects caused by air pollution and ensure accurate exposure assessments around ambient environments and inside human bodies. The collated articles employ a range of approaches—from epidemiological cohorts and toxicological studies—to elucidate the linkage between air pollutant exposure and the mechanisms related to health effects. The evidence presented in this Special Issue provides valuable insights for controlling air pollution and reducing the burden on public health.

2. An Overview of Published Articles

The eleven articles published in this Special Issue collectively advance our understanding of the health impacts of air pollution exposures, which can be categorized into four main research directions: elucidating underlying toxicity mechanisms, identifying critical exposure windows and vulnerable populations in epidemiological studies, exploring the impact on postoperative populations, and estimating the association between air pollutant exposure and health effects.

Firstly, several studies delve into the molecular mechanisms that may mediate the link between air pollution exposures and adverse health outcomes. Wang et al. (Contribution 1) indicated that $PM_{2.5}$ induced glomerular hyperfiltration in female mice by affecting RAS/KKS imbalances and the regulation of TGF. They innovatively unveiled the association between subchronic exposure to $PM_{2.5}$ and early kidney injury, highlighting its gender dependence. Gao et al. (Contribution 2) revealed that diesel exhaust caused disrupted lipid metabolism, acute liver injury, and more severe inhibition of cell proliferation and oxidative damage compared to gasoline exhaust particles. Fu et al. (Contribution 3) emphasized that cooking oil fumes (COFs), fine particulate matter ($PM_{2.5}$), and cigarette smoke (CS) could decrease the viability of epidermal HaCaT cells and dermal fibroblast (FB) cells, promote the secretion of pro-inflammatory cytokines IL-1α and TNF-α in HaCaT cells, increase intracellular ROS levels, and downregulate the mRNA expression of collagen I, III, IV, and VII in FB cells, thus leading to skin damage. Yan et al. (Contribution 4) summarized the molecular mechanisms involved in the health effects of $PM_{2.5}$ on adverse birth outcomes regarding cardiopulmonary and neurological developments, primarily including transcriptional and translational regulation, oxidative stress, inflammatory response, and epigenetic modulation.

Secondly, three papers assess the health impact of air pollution exposure by human epidemiology, highlighting critical susceptibility windows, vulnerable subpopulations, and the interactions of mixed exposures. Chen et al. (Contribution 5) found that prenatal exposure to incense-burning smoke (IBS) increased the risk of the presence of obesity in preschoolers, prenatal exposure to IBS combined with a lower frequency of early outdoor activity or a shorter duration of outdoor activity from the ages of 1 to 3 years increased the risk of obesity in preschoolers, and there were additive interactions between prenatal exposure to IBS and postnatal outdoor activity on obesity. Yang et al. (Contribution 6) employed a two-sample Mendelian randomization (MR) analysis that provided genetic evidence for a null causal relationship between air pollutants and NAFLD in the European population. The associations observed in epidemiological studies could be partly attributed to confounders. Han et al. (Contribution 7) illustrated that O_3 exposure was negatively associated with vision disorder. In addition, subgroup analyses revealed that $PM_{2.5}$ exposure was significantly correlated with the risk of glaucoma and age-related macular degeneration and that children and adolescents were more susceptible to NO_2 and $PM_{2.5}$ than adults.

Thirdly, two papers evaluate the impact of air pollutant exposure in postoperative populations. Urbanowicz et al. (Contribution 8) suggested that chronic exposure to ambient air pollutants such as $PM_{2.5}$ may be regarded as an additional risk factor in patients after surgical revascularization with left ventricular dysfunction. Zhang et al. (Contribution 9) found that the presence of the heavy metal of cadmium (Cd) in an atmospheric milieu acts as a catalyst in the progression of tumorigenesis within murine models of colon cancer (CC). The implementation of intestinal stents demonstrates a mitigating effect on tumor incidence within these CC murine models. The effect of Cd on the invasive effect of intestinal stents in the cancerous colon is not significant.

Finally, two papers assess the health effects of air pollutant exposure by modeling approaches. Wang et al. (Contribution 10) used the VSL (value of statistical life) method to find that the number of deaths attributed to $PM_{2.5}$ in Beijing in 2021 fell by 33.74 percent from 2016, while health economic losses will increase by USD 4.4 billion as per capita disposable income increases annually. Wu et al. (Contribution 11) developed spatial models for NO_2 and $PM_{2.5}$ and conducted exposure assessment in Beijing, China. The results showed that the partial least squares (PLS)–ordinary kriging (OK) models for NO_2 and $PM_{2.5}$ had the best performance compared to other spatial modeling algorithms. Hence, the exposure misclassification made by choosing different modeling approaches should be carefully considered, and the resulting bias needs to be evaluated in epidemiological studies.

3. Conclusions

The studies in this Special Issue provide a new understanding of the health impacts of air pollution. They elucidate toxicity mechanisms, identify critical windows and vulnerable populations in epidemiological studies, assess effects on postoperative patients, and estimate health impacts via modeling approaches.

The molecular mechanisms linking air pollution were related to kidney injury, liver damage, and skin aging through oxidative stress, inflammation, and epigenetic changes. Epidemiological research identified early life as a critical exposure window, with air pollution associated with childhood obesity and vision disorders. Postoperative studies indicate that chronic $PM_{2.5}$ exposure worsened outcomes in patients with heart failure, and heavy metals like cadmium may accelerate tumor progression. Epidemiological studies show that despite reduced $PM_{2.5}$-attributable deaths in Beijing, economic costs have risen, emphasizing the necessity for careful exposure assessment in future studies.

This Special Issue highlights the multifaceted health threats of air pollution while underscoring methodological considerations in exposure assessment and the importance of protecting vulnerable subgroups.

Data Availability Statement: The data presented in this manuscript will be made available by the authors upon request.

Acknowledgments: The Guest Editor would like to express sincere gratitude to all the authors for their valuable contributions to this Special Issue, as well as to the reviewers for their time and expertise in evaluating the manuscripts. The editorial team of *Toxics* is also acknowledged for the administrative and technical support they provided throughout the process.

Conflicts of Interest: The authors declare no conflict of interest.

List of Contributions:

1. Wang, H.; Ma, L.; Guo, Y.; Ren, L.; Li, G.; Sang, N. $PM_{2.5}$ Exposure Induces Glomerular Hyperfiltration in Mice in a Gender-Dependent Manner. *Toxics* **2024**, *12*, 878. https://doi.org/10.3390/toxics12120878.
2. Gao, Y.; Zhang, X.; Li, X.; Zhang, J.; Lv, Z.; Guo, D.; Mao, H.; Wang, T. Lipid Dysregulation Induced by Gasoline and Diesel Exhaust Exposure and the Interaction with Age. *Toxics* **2024**, *12*, 303. https://doi.org/10.3390/toxics12040303.
3. Fu, M.; Yang, Y.; Zhang, X.; Lei, B.; Chen, T.; Chen, Y. In Vitro Profiling of Toxicity Effects of Different Environmental Factors on Skin Cells. *Toxics* **2024**, *12*, 108. https://doi.org/10.3390/toxics12020108.
4. Yan, R.; Ma, D.; Liu, Y.; Wang, R.; Fan, L.; Yan, Q.; Chen, C.; Wang, W.; Ren, Z.; Ku, T.; et al. Developmental Toxicity of Fine Particulate Matter: Multifaceted Exploration from Epidemiological and Laboratory Perspectives. *Toxics* **2024**, *12*, 274. https://doi.org/10.3390/toxics12040274.
5. Chen, M.; Strodl, E.; Yang, W.; Yin, X.; Wen, G.; Sun, D.; Xian, D.; Zhao, Y.; Chen, W. Independent and Joint Effects of Prenatal Incense-Burning Smoke Exposure and Children's Early Outdoor Activity on Preschoolers' Obesity. *Toxics* **2024**, *12*, 329. https://doi.org/10.3390/toxics12050329.
6. Yang, J.; Zhang, Y.; Yuan, Y.; Xie, Z.; Li, L. Investigation of the Association between Air Pollution and Non-Alcoholic Fatty Liver Disease in the European Population: A Mendelian Randomization Study. *Toxics* **2024**, *12*, 228. https://doi.org/10.3390/toxics12030228.
7. Han, Z.; Zhao, C.; Li, Y.; Xiao, M.; Yang, Y.; Zhao, Y.; Liu, C.; Liu, J.; Li, P. Ambient Air Pollution and Vision Disorder: A Systematic Review and Meta-Analysis. *Toxics* **2024**, *12*, 209. https://doi.org/10.3390/toxics12030209.
8. Urbanowicz, T.; Skotak, K.; Olasińska-Wiśniewska, A.; Filipiak, K.J.; Płachta-Krasińska, A.; Piecek, J.; Krasińska, B.; Krasiński, Z.; Tykarski, A.; Jemielity, M. The Possible Role of $PM_{2.5}$ Chronic Exposure on 5-Year Survival in Patients with Left Ventricular Dysfunction Following Coronary Artery Bypass Grafting. *Toxics* **2024**, *12*, 697. https://doi.org/10.3390/toxics12100697.
9. Zhang, S.; Li, R.; Xu, J.; Liu, Y.; Zhang, Y. The Impact of Atmospheric Cadmium Exposure on Colon Cancer and the Invasiveness of Intestinal Stents in the Cancerous Colon. *Toxics* **2024**, *12*, 215. https://doi.org/10.3390/toxics12030215.

10. Wang, X.; Dewancker, B.J.; Tian, D.; Zhuang, S. Exploring the Burden of $PM_{2.5}$-Related Deaths and Economic Health Losses in Beijing. *Toxics* **2024**, *12*, 377. https://doi.org/10.3390/toxics12060377.
11. Wu, Y.; Xu, J.; Liu, Z.; Han, B.; Yang, W.; Bai, Z. Comparison of Population-Weighted Exposure Estimates of Air Pollutants Based on Multiple Geostatistical Models in Beijing, China. *Toxics* **2024**, *12*, 197. https://doi.org/10.3390/toxics12030197.

References

1. Xia, X.; Du, Z.; Liu, T.; Xu, K.; Yuan, C. The influence of meteorological factors and air pollution on acute cardiovascular and cerebrovascular events in Western Guizhou. *Sci. Rep.* **2025**, *15*, 22676. [CrossRef] [PubMed]
2. Jia, Y.; Lin, Z.; He, Z.; Li, C.; Zhang, Y.; Wang, J.; Liu, F.; Li, J.; Huang, K.; Cao, J.; et al. Effect of Air Pollution on Heart Failure: Systematic Review and Meta-Analysis. *Environ. Health Perspect.* **2023**, *131*, 076001. [CrossRef] [PubMed]
3. Shang, Y.; Sun, Z.; Cao, J.; Wang, X.; Zhong, L.; Bi, X.; Li, H.; Liu, W.; Zhu, T.; Huang, W. Systematic review of Chinese studies of short-term exposure to air pollution and daily mortality. *Environ. Int.* **2013**, *54*, 100–111. [CrossRef] [PubMed]
4. World Health Organization. *WHO Global Air Quality Guidelines: Particulate Matter ($PM_{2.5}$ and PM_{10}), Ozone, Nitrogen Dioxide, Sulfur Dioxide and Carbon Monoxide*; World Health Organization: Geneva, Switzerland, 2021.
5. Health Effects Institute. *State of Global Air Report 2024*; Health Effects Institute: Boston, MA, USA, 2024; Available online: www.stateofglobalair.org/resources/report/state-global-air-report-2024 (accessed on 19 June 2024).
6. Liang, D.; Li, Z.; Vlaanderen, J.; Tang, Z.; Jones, D.P.; Vermeulen, R.; Sarnat, J.A. A State-of-the-Science Review on High-Resolution Metabolomics Application in Air Pollution Health Research: Current Progress, Analytical Challenges, and Recommendations for Future Direction. *Environ. Health Perspect.* **2023**, *131*, 056002. [CrossRef]
7. Lai, Y.; Koelmel, J.P.; Walker, D.I.; Price, E.J.; Papazian, S.; Manz, K.E.; Castilla-Fernández, D.; Bowden, J.A.; Nikiforov, V.; David, A.; et al. High-Resolution Mass Spectrometry for Human Exposomics: Expanding Chemical Space Coverage. *Environ. Sci. Technol.* **2024**, *58*, 12784–12822. [CrossRef] [PubMed]

toxics

MDPI

Review

Ambient Air Pollution and Vision Disorder: A Systematic Review and Meta-Analysis

Zhuo Han [1,2,†], Chao Zhao [3,†], Yuhua Li [4], Meng Xiao [1,2], Yuewei Yang [1,2], Yizhuo Zhao [1,2], Chunyu Liu [1,2], Juan Liu [1,2,*] and Penghui Li [1,2,*]

[1] School of Environmental Science and Safety Engineering, Tianjin University of Technology, Tianjin 300384, China; hzzzz1pajk@163.com (Z.H.); 18835547676@163.com (M.X.); yyw15133010732@163.com (Y.Y.); zyz@stud.tjut.edu.cn (Y.Z.); liuchunyu981002@163.com (C.L.)

[2] Tianjin Key Laboratory of Hazardous Waste Safety Disposal and Recycling Technology, Tianjin 300384, China

[3] School of Chemical Engineering and Technology, Tianjin University, Tianjin 300072, China; zhao_chao@tju.edu.cn

[4] Shandong Provincial Eco-Environment Monitoring Center, Jinan 250100, China; liyuhua01@shandong.cn

* Correspondence: emptylj@126.com (J.L.); lipenghui406@163.com (P.L.)

† These authors contributed equally to this work.

Abstract: The effects of air pollution on physical health are well recognized, with many studies revealing air pollution's effects on vision disorder, yet no relationship has been established. Therefore, a meta-analysis was carried out in this study to investigate the connection between vision disorder and ambient particles (diameter $\leq$ 2.5 μm ($PM_{2.5}$), diameter $\leq$ 10 μm (PM_{10})) and gaseous pollutants (nitrogen dioxide (NO_2), sulfur dioxide (SO_2), carbon monoxide (CO), Ozone (O_3)). Twelve relevant studies published by 26 February 2024 were identified in three databases. A pooled odds ratios (ORs) of 95% confidence intervals (CIs) were obtained using random-effects meta-analysis models. Meta-analysis results revealed that for every 10 $\mu g/m^3$ increase in $PM_{2.5}$ and NO_2 exposure, a substantially higher incidence of vision disorder was observed (OR = 1.10; 95% CI: 1.01, 1.19; OR = 1.08, 95% CI: 1.00, 1.16). No significant correlation existed between exposure to PM_{10}, SO_2 and CO and vision disorder. However, O_3 exposure was negatively associated with vision disorder. In addition, subgroup analyses revealed that $PM_{2.5}$ exposure was significantly correlated with the risk of glaucoma and age-related macular degeneration and that children and adolescents were more susceptible to NO_2 and $PM_{2.5}$ than adults. Overall, exposure to air pollutants, especially $PM_{2.5}$ and NO_2, may increase the incidence of vision disorder.

Keywords: air pollution; $PM_{2.5}$; NO_2; vision disorder; meta-analysis; odds ratio

1. Introduction

Globally, vision disorder has become an issue with serious adverse effects on people's health and affects people's opportunities in the workplace and school [1]. Vision disorder refers to a limited ability to visually respond to light and structural stimuli due to lesions in the eye or central visual pathways [2]. The most common clinical symptoms include refractive errors (such as nearsightedness, farsightedness, or astigmatism), glaucoma, cataracts, age-related macular degeneration (AMD), and retinal damage caused by diabetes (diabetic retinopathy). According to the included articles, common and severe vision disorders include glaucoma, cataract and AMD, which were taken as the outcome criteria for vision disorder in this study. Age-related degenerative neuropathy glaucoma is a significant contributor to vision disorder and blindness worldwide [3]. Besides increased intraocular pressure, a sufficient but not necessary causing factor for glaucoma greater exposure to $PM_{2.5}$ has been revealed by studies to be associated with its adverse structural features. Thus, air pollution could be a possible risk factor for glaucoma. Cataracts, opacification of the ocular lens, are major reason of functional vision loss [4]. Air related factors such as ultraviolet light, high temperatures, and lack of oxygen may contribute to the formation of cataracts. AMD is a disorder with a late start that results in lipid-rich extracellular deposits, localized inflammation, and eventually neurodegeneration in the macula, the center of the retina [5]. Glaucoma, cataracts, and AMD share some common pathophysiological mechanisms, including increased inflammation and oxidative stress. Should there be a negative correlation between air pollution and vision disorder, then air pollution may be a novel and potentially modifiable risk factor.

Today, air pollution ranks fifth in terms of risks to public health and is an environmental threat to well-being at the global scale, affecting all populations to some extent [6,7]. The World Health Organization (WHO) lists PM (Particulate Matter), O_3 (Ozone), NO_2 (nitrogen dioxide), and SO_2 (sulfur dioxide) as the four most significant air pollutants [8]. Air pollution has long been a serious environmental concern because it can cause a wide range of health problems at different stages of life [9]. Our eyes are continuously taking in the world around us, also various air pollutants [9,10]. Conjunctivitis and dry eye risks are increased by air pollution, and oxidative stress from air pollutants also affect other eye illnesses, according to previous research [5,11].

Recent epidemiological studies have assessed how air pollution exposure and vision disorders are related [10,12,13]. However, our analysis of the pertinent literature revealed that racial disparities, pollution levels, lifestyle choices, and recognized risk factors for vision disorder, such as age, region (The research regions included in this study include China, South Korea, the United Kingdom and Canada), and gender, may have an impact on the findings [14,15]. According to one research exposure to SO_2 and CO (carbon monoxide) was positively related to the prevalence of vision disorder in children [13]. Meanwhile, in another study, PM_{10} (inhalable particles), NO_2, and SO_2 levels were not associated with cataracts [10]. It follows that these associations are heterogeneous. A summary of the connection between ambient air pollution and vision disorder is thus necessary. To evaluate the state of the art and point the way toward further exploration, a meta-analysis was carried out.

2. Materials and Methods

2.1. Search Strategy

As of 26 February 2024, two reviewers independently conducted literature searches on the risk of air pollution and vision disorder outcomes in electronic databases, including PubMed, Embase, and Web of Science. The search strategy is based on a combination of vision disorder (visual impairment, visual disorders, 'disorder, visual', visual disorder, macropsia, visual impairment, micropsia, vision disability, hemeralopia, metamorphopsia) and ambient air pollutants (air pollutants, atmospheric pollutants, sulfur dioxide, nitrogen dioxide, carbon monoxide, ozone, particulate matter, PM, PM_{10}, $PM_{2.5}$, VOCs) keywords. Specific search strategies are provided in Supplementary Table S1.

2.2. Inclusion and Exclusion Criteria

All studies were independently reviewed by two investigators (ZH and MX), and a third independent investigator (YY) was called upon to reach a consensus in case of any disputes. The following are the inclusion requirements: (1) original research; (2) population-based studies; (3) studies that observe something, such as a cohort, a case–control study, or a cross-sectional study; (4) exposure to particle and gaseous contaminants in the air, including PM_1, $PM_{2.5}$, PM_{10}, NO_2, SO_2, CO and O_3; (5) studies providing ORs, relative risk (RR), or hazard ratios (HRs) with 95% CIs for the visual impairment outcomes associated with any air pollutants; and (6) articles in English.

The following were the exclusion requirements: (1) studies in which no data can be retrieved; (2) studies involving animal experiments; (3) studies of poor quality; (4) comments, letters, responses to review articles, and meta-analyses.

2.3. Quality Assessment

The following techniques were employed to assess the quality of the literature by the study types of the included articles: (1) Cross-sectional study statistics assessment and review instrument meta-analysis by the Joanna Briggs Institute (JBI) (Table S2) [16]; (2) 9-star Newcastle–Ottawa Scale (NOS) (Table S3) for cohort studies and case–control studies [17]. In our study, the JBI scale contained 10 items on a scale of 0 to 20, each rated on a scale of 2 (detailed, comprehensive, and correctly described); 1 (mentioned but not described in detail); and 0 (not met). Studies are categorized as "high quality" if they receive a JBI score of at least 16, as opposed to "low quality" otherwise [16]. The NOS scale had a total score that ranged from 0 to 9, and the study's quality was determined by its selection (0–4 points), comparability (0–2 points), and outcome (0–3 points) quality factors. The study quality was rated on a scale of 0–3 as low, 4–6 as medium, and 7–9 as high [17]. Supplementary Tables S4 and S5 of the Supplementary Materials detailed the grading system.

2.4. Data Extraction

Two investigators retrieved data from all included studies separately and in a defined way, and third investigator resolved disagreements through discussion. For every eligible study, we extracted the initial author's name, publication year, study site, time frame, study design, sample size, population characteristics, pollution characteristics, assessment method, adjusted variables, outcome definition, time of assessment, type of outcome and subgroup analysis results, effect size (OR, RR or HR, 95% CI) of the correlation between air pollutants and vision disorder.

We transformed all air pollutant measurement units to $\mu g/m^3$ to standardize impact sizes: (1) 1 ppm = 1000 ppb, 1 mg/m^3 = 1000 $\mu g/m^3$; (2) NO_2: 1 ppb = 46/22.4 $\mu g/m^3$; (3) O_3: 1 ppb = 48/22.4 $\mu g/m^3$; (4) SO_2: 1 ppb = 64/22.4 $\mu g/m^3$; (5) CO: 1 ppb = 28/22.4 $\mu g/m^3$ [15]. After that, all effect estimates were combined for a 10 $\mu g/m^3$ rise in pollutant concentration. The following formulas were used to transform the standard risks for each investigation [18]:

$$OR_{(standardized)} = OR_{(original)}^{Increment(10)/Increment(original)}$$

2.5. Statistical Analysis

Statistical analysis was carried out using Stata 17.0. ORs and their 95% CIs, which were mostly used in studies with various designs, populations, and follow-up times, were used to present pooled data. Other effect sizes were converted into ORs. Forest plots and standard cut-offs for I^2 statistics were used to assess heterogeneity across studies. Heterogeneity was ranked as low ($I^2 \leq 25\%$), medium ($25\% < I^2 < 75\%$), and high ($I^2 \geq 75\%$) at those percentages. Subgroup and sensitivity analyses were done to look into the causes of heterogeneity. When the values of I^2 were greater than 50%, the random-effects inverse-variance model was used to compute the combined estimates. Moreover, statistical significance was assumed when the p-value of a two-tailed test was less than 0.05 [19].

3. Result

3.1. Study Results

Using three electronic databases, we screened 2007 articles in total and eliminated 390 duplicates. The titles and abstracts of the remaining 1617 articles were preliminarily screened, of which 1555 were excluded after the initial screening, and a total of 62 articles were screened for full-text reading. Considering the inclusion and exclusion standards, 50 studies were excluded, of which four were reviews, one was an animal study, three were non-English articles, and 42 did not meet the inclusion criteria (Figure 1). Twelve studies [3,5,10,12,13,20–26] evaluating the relationship between air pollutant exposure and the risk of vision disorder outcomes were included in this meta-analysis.

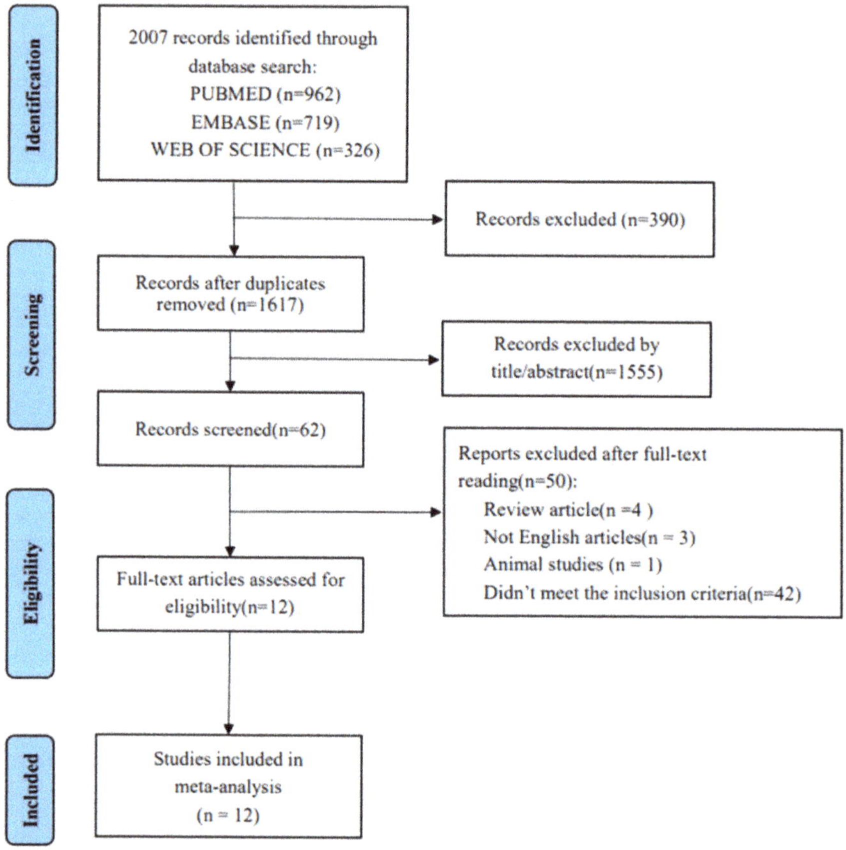

Figure 1. Flow chart of the literature search and selection for meta-analysis.

3.2. Study Characteristics

The characteristics of the included studies are summarized in Table 1. Twelve studies were published between 2018 and 2022, with the studies covering the period from 2000 to 2021. Seven were cross-sectional, three were cohort, and two were case-crossover studies. The studies were carried out in four nations: China (n = 6), South Korea (n = 3), the United Kingdom (n = 2), and Canada (n = 1), and they involved a large number of participants, ranging from 3225 to 340,313. Our review included the following number of studies on various pollutants: PM_{10} (n = 6), $PM_{2.5}$ (n = 10), PM_1 (n = 1), NO_2 (n = 7), SO_2 (n = 4), CO (n = 5), and O_3 (n = 3). Regarding quality assessment, twelve studies met the criteria for good quality (Supplementary Tables S3 and S5). Most included studies estimated the correlations between air pollution and vision disorder outcomes by multivariable multiple logistic regression and multiple cox proportional hazards regression models, and evaluated OR, RR or HR with 95% CIs for each air pollutant selected.

Table 1. Characteristics of studies included in the systematic review and meta-analysis.

Study	Location	Data Period	Design	Sample Size	Age	Exposure Pollutant(s)	Statistical Model	Outcome Type	Quality
Choi et al., 2018 [10]	Republic of Korea	2006–2012	Cross-sectional study	18,622	40+	O_3, NO_2, SO_2, PM_{10}	Multiple logistic regression analyses	Cataract	17/20
Chua et al., 2019 [3]	United Kingdom	2006–2010	Cross-sectional study	111,370	40–69	$PM_{2.5}$	Multiple logistic regression analyses	Glaucoma	18/20
Chang et al., 2019 [5]	China-Taiwan	2000–2010	Longitudinal population-based study	39,819	50+	NO_2, CO	Multiple Cox proportional hazards regression	AMD	6/9
Shin et al., 2020 [21]	Republic of Korea	2002–2015	Longitudinal population-based study	115,728	50+	$PM_{2.5}$, PM_{10}, NO_2, CO, SO_2, O_3	Multiple Cox proportional hazards regression	Cataract	9/9
Yang et al., 2021 [23]	China	2010–2013	Cross-sectional study	61,995	6–18	PM_1, $PM_{2.5}$, PM_{10}, NO_2	SAS PROC SURVEYLOGISTIC, SAS PROC SURVEYREG	Visual impairment	16/20
Grant et al., 2021 [20]	Canada	2011–2015	Cross-sectional population-based study	30,097	45–85	$PM_{2.5}$, O_3, SO_2, NO_2	Multiple logistic regression analyses	AMD, Cataract, Glaucoma, Visual impairment	19/20
Sun et al., 2021 [22]	China-Taiwan	2008–2013	Nested case–control study	3225	65+	$PM_{2.5}$	Multiple logistic regression analyses	Glaucoma	6/9
Yang et al., 2021 [24]	China	2000–2016	Cross-sectional study	33,701	40+	$PM_{2.5}$	Multiple logistic regression analyses	Glaucoma	16/20
Chen et al., 2022 [13]	China	2005–2018	Longitudinal, two-center cohort study	340,313	SD: 11.30 (±2.64)	SO_2, CO	Multiple Cox proportional hazards regression	Visual impairment	8/9
Li et al., 2022 [26]	China	2015–2021	Case-crossover study	14,385	SD: 56.79 (±15.33)	$PM_{2.5}$, PM_{10}, NO_2, CO	Conditional logistic regression model	Glaucoma	7/9
Chua et al., 2022 [12]	United Kingdom	2006–2010	Cross-sectional study	115,954	40–69	$PM_{2.5}$, PM_{10}, NO_2	Multiple logistic regression analyses	AMD	17/20
Ju et al., 2022 [25]	Republic of Korea	2008–2012	Cross-sectional study	15,115	40+	NO_2, CO, O_3	Survey-logistic regression models	AMD	16/20

Abbreviations: PM_1: particle with aerodynamic diameter ≤ 1 μm; SD: The mean age.

3.3. The Association between Environmental Air Pollutants Exposure and Vision Disorder

Twelve studies looked into the connection between exposure to air pollution and vision disorder; nine reported ORs with 95% CIs, two supplied HRs with 95% CIs, and one reported RRs with 95% CIs. We estimated the pooled ORs for vision disorders (cataract, glaucoma, AMD and visual impairment) associated with each air pollutant. Three, five, four and two studies assessed the relationship between air pollutant exposure and cataract, glaucoma, AMD and visual impairment, respectively. The correlations of vision disorder with exposure to PM_{10}, $PM_{2.5}$, PM_1, SO_2, NO_2, O_3 and CO were reported in studies (Tables 2 and 3).

Table 2. Summary effects and 95% confidence intervals for vision disorder associated with PM.

Air Pollutant	Author (Year)	Outcome Type	Incremental Scale	Original OR/HR	Transformed OR
PM_{10}	Choi et al. (2018) [10]	Cataract	5 μg/m^3	OR: 0.91 (95% CI, 0.78–1.07)	OR: 0.83 (95% CI, 0.61–1.14)
	Shin et al. (2020) [21]	Cataract	IQR: 9.1 μg/m^3	HR: 1.069 (95% CI, 1.025–1.115)	OR: 1.076 (95% CI, 1.028–1.127)
	Yang et al. (2021) [23]	Visual impairment	IQR: 16.11 μg/m^3	OR: 1.142 (95% CI, 1.019–1.281)	OR: 1.086 (95% CI, 1.012–1.166)
	Li et al. (2022) [26]	Glaucoma	IQR: 35 μg/m^3	OR: 1.03 (95% CI, 1.01–1.05)	OR: 1.01 (95% CI, 1.00–1.01)
	Chua et al. (2022) [12]	AMD	IQR: 2.67 μg/m^3	OR: 0.94 (95% CI, 0.86–1.02)	OR: 0.79 (95% CI, 0.57–1.08)
	Ju et al. (2022) [25]	AMD	IQR: 8 μg/m^3	OR: 1.13 (95% CI, 0.99–1.34)	OR: 1.17 (95% CI, 0.99–1.44)
$PM_{2.5}$	Chua et al. (2019) [3]	Glaucoma	IQR: 1.12 μg/m^3	OR: 1.06 (95% CI, 1.01–1.12)	OR: 1.68 (95% CI, 1.09–2.75)
	Shin et al. (2020) [21]	Cataract	IQR: 7.0 μg/m^3	HR: 0.905 (95% CI, 0.772–1.062)	OR: 0.905 (95% CI, 0.867–1.090)
	Yang et al. (2021) [23]	Visual impairment	14.79 μg/m^3	OR: 1.267 (95% CI, 1.082–1.484)	OR: 1.174 (95% CI, 1.055–1.306)
	Grant et al. (2021) [20]	Glaucoma	IQR: 2.9 μg/m^3	OR: 1.24 (95% CI, 1.05–1.46)	OR: 2.10 (95% CI, 1.18–3.69)
	Grant et al. (2021) [20]	AMD (with visual impairment)	IQR: 2.9 μg/m^3	OR: 1.41 (95% CI, 0.96–2.08)	OR:3.27 (95% CI, 0.87–12.49)
	Grant et al. (2021) [20]	Cataract	IQR: 2.9 μg/m^3	OR: 0.98 (95% CI, 0.90–1.07)	OR: 0.93 (95% CI, 0.70–1.26
	Sun et al. (2021) [22]	Glaucoma	10 μg/m^3	OR: 1.19 (95% CI, 1.05–1.36)	OR: 1.19 (95% CI, 1.05–1.36)
	Yang et al. (2021) [24]	Glaucoma	10 μg/m^3	OR: 1.07 (95% CI, 1.00–1.15)	OR: 1.07 (95% CI, 1.00–1.15)
	Li et al. (2022) [26]	Glaucoma	IQR: 26 μg/m^3	OR: 1.07 (95% CI, 1.03–1.11)	OR: 1.03(95% CI, 1.01–1.04)
	Chua et al. (2022) [12]	AMD	IQR: 1.07 μg/m^3	OR: 1.08 (95% CI, 1.01–1.16)	OR: 2.05(95% CI, 1.10–4.00)
PM_1	Yang et al. (2021) [23]	Visual impairment	10.24 μg/m^3	OR: 1.133 (95% CI, 1.035–1.240)	OR: 1.130 (95% CI, 1.034–1.234)

Table 3. Summary effects and 95% confidence intervals for vision disorder associated with SO_2, NO_2, O_3, CO.

Air Pollutant	Author (Year)	Outcome Type	Incremental Scale	Original OR/HR	Transformed OR
SO_2	Choi et al. (2018) [10]	Cataract	0.003 ppm	OR: 0.90 (95% CI, 0.62–1.30)	OR: 0.88 (95% CI, 0.56–1.37)
	Shin et al. (2020) [21]	Cataract	IQR: 0.7 ppb	HR: 1.027 (95% CI, 0.984 1.073)	OR: 1.147 (95% CI, 0.920–1.439)
	Chen et al. (2022) [13]	Visual impairment	IQR: 16.16 μg/m^3	RR: 2.26 (95% CI, 2.22–2.29)	OR: 1.66 (95% CI, 1.64–1.67)
	Ju et al. (2022) [25]	AMD	IOR: 1 ppb	OR: 0.99 (95% CI, 0.92–1.06)	OR: 0.96 (95% CI, 0.74–1.23)
NO_2	Choi et al. (2018) [10]	Cataract	0.003 ppm	OR: 0.93 (95% CI, 0.85–1.02)	OR: 0.92 (95% CI, 0.82–1.02)
	Chang et al. (2019) [5]	AMD	IQR: 9825.5 ppb	HR: 1.91 (95% CI, 1.64–2.23)	OR: 1.00 (95% CI, 1.00–1.00)
	Shin et al. (2020) [21]	Cataract	IQR: 2.1 ppb	HR: 1.080 (95% CI, 1.030–1.133)	OR: 1.205 (95% CI, 1.074–1.354)
	Yang et al. (2021) [23]	Visual impairment	9.78 μg/m^3	OR: 1.276 (95% CI, 1.173–1.388)	OR: 1.283 (95% CI, 1.177–1.398)
	Li et al. (2022) [26]	Glaucoma	IQR: 27 μg/m^3	OR: 1.12 (95% CI, 1.08–1.17)	OR: 1.04 (95% CI, 1.03–1.06)
	Chua et al. (2022) [12]	Glaucoma	10 μg/m^3	OR: 0.99 (95% CI, 0.91–1.08)	OR: 0.99 (95% CI, 0.91–1.08)
	Ju et al. (2022) [25]	AMD	IQR: 12 ppb	OR:1.24 (95% CI, 1.05–1.46)	OR: 1.09 (95% CI, 1.01–1.17)
O_3	Choi et al. (2018) [10]	Cataract	0.003 ppm	OR: 0.80 (95% CI, 0.69–0.93)	OR: 0.71 (95% CI, 0.56–0.89)
	Shin et al. (2020) [21]	Cataract	IQR: 5.4 ppb	HR: 0.931 (95% CI, 0.888–0.977)	OR: 0.940 (95% CI, 0.902–0.980)
	Ju et al. (2022) [25]	AMD	IQR: 5 ppb	OR: 0.80 (95% CI, 0.70–0.92)	OR: 0.81 (95% CI, 0.72–0.93)
CO	Chang et al. (2019) [5]	AMD	IQR: 297.1 ppm	HR: 1.84 (95% CI, 1.57–2.15)	OR: 1.00 (95% CI, 1.00–1.00)
	Shin et al. (2020) [21]	Cataract	11 ppm	HR: 0.991 (95% CI, 0.949–1.035)	OR: 0.999 (95% CI, 0.999–1.000)
	Chen et al. (2022) [13]	Visual impairment	1.28 mg/m^3	RR: 2.30 (95% CI, 2.26–2.35)	OR: 1.01 (95% CI, 1.01–1.01)
	Li et al. (2022) [26]	Glaucoma	IQR: 0.5 mg/m^3	OR: 1.04 (95% CI, 1.01–1.07)	OR: 1.00 (95% CI, 1.00–1.00)
	Ju et al. (2022) [25]	AMD	IQR: 100 ppb	OR: 1.22 (95% CI, 1.09–1.38)	OR: 1.02 (95% CI, 1.01–1.03)

The combined results suggested that air pollutants could boost the likelihood of having a vision disorder, with the combined OR (95% CI) of 1.10 (1.01–1.19) and 1.08 (1.00–1.16) per 10 μg/m^3 increment in exposure to $PM_{2.5}$ and NO_2, respectively (Figure 2). But the results showed that PM_{10} (OR = 1.04, 95% CI: 0.99, 1.10; I^2 = 71.1%, p = 0.004) (Figure 2A), SO_2 (OR = 1.16, 95% CI: 0.82, 1.64; I^2 = 97.1%, p = 0.000) (Figure 2C) and CO (OR = 1.01, 95% CI: 0.99, 1.03; I^2 = 94.2%, p = 0.000) (Figure 2F) were not significantly associated with vision disorder. The pooled OR from all studies between O_3 exposure and vision disorder was 0.84 (95% CI: 0.72, 0.98) with significant heterogeneity (I^2 = 79.3%, p = 0.008) (Figure 2E).

To further investigate the causes of this variation, we performed a meta-regression and a subgroup analysis.

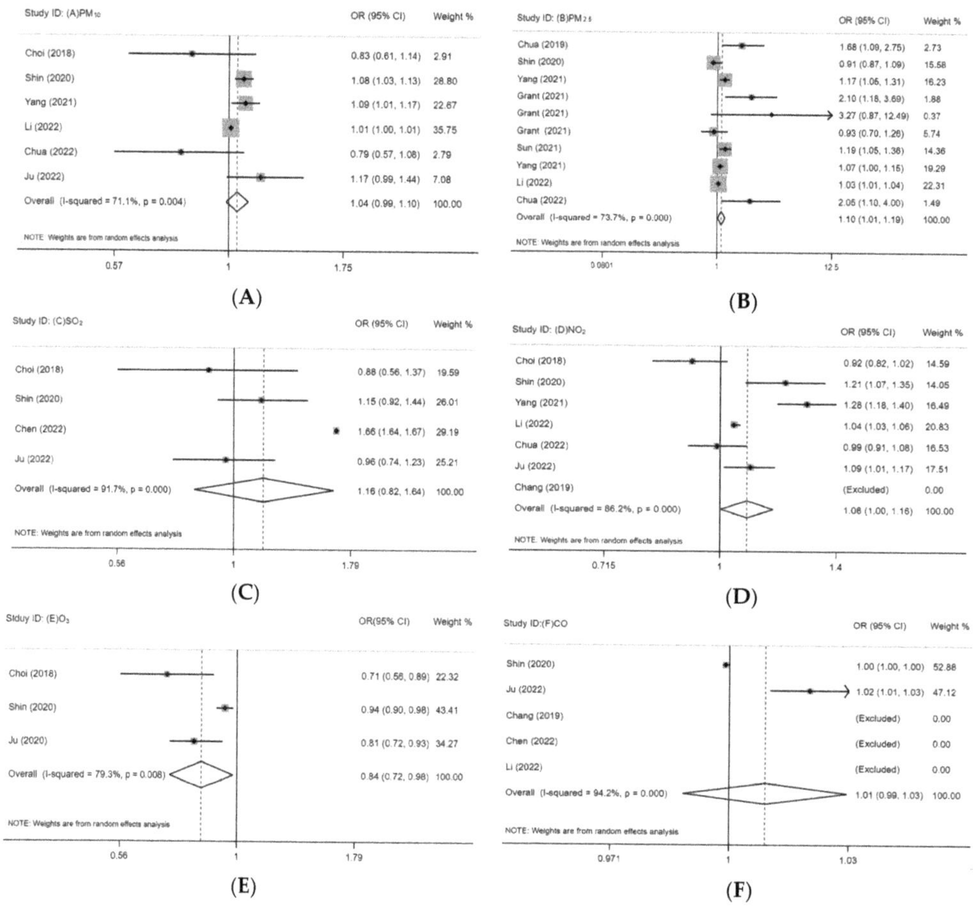

Figure 2. Associations of PM_{10} (**A**), $PM_{2.5}$ (**B**), SO_2 (**C**), NO_2 (**D**), O_3 (**E**) and CO (**F**) with vision disorder. (1. A solid line perpendicular to the X-axis and with a horizontal axis of 1 is an invalid line; 2. Multiple line segments parallel to the horizontal axis represent the 95% CI of each included study, and black dots represent the OR value of each study; 3. Arrow: The 95% CI of the OR value in this study exceeds the display range of the graph; 4. The diamond represents the summary results of multiple studies, where the dashed line perpendicular to the X-axis and passing through the center of the diamond represents the merged effect value, and the width of the diamond represents 95% CI of the merged results; 5. The area of gray squares represents weight, and the larger the weight, the larger the square area) [3,5,10,12,13,20–26].

3.4. Subgroup Analyses

We first performed a subgroup study based on how NO_2 affected different regions (China, Korea and the United Kingdom) and age (6–18, 40+) (Figure 3). Secondly, we conducted a subgroup analysis of age and different common diseases of vision disorder according to $PM_{2.5}$ (Figure 3). The findings demonstrated that there was no statistically strong correlation between elevated NO_2 concentrations and the risk of vision disorder in China, Korea, and the United Kingdom, with combined ORs of 1.15 (95% CI: 0.94, 1.41), 1.07 (95% CI: 0.93, 1.22) and 0.99 (95% CI: 0.91, 1.08). Additionally, the impact of $PM_{2.5}$ on various glaucoma, cataract, and AMD diseases was revealed by subgroup analysis. We can obtain the combined effect of studies with the risk of glaucoma (OR = 1.12, 95% CI: 1.02, 1.23), cataract (OR = 0.91, 95% CI: 0.82, 1.01), AMD (OR = 2.24, 95% CI: 1.25, 4.00). It can be concluded that $PM_{2.5}$ is positively correlated with glaucoma and AMD, while there is no significant correlation between cataract. Finally, subgroup analysis by age level showed that $PM_{2.5}$ (OR = 1.17, 95% CI: 1.06, 1.31) and NO_2 (OR = 1.28, 95% CI: 1.18, 1.40) were positively correlated with vision disorder in children and adolescents, but not significantly correlated with adults over 40 years of age.

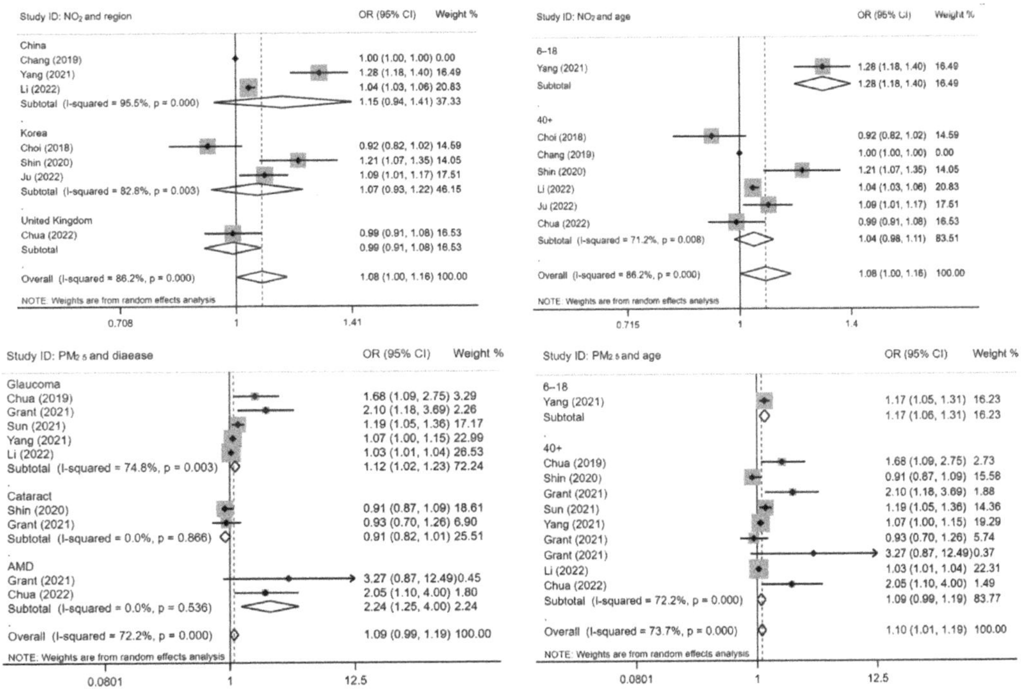

Figure 3. The effect of NO_2 and $PM_{2.5}$ on vision disorder, stratified by region, disease and age. (1. A solid line perpendicular to the X-axis and with a horizontal axis of 1 is an invalid line; 2. Multiple line segments parallel to the horizontal axis represent the 95% CI of each included study, and black dots represent the OR value of each study; 3. Arrow: The 95% CI of the OR value in this study exceeds the display range of the graph; 4. The diamond represents the summary results of multiple studies, where the dashed line perpendicular to the X-axis and passing through the center of the diamond represents the merged effect value, and the width of the diamond represents 95% CI of the merged results; 5. The area of gray squares represents weight, and the larger the weight, the larger the square area) [3,5,10,12,20–26].

3.5. Sensitivity Analysis and Publication Bias

The stability of the pooled data was evaluated using the one-study deletion sensitivity analysis, which involved repeatedly combining estimations and removing one study at a time. Supplementary Figures S1–S6 of the results reveal that the majority of the pollutant consolidation results are steady. We also evaluated the potential publication bias with funnel plots (Supplementary Figures S7–S12) when 10 or more studies were included [27]. The funnel plot can be used to evaluate publication bias visually. Additionally, we used an Egger test to evaluate publication bias. Egger's tests suggested that there occurred no significant publication bias in PM_{10}, NO_2, and O_3 exposure on vision disorder (p-value of the Egger's test > 0.05), while $PM_{2.5}$ and SO_2 exposure had publication bias on vision disorder ($p < 0.05$) (Supplementary Table S6).

4. Discussion

To our knowledge, this study is the first to thoroughly evaluate the link between exposure to air pollution and vision disorder. Although a similar systematic review has been conducted, it compares the age-related burden of eye disease in adults exposed to ambient air pollutants [28]. Our study differs from previous studies in that we included literature on children and adolescents in addition to adults, and estimated the combined effect of ambient air pollution on their vision disorders. Twelve studies were included after being retrieved from the system. After pooling the effect estimates from the 12 studies, it is found that the increased concentration of $PM_{2.5}$ and NO_2 may increase the incidence of vision disorder, whereas no significant association between PM_{10}, SO_2, CO and vision disorder was observed. In addition, earlier research indicated that exposure to O_3 was positively correlated with the risk of vision disorder. However, this investigation found that O_3 was negatively associated with vision disorder. The explanation for the results of this meta-analysis might be due to the inclusion of different studies and study designs in the included articles. Therefore, further research is needed to understand this relationship fully.

Exposure to air pollutants raises the chance of vision disorder, and previous research has shown that air pollution may directly irritate the eyes, especially in the cornea and conjunctiva [9,29,30]. This study showed that exposure to $PM_{2.5}$ and NO_2 was positively correlated with vision disorder. Previous researchers used fluorescent $PM_{2.5}$ tracers to understand how $PM_{2.5}$ enters the eye. They discovered that particles of a size between 10 and 500 nm entered the anterior chamber via the cornea and were mostly deposited in the outflow tissue, with the majority of the particles staying in the ciliary body. This study suggests that $PM_{2.5}$ exposure may impact the cornea's connective tissue biomechanical capabilities [3,20]. The positive correlation between NO_2 and vision disorder may be explained by the slow hydrolysis of NO_2 into nitrous and nitric acid after respiratory inhalation, which causes lipid peroxidation and oxidative stress [5]. In addition, since the retina is a component of the central nervous system, it makes biological sense that it may be susceptible to NO_2 poisoning [5].

In a prior study, higher ozone concentrations were linked to dry eye disease [31], and other research demonstrated that ozone exposure causes ocular surface degradation and an inflammatory state [11]. Therefore, we expected that there might be a positive association between ozone and vision disorder. Contrary to our expectations, this study found a negative correlation between ozone and vision disorder. A possible explanation is that ozone is a well-known polar molecule, that may not penetrate the cornea easily [10]. Therefore, the lens may be immune to the oxidative damage caused by ozone [10]. Another possible explanation is that exposure to ultraviolet (UV) radiation is the major cause of oxidative stress and the most significant risk factor for cataract development [32]. Less UV radiation may reach the surface and enter the eye due to the stratospheric ozone layer's filtering of UV rays [10]. It also reduces the vision disorder caused by oxidative stress caused by ultraviolet light.

Subgroup analyses were conducted to investigate possible causes of heterogeneity in the meta-analysis. The findings showed that study region, disease and age are the primary causes. Subgroup analysis showed no significant correlation between NO_2 exposure and vision disorder in China, South Korea and the United Kingdom. Possible explanations are the limited number of studies and potential sources of heterogeneity such as demographics, participant characteristics, sample size, and regional environmental air pollution monitoring. In addition, subgroup analysis of diseases found that $PM_{2.5}$ exposure was significantly correlated with the risk of glaucoma and AMD. With glaucoma and AMD being multifactorial neurodegenerative illnesses that may result in the death of retinal ganglion cells and visual field abnormalities, there is growing evidence that air pollution may have a role in the development of neurodegenerative disorders [33,34]. Therefore, this may be why $PM_{2.5}$ in the subgroup analysis is positively correlates with glaucoma and AMD. Cataracts develop from many factors: metabolic disorders, dietary deficiency, or environmental stressors, including severe cold or heat, radiation, metal ions, and toxins [10,12]. The subgroup analysis results show that the correlation between $PM_{2.5}$ and the incidence of cataracts is insignificant, possibly because $PM_{2.5}$ in the air is not a crucial factor affecting cataract occurrence among the above-mentioned factors. Finally, we found that air pollution affects children and adolescents more than adults due to their exposure level and physiological characteristics. Due to their increased ventilation rates and frequent outside activity, children and adolescents may be exposed to air contaminants more often [35]. In addition, the bodies of children and adolescents are still growing and their immune systems are still underdeveloped, which makes them less resistant to air pollution than adults.

No gender-based subgroup analyses were carried out in this study due to data limitations, although recent research has indicated gender variations. The gender-specific effects can be attributable to socially derived air pollution exposures. In addition, there are also gender differences in the human body's gas-blood barrier permeability, particle deposition, and gas absorption [36]. For example, Studies have shown that many human organs may be affected by indoor air pollution, where the eyes are directly exposed to emissions from the burning of solid fuels, including high levels of fine $PM_{2.5}$ and CO [37]. The higher association between cataracts in women than men, considering the mixed effects of women's exposure to indoor cooking fuels and outdoor activities on cataracts [38]. On the contrary, for children, boys spend more time outside and are more active than girls, which exposes them to more air pollution and may make them more vulnerable to its effects [23].

Several mechanisms have been suggested to explain these findings. Studies have shown that for cataracts, oxidative stress of reactive oxygen species and reactive nitrogen (ROS/RNS) is considered the main formation mechanism [39]. Oxidative stress caused by air pollution is the stressor inducing cataracts, which may harm the membrane cavity and secreted proteins [10]. The integrity of the cornea's barrier may be altered by PM and NO_x, which may also encourage the creation of ROS and cause inflammation of the retina and ocular surface [9,40]. As was previously discussed, atmospheric particulate matter and NO_2 may produce ROS/RNS and trigger oxidative damage to a wide range of biomolecules [40]. Therefore, oxidative stress and inflammation are mechanisms that explain the effect of air pollutants on the occurrence of eye diseases. The corresponding reduction of air pollutants may affect the pathogenesis of vision disorder and thus reduce the incidence of vision disorder.

The results suggested that air pollution is correlated with vision disorder, in which $PM_{2.5}$ and NO_2 exposure may be positively correlated with vision disorder-related risk, PM_{10}, SO_2 and CO exposure have no significant effect on vision disorder, and O_3 exposure is negatively associated with vision disorder. The association varied by region, disease and age. $PM_{2.5}$ exposure was significantly correlated with the risk of glaucoma and AMD, but with cataracts not significant. Children and adolescents are more vulnerable to the impacts of air pollution than adults. In addition, the OR value can reflect the strength of the association between air pollutants and vision disorder. In Figure 2, the middle vertical line is the invalid line, OR = 1. When the combined OR value is on the right side of the invalid line, it means that the study factor (air pollutant) and the outcome (vision disorder) are in a positive relationship, and the farther away from the invalid line, the OR value is greater than 1, and the greater the correlation strength. Therefore, $PM_{2.5}$ is more strongly associated with vision disorder than NO_2.

This systematic review and meta-analysis have some limitations. First, the cross-sectional nature does not determine causality between studies [23]. Second, the dearth of research made it impossible to analyze the potential sources of heterogeneity thoroughly. This suggests that variations in population factors, participant characteristics, sample size, and geographical location may be at play. Third, considering heterogeneity and the small amount of studies for every air contaminant, care should be exercised when interpreting the findings. Fourth, we classified the diseases associated with vision disorders. However, in the included articles, only cataracts, glaucoma, age-related macular degeneration and visual impairment were studied as outcomes, and no mention was made of hyperopia, myopia, night blindness and deformities. Above all, misclassification of exposures was unavoidable since data from monitoring stations was utilized in practically all research. In addition, we did not analyze PM_1 based to the limitations of the available literature.

Based on previous studies, to better understand the relationship between air pollutants and vision disorder, here are some ideas on where to take subsequent studies: (1) Additional large-scale, long-term cohort studies are required for a more accurate and trustworthy evaluation. (2) More careful monitoring of exposure levels. (3) More research is needed to determine the effects of air pollution on vision disorders in terms of genetics, demographics, social variables, and behaviors. (4) Multiple pollutant interactions and their consequences on vision disorder have yet to be quantified.

5. Conclusions

In conclusion, ambient air pollution may contribute to vision disorder. $PM_{2.5}$ and NO_2 are air pollutants correlated with an increased risk of vision disorder. The correlation varied by region, disease and age. The results indicate that policymakers might anticipate the likelihood of vision disorder due to air pollution and adopt targeted preventative actions in advance. In the future, more relevant research is necessary to provide a more accurate and reliable assessment.

Supplementary Materials: The following supporting information can be downloaded at: https://www.mdpi.com/article/10.3390/toxics12030209/s1, Table S1: Literature search terms; Table S2: JBI evaluation criteria for cross-sectional studies; Table S3: NOS evaluation criteria for cohort studies and case-control studiesQuality; Table S4: assessment for the cross-sectional studies using JBI; Table S5: Quality assessment for the cohort studies and case-control studies using NOS; Table S6: Egger's test for publication bias of studies exploring exposure to different pollutants and vision disorder; Figure S1: Sensitivity analysis results of PM_{10}; Figure S2: Sensitivity analysis results of $PM_{2.5}$; Figure S3: Sensitivity analysis results of SO_2; Figure S4: Sensitivity analysis results of NO_2; Figure S5: Sensitivity analysis results of O_3; Figure S6: Sensitivity analysis results of CO; Figure S7: Funnel plot for publication bias of studies exploring exposure to PM_{10} and vision disorder; Figure S8: Funnel plot for publication bias of studies exploring exposure to $PM_{2.5}$ and vision disorder; Figure S9: Funnel plot for publication bias of studies exploring exposure to SO_2 and vision disorder; Figure S10: Funnel plot for publication bias of studies exploring exposure to NO_2 and vision disorder; Figure S11: Funnel plot for publication bias of studies exploring exposure to O_3 and vision disorder; Figure S12: Funnel plot for publication bias of studies exploring exposure to CO and vision disorder.

Author Contributions: Z.H.: methodology, formal analysis, investigation, data curation, writing—original draft, writing—review and editing; C.Z. and Y.L.: writing—review and editing, supervision. M.X.: methodology, investigation, data curation; Y.Y.: methodology, investigation, data curation; Y.Z.: Writing—review and editing, supervision; C.L. and J.L.: writing—review and editing, supervision; P.L.: writing—review and editing, supervision, project administration, funding acquisition. All authors have read and agreed to the published version of the manuscript.

Funding: This work was supported by China Postdoctoral Science Foundation (2020M670667), Tianjin Research Program (22ZYCGCG00920, 21YFSNSN00030).

Institutional Review Board Statement: Not applicable.

Informed Consent Statement: Not applicable.

Data Availability Statement: The original data presented in the study are included in the article/Supplementary Materials; further inquiries can be directed to the corresponding authors.

Conflicts of Interest: The authors declare no conflicts of interest.

References

1. Eckert, K.A.; Carter, M.J.; Lansingh, V.C.; Wilson, D.A.; Furtado, J.M.; Frick, K.D.; Resnikoff, S. A Simple Method for Estimating the Economic Cost of Productivity Loss Due to Blindness and Moderate to Severe Visual Impairment. *Ophthalmic Epidemiol.* **2015**, *22*, 349–355. [CrossRef]
2. Dale, N.; Sakkalou, E.; O'Reilly, M.; Springall, C.; De Haan, M.; Salt, A. Functional vision and cognition in infants with congenital disorders of the peripheral visual system. *Dev. Med. Child Neurol.* **2017**, *59*, 725–731. [CrossRef] [PubMed]
3. Chua, S.; Khawaja, A.P.; Morgan, J.; Strouthidis, N.; Reisman, C.; Dick, A.D.; Khaw, P.T.; Patel, P.J.; Foster, P.J.; Atan, D.; et al. The Relationship Between Ambient Atmospheric Fine Particulate Matter (PM2.5) and Glaucoma in a Large Community Cohort. *Investig. Ophthalmol. Vis. Sci.* **2019**, *60*, 4915–4923. [CrossRef] [PubMed]
4. Asbell, P.A.; Dualan, L.; Mindel, J.; Brocks, D.; Ahmad, M.; Epstein, S. Age-related cataract. *Lancet* **2005**, *365*, 599–609. [CrossRef]
5. Chang, K.H.; Hsu, P.Y.; Lin, C.J.; Lin, C.L.; Juo, S.; Liang, C.L. Traffic-related air pollutants increase the risk for age-related macular degeneration. *J. Investig. Med.* **2019**, *67*, 1076–1081. [CrossRef] [PubMed]
6. Cohen, A.J.; Brauer, M.; Burnett, R.; Anderson, H.R.; Frostad, J.; Estep, K.; Balakrishnan, K.; Brunekreef, B.; Dandona, L.; Dandona, R.; et al. Estimates and 25-year trends of the global burden of disease attributable to ambient air pollution: An analysis of data from the Global Burden of Diseases Study 2015. *Lancet* **2017**, *389*, 1907–1918. [CrossRef]
7. World Health Organization. *Ambient Air Pollution: A Global Assessment of Exposure and Burden of Disease*; World Health Organization: Geneva, Switzerland, 2016.
8. World Health Organization. *WHO Global Air Quality Guidelines: Particulate Matter (PM2.5 and PM10), Ozone, Nitrogen Dioxide, Sulfur Dioxide and Carbon Monoxide*; World Health Organization: Geneva, Switzerland, 2021.
9. Wei, C.C.; Lin, H.J.; Lim, Y.P.; Chen, C.S.; Chang, C.Y.; Lin, C.J.; Chen, J.; Tien, P.T.; Lin, C.L.; Wan, L. PM2.5 and NOx exposure promote myopia: Clinical evidence and experimental proof. *Environ. Pollut.* **2019**, *254*, 113031. [CrossRef] [PubMed]
10. Choi, Y.H.; Park, S.J.; Paik, H.J.; Kim, M.K.; Wee, W.R.; Kim, D.H. Unexpected potential protective associations between outdoor air pollution and cataracts. *Environ. Sci. Pollut. Res.* **2018**, *25*, 10636–10643. [CrossRef] [PubMed]
11. Nita, M.; Grzybowski, A. The Role of the Reactive Oxygen Species and Oxidative Stress in the Pathomechanism of the Age-Related Ocular Diseases and Other Pathologies of the Anterior and Posterior Eye Segments in Adults. *Oxid. Med. Cell. Longev.* **2016**, *2016*, 3164734. [CrossRef]
12. Chua, S.; Warwick, A.; Peto, T.; Balaskas, K.; Moore, A.T.; Reisman, C.; Desai, P.; Lotery, A.J.; Dhillon, B.; Khaw, P.T.; et al. Association of ambient air pollution with age-related macular degeneration and retinal thickness in UK Biobank. *Br. J. Ophthalmol.* **2022**, *106*, 705–711. [CrossRef]
13. Chen, L.; Wei, J.; Ma, T.; Gao, D.; Wang, X.J.; Wen, B.; Chen, M.M.; Li, Y.H.; Jiang, J.; Wu, L.J. Ambient gaseous pollutant exposure and incidence of visual impairment among children and adolescents: Findings from a longitudinal, two-center cohort study in China. *Environ. Sci. Pollut. Res.* **2022**, *29*, 73262–73270. [CrossRef]
14. Nam, G.E.; Han, K.; Ha, S.G.; Han, B.D.; Kim, D.H.; Kim, Y.H.; Cho, K.H.; Park, Y.G.; Ko, B.J. Relationship between socioeconomic and lifestyle factors and cataracts in Koreans: The Korea National Health and Nutrition Examination Survey 2008–2011. *Eye* **2015**, *29*, 913–920. [CrossRef]
15. Shin, J.; Han, S.H.; Choi, J. Exposure to Ambient Air Pollution and Cognitive Impairment in Community-Dwelling Older Adults: The Korean Frailty and Aging Cohort Study. *Int. J. Environ. Res. Public Health* **2019**, *16*, 3767. [CrossRef]
16. Fan, S.J.; Heinrich, J.; Bloom, M.S.; Zhao, T.Y.; Shi, T.X.; Feng, W.R.; Sun, Y.; Shen, J.C.; Yang, Z.C.; Yang, B.Y.; et al. Ambient air pollution and depression: A systematic review with meta-analysis up to 2019. *Sci. Total Environ.* **2020**, *701*, 134721. [CrossRef]
17. Deji, Z.M.; Liu, P.; Wang, X.; Zhang, X.; Luo, Y.H.; Huang, Z.Z. Association between maternal exposure to perfluoroalkyl and polyfluoroalkyl substances and risks of adverse pregnancy outcomes: A systematic review and meta-analysis. *Sci. Total Environ.* **2021**, *783*, 146984. [CrossRef] [PubMed]
18. Yang, B.; Qian, Z.; Howard, S.W.; Vaughn, M.G.; Fan, S.; Liu, K.; Dong, G. Global association between ambient air pollution and blood pressure: A systematic review and meta-analysis. *Environ. Pollut.* **2018**, *235*, 576–588. [CrossRef] [PubMed]
19. Ye, J.J.; Wang, S.S.; Fang, Y.; Zhang, X.J.; Hu, C.Y. Ambient air pollution exposure and risk of chronic kidney disease: A systematic review of the literature and meta-analysis. *Environ. Res.* **2021**, *195*, 110867. [CrossRef] [PubMed]
20. Grant, A.; Leung, G.; Aubin, M.J.; Kergoat, M.J.; Li, G.; Freeman, E.E. Fine Particulate Matter and Age-Related Eye Disease: The Canadian Longitudinal Study on Aging. *Investig. Ophthalmol. Vis. Sci.* **2021**, *62*, 7. [CrossRef] [PubMed]
21. Shin, J.; Lee, H.; Kim, H. Association between Exposure to Ambient Air Pollution and Age-Related Cataract: A Nationwide Population-Based Retrospective Cohort Study. *Int. J. Environ. Res. Public Health* **2020**, *17*, 9231. [CrossRef] [PubMed]
22. Sun, H.; Luo, C.; Chiang, Y.; Li, K.Y.Y.; Ho, Y.; Lee, S.; Chen, W.; Chen, C.; Kuan, Y. Association Between PM2.5 Exposure Level and Primary Open-Angle Glaucoma in Taiwanese Adults: A Nested Case–control Study. *Int. J. Environ. Res. Public Health* **2021**, *18*, 1714. [CrossRef] [PubMed]
23. Yang, B.Y.; Guo, Y.M.; Zou, Z.Y.; Gui, Z.H.; Bao, W.W.; Hu, L.W.; Chen, G.B.; Jing, J.; Ma, J.; Li, S.S.; et al. Exposure to ambient air pollution and visual impairment in children: A nationwide cross-sectional study in China. *J. Hazard. Mater.* **2021**, *407*, 124750. [CrossRef]
24. Yang, X.; Yang, Z.; Liu, Y.; Chen, X.; Yao, B.; Liang, F.; Shan, A.; Liu, F.; Chen, S.; Yan, X. The association between long-term exposure to ambient fine particulate matter and glaucoma: A nation-wide epidemiological study among Chinese adults. *Int. J. Hyg. Environ. Health* **2021**, *238*, 113858. [CrossRef]

25. Ju, M.J.; Kim, J.; Park, S.K.; Kim, D.H.; Choi, Y. Long-term exposure to ambient air pollutants and age-related macular degeneration in middle-aged and older adults. *Environ. Res.* **2022**, *204*, 111953. [CrossRef]
26. Li, L.; Zhu, Y.; Han, B.; Chen, R.; Man, X.; Sun, X.; Kan, H.; Lei, Y. Acute exposure to air pollutants increase the risk of acute glaucoma. *BMC Public Health* **2022**, *22*, 1782. [CrossRef]
27. Sterne, J.; Gavaghan, D.; Egger, M. Publication and related bias in meta-analysis: Power of statistical tests and prevalence in the literature. *J. Clin. Epidemiol.* **2000**, *53*, 1119–1129. [CrossRef]
28. Grant, A.; Leung, G.; Freeman, E.E. Ambient Air Pollution and Age-Related Eye Disease: A Systematic Review and Meta-Analysis. *Investig. Ophthalmol. Vis. Sci.* **2022**, *63*, 17. [CrossRef]
29. Cui, Y.H.; Hu, Z.X.; Gao, Z.X.; Song, X.L.; Feng, Q.Y.; Yang, G.; Li, Z.J.; Pan, H.W. Airborne particulate matter impairs corneal epithelial cells migration via disturbing FAK/RhoA signaling pathway and cytoskeleton organization. *Nanotoxicology* **2018**, *12*, 312–324. [CrossRef] [PubMed]
30. West, S.K.; Bates, M.N.; Lee, J.S.; Schaumberg, D.A.; Lee, D.J.; Adair-Rohani, H.; Chen, D.F.; Araj, H. Is Household Air Pollution a Risk Factor for Eye Disease? *Int. J. Environ. Res. Public Health* **2013**, *10*, 5378–5398. [CrossRef] [PubMed]
31. Hwang, S.H.; Choi, Y.H.; Paik, H.J.; Wee, W.R.; Kim, M.K.; Kim, D.H. Potential Importance of Ozone in the Association Between Outdoor Air Pollution and Dry Eye Disease in South Korea. *JAMA Ophthalmol.* **2016**, *134*, 503–510. [CrossRef] [PubMed]
32. Phaniendra, A.; Jestadi, D.B.; Periyasamy, L. Free Radicals: Properties, Sources, Targets, and Their Implication in Various Diseases. *Indian J. Clin. Biochem.* **2015**, *30*, 11–26. [CrossRef]
33. Khreis, H.; Bredell, C.; Wai Fung, K.; Hong, L.; Szybka, M.; Phillips, V.; Abbas, A.; Lim, Y.; Jovanovic Andersen, Z.; Woodcock, J.; et al. Impact of long-term air pollution exposure on incidence of neurodegenerative diseases: A protocol for a systematic review and exposure-response meta-analysis. *Environ. Int.* **2022**, *170*, 107596. [CrossRef]
34. Okamoto, Y.; Akagi, T.; Suda, K.; Kameda, T.; Miyake, M.; Ikeda, H.O.; Nakano, E.; Uji, A.; Tsujikawa, A. Longitudinal changes in superficial microvasculature in glaucomatous retinal nerve fiber layer defects after disc hemorrhage. *Sci. Rep.* **2020**, *10*, 22058. [CrossRef]
35. Deflorio-Barker, S.; Zelasky, S.; Park, K.; Lobdell, D.T.; Stone, S.L.; Rappazzo, K.M. Are the adverse health effects of air pollution modified among active children and adolescents? A review of the literature. *Prev. Med.* **2022**, *164*, 107306. [CrossRef]
36. Clougherty, J.E. A Growing Role for Gender Analysis in Air Pollution Epidemiology. *Environ. Health Perspect.* **2010**, *118*, 167–176. [CrossRef] [PubMed]
37. Jiang, Q.Q.; Wang, S.Q.; Zhang, H.; Guo, Y.; Lou, Y.L.; Huang, S.; You, Q.Q.; Cao, S.Y. The Association Between Solid Fuel Use and Visual Impairment Among Middle-Aged and Older Chinese Adults: Nationwide Population-Based Cohort Study. *JMIR Public Health Surveill.* **2023**, *9*, e43914. [CrossRef] [PubMed]
38. Ravilla, T.D.; Gupta, S.; Ravindran, R.D.; Vashist, P.; Krishnan, T.; Maraini, G.; Chakravarthy, U.; Fletcher, A.E. Use of Cooking Fuels and Cataract in a Population-Based Study: The India Eye Disease Study. *Environ. Health Perspect.* **2016**, *124*, 1857–1862. [CrossRef] [PubMed]
39. Beebe, D.C.; Holekamp, N.M.; Shui, Y.B. Oxidative Damage and the Prevention of Age-Related Cataracts. *Ophthalmic Res.* **2010**, *44*, 155–165. [CrossRef] [PubMed]
40. Torricelli, A.; Novaes, P.; Matsuda, M.; Alves, M.R.; Monteiro, M. Ocular surface adverse effects of ambient levels of air pollution. *Arq. Bras. Oftalmol.* **2011**, *74*, 377–381. [CrossRef]

toxics

MDPI

Review

Developmental Toxicity of Fine Particulate Matter: Multifaceted Exploration from Epidemiological and Laboratory Perspectives

Ruifeng Yan, Danni Ma, Yutong Liu, Rui Wang, Lifan Fan, Qiqi Yan, Chen Chen, Wenhao Wang, Zhihua Ren, Tingting Ku *, Xia Ning and Nan Sang

College of Environment and Resource, Research Center of Environment and Health, Shanxi University, Taiyuan 030006, China; yanruifeng@sxu.edu.cn (R.Y.); 18535704463@163.com (D.M.); 202313905002@email.sxu.edu.cn (Y.L.); wir010202@163.com (R.W.); 202223905001@email.sxu.edu.cn (L.F.); yqq13134680242@163.com (Q.Y.); 13347541630@163.com (C.C.); wwh11232002@163.com (W.W.); zhren@sxu.edu.cn (Z.R.); ningxia@sxu.edu.cn (X.N.); sangnan@sxu.edu.cn (N.S.)

* Correspondence: kutingting@sxu.edu.cn

Abstract: Particulate matter of size ≤ 2.5 μm ($PM_{2.5}$) is a critical environmental threat that considerably contributes to the global disease burden. However, accompanied by the rapid research progress in this field, the existing research on developmental toxicity is still constrained by limited data sources, varying quality, and insufficient in-depth mechanistic analysis. This review includes the currently available epidemiological and laboratory evidence and comprehensively characterizes the adverse effects of $PM_{2.5}$ on developing individuals in different regions and various pollution sources. In addition, this review explores the effect of $PM_{2.5}$ exposure to individuals of different ethnicities, genders, and socioeconomic levels on adverse birth outcomes and cardiopulmonary and neurological development. Furthermore, the molecular mechanisms involved in the adverse health effects of $PM_{2.5}$ primarily encompass transcriptional and translational regulation, oxidative stress, inflammatory response, and epigenetic modulation. The primary findings and novel perspectives regarding the association between public health and $PM_{2.5}$ were examined, highlighting the need for future studies to explore its sources, composition, and sex-specific effects. Additionally, further research is required to delve deeper into the more intricate underlying mechanisms to effectively prevent or mitigate the harmful effects of air pollution on human health.

Keywords: fine particulate matter; adverse birth outcomes; respiratory development; cardiovascular development; neurological development; mechanism

1. Introduction

Particulate matter of size ≤ 2.5 μm ($PM_{2.5}$) is defined as a type of fine PM with a diameter of <2.5 μm, which is distinguished by small particle dimensions, large relative surface area, and a capacity to adsorb heavy metals and toxic organic pollutants. These characteristics facilitate the infiltration of $PM_{2.5}$ into the human body, leading to various adverse reactions. Extensive research has consistently demonstrated the harmful health effects of prolonged $PM_{2.5}$ exposure, which predisposes individuals to an augmented risk of cardiovascular and respiratory ailments as well as neurological disorders such as Alzheimer's disease [1–3]. Moreover, outdoor air pollution, specifically that caused by ambient PM, has been officially classified as a Class I human carcinogen by the International Agency for Research on Cancer [4].

During early life, which is a pivotal stage of individual development, the body's system exhibits heightened sensitivity to environmental pollutants and is more prone to their toxic effects compared with adults. Therefore, there is a substantial interest in exploring the potential causal link between $PM_{2.5}$ exposure in early life and a wide array of diseases. An increasing amount of epidemiological research has established a correlation between developmental exposure to $PM_{2.5}$ and the heightened risk of birth defects and various diseases [5–8]. $PM_{2.5}$ exposure during pregnancy can lead to negative consequences such as preterm labor (PTB), low birth weight (LBW), and multiple facial defects [9–11]. Furthermore, prenatal and postnatal exposures to $PM_{2.5}$ reportedly impact lung development [12,13], heighten vulnerability to respiratory infections, and potentially contribute to the occurrence of respiratory ailments during early childhood [12]. The high level of maternal exposure to air pollution is also correlated with the increased chances of congenital heart defects (CHDs) in the offspring and has a detrimental effect on their neurodevelopment in early childhood [14–16]. Additionally, even minimal levels of air pollution exposure during pregnancy (levels that might not significantly affect adults) reportedly disrupt fetal development and result in long-term dysfunction [17].

Considering the escalating public concern regarding the health hazards associated with $PM_{2.5}$ during early life, the effects of prenatal exposure to $PM_{2.5}$ on fetal health remain uncertain. This review systematically investigates the detrimental biological effects of these pollutants on the developmental outcomes of humans by incorporating approximately 20 years of epidemiological and laboratory evidence, encompassing the latest research findings and advancements (epidemiological evidence is presented in Table 1). This review emphasizes the differences in the developmental toxicity of $PM_{2.5}$ from different regions and pollution sources as well as variations among different ethnicities, sexes, and socioeconomic levels, through the comprehensive analysis and comparison of various research outcomes.

Integrating and summarizing the commonalities found in these data reveal the complexity and diversity of $PM_{2.5}$ developmental toxicity, which can provide readers with a comprehensive background and foundation for better understanding the current status and trends in this field. Concurrently, this study comprehensively elucidates the possible molecular mechanisms underlying the health impairments triggered by $PM_{2.5}$ in various systems, mainly involving transcriptional and translational regulation, oxidative stress and inflammatory responses, and epigenetic regulation [18], providing deeper theoretical support and guidance for research in related fields. The primary conclusions and novel perspectives regarding the relation between public health and $PM_{2.5}$ are summarized in this review, which might offer insights into the prevention and treatment of environment-related illnesses, assist with the development of clinically applicable drugs, and serve as specific instructions for future research directions.

Table 1. Epidemiological studies on the adverse developmental outcomes of prenatal or postnatal $PM_{2.5}$ exposure.

Country	Contaminant	Exposure Period	Outcome	Supporting Statistics	References
China	$PM_{2.5}$	During the entire pregnancy	PROM	A substantial link between acute $PM_{2.5}$ exposure (per interquartile range increase) and the likelihood of PROM (OR = 1.11; 95% CI: 1.03, 1.19 for $PM_{2.5}$ on delivery day; OR = 1.10; 95% CI: 1.02, 1.18 for $PM_{2.5}$ 1 day before delivery)	Wang et al., 2022 [19]
USA	$PM_{2.5}$	During the entire pregnancy	PTB	High levels of $PM_{2.5}$ exposure were correlated with a 19% increase in PTB risk	Defranco et al., 2016 [20]
China	$PM_{2.5}$ and PM_{10}	During the entire pregnancy	PTB and near-term birth	Exposure to $PM_{2.5}$ or PM_{10} throughout pregnancy increased the likelihood of PTB and near-term birth (HR: 1.09 [95% CI: 1.08, 1.10] for a 10 $\mu g/m^3$ increase in $PM_{2.5}$)	Li et al., 2018 [21]

Table 1. *Cont.*

Country	Contaminant	Exposure Period	Outcome	Supporting Statistics	References
USA	$PM_{2.5}$ and NO_2	During the entire pregnancy	Declined birth weights	For each 10 μg/m^3 increase in $PM_{2.5}$ exposure, birth weights underwent a decline of 18.4, 10.5, 29.7, and 48.4 g during the first, second, and third trimesters, or throughout the entire pregnancy, respectively	Savitz et al., 2014 [22]
USA	$PM_{2.5}$	During the entire pregnancy	LBW	A mean concentration increase in $PM_{2.5}$ exposure was linked to a 3.2% (95% CI = −1.0%, 6.3%) increase in the probability of LBW among term births	Kirwa et al., 2019 [23]
Republic of Chile	$PM_{2.5}$ and PM_{10}	Gestational exposure	LBW	$PM_{2.5}$ exposure during the second trimester was associated with a higher likelihood of LBW (OR: 1.031; 95% CI: 1.004–1.059)	Rodríguez-Fernández et al., 2022 [24]
USA	$PM_{2.5}$, PM_{10}, CO	During 3 months prior to conception and gestational weeks 3–8	Orofacial defects, CP	The positive associations of $PM_{2.5}$ with CP were most eminent from gestational weeks 3–5	Zhu et al., 2015 [5]
USA	$PM_{2.5}$ and O_3	During early gestation (weeks 5–10 of gestation)	CP	Each 10 μg/m^3 increase in $PM_{2.5}$ concentration was accompanied by a 43% increase in the risk of developing CP	Zhou et al., 2017 [25]
China	$PM_{2.5}$	Elementary school students aged 5–12	Impaired respiratory health, increased airway inflammation, reduced lung function	Among all constituents of $PM_{2.5}$, organic carbon, elemental carbon, NO_3^-, and NH_4^+ had the consistent and strongest associations with airway inflammation biomarkers and lung function parameters, followed by metallic elements	Wu et al., 2021 [26]
Poland	$PM_{2.5}$	During the entire pregnancy	Increased susceptibility to respiratory infections in early childhood	The aOR for the occurrence of recurrent bronchopulmonary infections during the follow-up period significantly increased in a dose–response relationship with the prenatal $PM_{2.5}$ level (OR = 2.44, 95% CI: 1.12–5.36)	Jedrychowski et al., 2013 [12]
China	$PM_{2.5}$	During pregnancy and infancy	Asthma	The susceptible periods of developing asthma included gestational weeks 6–22 and 9–46 weeks following delivery	Jung et al., 2019 [27]
USA	$PM_{2.5}$	During the entire pregnancy	Asthma	Boys with higher prenatal exposure during midgestation (16–25-week gestation) exhibited an increased incidence of developing asthma by the age of 6 years	Hsu et al., 2015 [28]
USA	$PM_{2.5}$	During established morphogenic phases of prenatal lung development	Asthma	An increase in $PM_{2.5}$ by 2 μg/m^3 was found to have a connection with a 1.29-fold higher risk of developing asthma	Hazlehurst et al., 2021 [29]

Table 1. *Cont.*

Country	Contaminant	Exposure Period	Outcome	Supporting Statistics	References
USA	$PM_{2.5}$	Potential	Repeated wheezing	Heightened prenatal exposure to $PM_{2.5}$ during the later stages of pregnancy correlated with recurrent wheezing in early childhood	Chiu et al., 2022 [30]
Israeli	CO, NO_2, O_3, SO_2, PM_{10}, $PM_{2.5}$	During weeks 3–8 of pregnancy	Multiple CHDs	Higher maternal exposure to PM_{10} was linked to an elevated likelihood of multiple CHDs (aOR 1.05, 95% CI: 1.01–1.10 for a 10 $\mu g/m^3$ increment)	Agay-Shay et al., 2013 [31]
China	PM_{10}, $PM_{2.5}$, NO_2, CO, SO_2	During the entire pregnancy	CHDs	Markedly increasing the association of $PM_{2.5}$ exposure during the second and third trimesters with the occurrence of CHDs, with aORs of 1.228 and 1.236 (95% CI: 1.141–1.322, 1.154–1.324 individually) for each 10 $\mu g/m^3$ increase in $PM_{2.5}$ level	Sun et al., 2022 [16]
USA	Benzene and $PM_{2.5}$	During gestation	Selected heart defects	Exposure to elevated concentrations of $PM_{2.5}$ was linked to a higher risk of developing specific heart defects, including truncus arteriosus, the coarctation of the aorta, and interrupted aortic arch	Tanner et al., 2015 [32]
USA	$PM_{2.5}$	During pregnancy	Increased BP in children aged 3–9 years old	A 5 $\mu g/m^3$ rise in $PM_{2.5}$ during the third trimester was associated with a 3.49 percentile (95% CI: 0.71–6.26) elevation in child SBP or a 1.47 times (95% CI: 1.17–1.85) higher hazard of elevated BP	Zhang et al., 2018 [9]
USA	$PM_{2.5}$ and BC	Each trimester of pregnancy and within 2–90 days before birth	Elevated BP among newborns	Exposure to $PM_{2.5}$ and BC during the late pregnancy stage was associated with elevated BP among newborns (e.g., 1.0 mmHg; 95% CI: 0.1, 1.8 for a 0.32 $\mu g/m^3$ increase in mean 90-day residential BC)	Van Rossem et al., 2015 [33]
Spain	$PM_{2.5}$ and NO_2	Throughout the whole period of the pregnancies	Adverse impacts on memory and verbal abilities in boys	Boys being more susceptible between the ages of 4 and 6 years, particularly in areas associated with memory, verbal aptitude, and overall cognitive abilities	Lertxundi et al., 2019 [34]
USA	$PM_{2.5}$	Entire pregnancy	ID	The risks of ID associated with having daily average $PM_{2.5}$ concentrations over the current US NAAQS threshold (i.e., $\geq$12.0 $\mu g/m^3$) during the preconception and first trimester windows were substantial; the odds ratios were 1.8 and 2.4, respectively	Grineski et al., 2023 [35]

Table 1. *Cont.*

Country	Contaminant	Exposure Period	Outcome	Supporting Statistics	References
USA	$PM_{2.5}$	Prenatal	Slightly lower IQ in late childhood	A substantial correlation was observed between $PM_{2.5}$ exposure in the later stages of pregnancy (months 5–7) and the IQ of children	Holm et al., 2023 [36]
China	$PM_{2.5}$ and PM_{10}	Prenatal and early postnatal exposures	Decreased MDI and PDI scores	Exposure to $PM_{2.5}$ and PM_{10} in either of the two periods was linked to reduced scores of the MDI and PDI in the offspring	Wang et al., 2022 [14]
China	$PM_{2.5}$	Prenatal	SDDs	$PM_{2.5}$ exposure may elevate the risk of SDDs in both sexes (RR: 1.52, 95% CI: 1.19, 2.03, per 10 $\mu g/m^3$ increase in $PM_{2.5}$ exposure), particularly in problem-solving skills among girls (RR: 2.23, 95% CI: 1.22, 4.35)	Wang et al., 2021 [37]
China	$PM_{2.5}$	Prenatal and postnatal	Decreased LDCDQ scores and increased risk of DCD	Exposure to $PM_{2.5}$ was linked to diminished motor performance and a greater risk of DCD, with an aOR of 1.06 (95% CI: 1.01, 1.10) and 1.06 (95% CI: 1.01, 1.13) for every interquartile range elevation in $PM_{2.5}$ exposure during the first 3 months and the initial 3 years, separately	Cai et al., 2023 [38]
China	$PM_{2.5}$	During the prenatal and postnatal periods	Postponement in gross motor, fine motor, and personal–social development	Exposure during the second trimester of pregnancy was linked to an elevated probability of delayed neurodevelopment related to gross motor skills (aOR: 1.09 per 10 $\mu g/m^3$ increase). The delayed development of fine motor skills was revealed to be involved with $PM_{2.5}$ exposure in the second and third trimesters (aOR: 1.06)	Shih et al., 2023 [39]
USA	$PM_{2.5}$	From 3 months before pregnancy until the child's second birthday	ASD	A 50% rise in the risk of ASD when exposed to an average cumulative level of $PM_{2.5}$ from 3 months before conception through the child's second year (p = 0.046)	Talbott et al., 2015 [40]
USA	$PM_{2.5}$ and PM_{10}	From 9 months before pregnancy to 9 months after delivery	Greater odds of ASD	The relation between ASD and $PM_{2.5}$ exposure was more pronounced in the final trimester (OR = 1.42 per IQR raise in $PM_{2.5}$; 95% CI: 1.09, 1.86)	Raz et al., 2015 [41]

Table 1. *Cont.*

Country	Contaminant	Exposure Period	Outcome	Supporting Statistics	References
USA	$PM_{2.5}$, NO_2, O_3	During pregnancy	ASD	The sensitive periods of $PM_{2.5}$ exposure linked to ASD occurred early in pregnancy, demonstrating statistical significance over 1–27 weeks of gestation (cumulative HR = 1.14 [95% CI: 1.06, 1.23] per IQR [7.4 μg/m^3] increase)	Rahman et al., 2022 [42]
USA	Aircraft ultrafine particles	During pregnancy	ASD	A significant association was identified between the increased risk of ASD and maternal exposure to aircraft $PM_{0.1}$ throughout pregnancy (HR: 1.02, [95% CI: 1.01–1.03] per interquartile range [IQR] = 0.02 μg/m^3 rise)	Carter et al., 2023 [43]

Abbreviations: ASD, autism spectrum disorders; BC, black carbon; BP, blood pressure; CHDs, congenital heart diseases; CP, cleft palate alone; DCD, developmental coordination disorder; ID, intellectual disability; IQ, Intelligence Quotient; LDCDQ, Little DCD Questionnaire; MDI, Mental Developmental Index; PDI, Psychomotor Developmental Index; PROM, premature rupture of membranes; and SDD, suspected developmental delay.

2. Materials and Methods

2.1. Search Strategy

We performed a literature review using the PubMed database to identify articles published in the last 20 years (2003–2023) regarding the developmental toxicity of $PM_{2.5}$ exposure. We utilized various combinations of the following keywords: "air pollution" or "particulate matter" or "PM" and "pregnancy" or "child" or "offspring" or "developmental toxicity". Additionally, the studies identified through the aforementioned search strategy were examined.

2.2. Inclusion Criteria

Studies were included if they involved (1) epidemiological or clinical investigations evaluating the effect of maternal exposure to $PM_{2.5}$ on offspring development, exploring the association between $PM_{2.5}$ and various adverse outcomes such as neurological disorders and cardiopulmonary diseases in offspring; (2) research delving into the developmental toxicity and underlying mechanisms of $PM_{2.5}$ utilizing in vivo and in vitro models with commonly utilized laboratory materials (e.g., mice, rats, and zebrafish); or (3) comprehensive analysis of the mechanisms underlying developmental toxicity induced by $PM_{2.5}$, encompassing aspects such as transcriptional and translational regulation, oxidative stress, inflammatory responses, epigenetic modifications, and other pertinent factors.

2.3. Exclusion Criteria

The studies were excluded if they were (1) not written in English, (2) published before 2003, (3) if their full text was not available from PubMed, or (4) if they addressed irrelevant populations or exposures not during the developmental period.

3. Adverse Birth Outcomes Induced by $PM_{2.5}$

3.1. Epidemiological Studies

3.1.1. Preterm Birth

The present findings confirmed that maternal exposure to $PM_{2.5}$ was correlated with an increased probability of preterm labor. A nationwide survey in China revealed that maternal $PM_{2.5}$ exposure, whether acute or chronic, considerably heightened the likelihood of PROM, resulting in a heightened risk of negative outcomes for mothers and newborns, including preterm birth, intrauterine infection, and abruptio placentae [19]. A substantial link has been reported between acute $PM_{2.5}$ exposure (per interquartile range increase) and the likelihood of PROM (odds ratio [OR] = 1.11; 95% confidence interval [CI]: 1.03, 1.19 for $PM_{2.5}$ on delivery day; OR = 1.10; 95% CI: 1.02, 1.18 for $PM_{2.5}$ one day before delivery).

Women with lower levels of education or obesity or who gave birth during colder seasons appeared to be more sensitive to the effects of ambient $PM_{2.5}$ [19]. In a cohort study conducted in Ohio, high levels of $PM_{2.5}$ exposure during pregnancy were correlated with a 19% increase in PTB risk, with the highest risk occurring during late pregnancy [20]. This study also employed a logistic regression model to identify other factors linked to preterm birth, notably maternal race. After accounting for other variables, non-Hispanic black mothers demonstrated a heightened risk of preterm birth (aOR 1.46) compared to non-Hispanic white mothers (aOR 1.00), with a statistically significant association. Moreover, a cohort comprising >1.28 million births in China demonstrated that exposure to $PM_{2.5}$ or PM_{10} throughout pregnancy increased the likelihood of PTB and near-term birth (hazard ratio [HR]: 1.09 [95% CI: 1.08, 1.10] for a 10 μg/m^3 increase in $PM_{2.5}$). Women with poor socioeconomic backgrounds, obesity, and smoking habits were more susceptible to PM exposure [21]. Taken together, these findings highlight the significance of considering the actual background of pregnant women, such as income levels and racial differences, in analyzing the toxic effects of $PM_{2.5}$.

3.1.2. Low Birth Weight and Reduced Fetal Growth

Birth weight is a well-known predictor of overall neonatal health. There is a well-established link between LBW and elevated neonatal mortality and morbidity rates [7]. In recent years, researchers have accumulated evidence indicating a direct association between increased prenatal exposure to $PM_{2.5}$ and higher probability of LBW. A study including 252,967 births conducted from 2008 to 2010 reported that for each 10 μg/m^3 increase in $PM_{2.5}$ exposure, birth weights underwent a decline of 18.4, 10.5, 29.7, and 48.4 g during the first, second, and third trimesters, or throughout the entire pregnancy, respectively [22]. An extensive analysis involving >330,000 births to Hispanic and Black mothers spanning 14 years in Puerto Rico noted that a mean concentration increase in $PM_{2.5}$ exposure was linked to a 3.2% (95% CI = −1.0%, 6.3%) increase in the probability of LBW among term births [23].

A cross-sectional analytical project comprising 595,369 Chilean newborns investigated the connection between LBW and gestational exposure to $PM_{2.5}$ and PM_{10}. The investigation concluded that $PM_{2.5}$ exposure during the second trimester was associated with a higher likelihood of LBW (OR: 1.031; 95% CI: 1.004–1.059), whereas PM_{10} had an impact on the entire duration of pregnancy [24]. These findings strongly support the correlation between urban air pollution exposure and LBW as well as diminished fetal growth.

3.1.3. Facial Defects

While there is supporting evidence demonstrating a correlation between maternal ambient air pollution exposure and the occurrence of congenital orofacial clefts in children, epidemiologic research has produced inconclusive findings. A large retrospective cohort in the US investigated substantial and positive relevance between ambient air pollution and the risk of orofacial defects in the offspring of mothers who were exposed to $PM_{2.5}$ during the 3 months before conception [5]. Specifically, the positive associations of $PM_{2.5}$ with cleft palate were most eminent from gestational weeks 3–5 when analyzed in terms of individual week [5]. According to a comparable study, each 10 μg/m^3 increase in $PM_{2.5}$ concentration was accompanied by a 43% increase in the risk of developing cleft palate [25]. Conversely, no substantial correlation was detected between the concentration of $PM_{2.5}$ and the incidence of cleft lip [25], which also indicates potential uncertainty regarding facial defects in relation to $PM_{2.5}$ exposure. In addition to facial defects, it is crucial to further explore other types of birth defects associated with $PM_{2.5}$ exposure to address existing gaps in knowledge.

3.2. Experimental Research

Experimental studies demonstrated that $PM_{2.5}$ exposure inhibited embryonic development, which aligned with the aforementioned epidemiological observations. Offspring birth weight was substantially reduced owing to maternal exposure to concentrated ambient $PM_{2.5}$ (CAP), while the body weight of adult male descendants showed an increase [44]. Similarly, a substantial decrease in body weight and crown-rump length on GD13 (gestation day) and GD18 was revealed in another study that evaluated fetal and placenta development exposure in utero in mice, which was concomitant with abnormal placental structure and aberrant placental functional gene expression [45]. The detrimental effects of $PM_{2.5}$ on birth outcomes have also been extensively investigated through numerous zebrafish experiments. $PM_{2.5}$ exposure caused developmental toxicity that varied with dose and duration [46], leading to increased mortality and malformations as well as decreased hatchability rate and body length [47]. These findings underscore the potential association between $PM_{2.5}$ exposure during pregnancy and embryo growth restriction. However, as experimental model organisms, mice exhibit differences from humans or other animals in aspects such as physiological structure, metabolic pathways, and behavioral patterns, making it inappropriate to directly extrapolate findings to other species or natural ecosystems. Subsequent epidemiological and toxicological investigations are required to examine the consequences of $PM_{2.5}$ on other species.

4. Adverse Effects of $PM_{2.5}$ on Respiratory Development

4.1. Epidemiological Studies

The development of lungs is a complex process that spans from conception to the postnatal period [27]; particulate air pollution impacts lung development during the prenatal and postnatal period [12,13], increases the likelihood of contracting respiratory infections, and could cause respiratory health issues during early childhood [12]. An increasing number of studies have associated $PM_{2.5}$ exposure with children's respiratory health, with findings revealing that developmental exposure can disrupt alveolarization, compromise lung function, and alter pulmonary immune differentiation, potentially impacting short- and long-term health conditions [48,49]. According to a longitudinal panel investigation with repeated health assessments conducted in Shanghai involving 62 children, short-term $PM_{2.5}$ exposure can compromise children's respiratory health, increasing airway inflammation, reducing lung function, and altering the microbial colonization of the buccal mucosa [26]. In a separate study involving 214 children monitored over 7 years, the adjusted OR (aOR) for the occurrence of recurrent bronchopulmonary infections during the follow-up period significantly increased in a dose–response relationship with the prenatal $PM_{2.5}$ level (OR = 2.44, 95% CI: 1.12–5.36) [12]. This study also reported that setting the 24 h average $PM_{2.5}$ concentration at 20 $\mu g/m^3$ as a target value can offer superior protection for unborn babies compared with the previously established EPA guidelines.

In addition, clinical respiratory symptoms of particulate pollution aggravate asthma [50]. According to a large birth cohort study conducted in Taichung City, there is a notable association between augmented prenatal and postnatal exposure to $PM_{2.5}$ and an elevated risk of developing asthma. The susceptible periods included gestational weeks 6–22 and 9–46 weeks following delivery [27]. Boys with higher prenatal exposure during midgestation (16–25-week gestation) exhibited an increased incidence of developing asthma by the age of 6 years [28]. In a combined analysis of two pregnancy cohorts, children living with higher $PM_{2.5}$ concentrations during the saccular stage of fetal lung development were more likely to develop asthma. An increase in $PM_{2.5}$ by 2 $\mu g/m^3$ was found to have a connection with a 1.29-fold higher risk of developing asthma [29]. The potential impact of $PM_{2.5}$ on offspring may exhibit sex-specific and time-dependent consequences, which appear to differ based on ethnicity and level of maternal antioxidant intake. Research on a multiethnic inner-city population revealed that heightened prenatal exposure to $PM_{2.5}$ during the later stages of pregnancy correlated with recurrent wheezing in early childhood, specifically among male infants born to Black mothers with low levels of antioxidant consumption [30].

Existing research has provided valuable insights into the association between $PM_{2.5}$ exposure and respiratory health by considering gender and racial differences.

4.2. Experimental Research

Animal studies revealed that maternal exposure to $PM_{2.5}$ during the sensitive windows resulted in fetal pulmonary dysfunction and increased the risk of lung diseases. In a rat model, prolonged exposure during pregnancy substantially modified the structure and function of the lungs in the offspring [51], characterized by heightened lung consolidation, airway inflammation, and diminished lung volume and compliance [52]. Another study reported various changes, such as interstitial proliferation in the lungs, notable oxidative stress, and enhancement of epithelial–mesenchymal transition (EMT) [53]. Moreover, previous findings revealed that male descendants experienced a dysplasia-like syndrome, encompassing hypoalveolarization, diminished secretory function, delayed microvascular development, and inflammation within the lungs. Nonetheless, female offspring exhibited only slight changes in alveolarization and lung inflammation, indicating that male offspring were more vulnerable to maternal $PM_{2.5}$ exposure. Interestingly, these negative effects were nearly reversed during postnatal development [54]. There are physiological, immunological, and metabolic differences between genders that may result in divergent responses to $PM_{2.5}$ exposure. However, current research predominantly focuses on the general population, without fully considering the impact of gender differences on susceptibility to $PM_{2.5}$. There is a lack of comprehensive understanding regarding the gender-specific respiratory diseases of $PM_{2.5}$.

5. Cardiovascular Diseases Induced by $PM_{2.5}$

5.1. Epidemiological Studies

5.1.1. Heart Defects

There is considerable evidence suggesting that maternal exposure to air pollution is positively correlated with the risk of CHD in offspring [55,56]. A cohort study based on registries employed a spatiotemporal approach using Geographic Information System data and weekly inverse distance weighting modeling to examine the potential connections between exposure to ambient air pollution during week 3–8 of pregnancy and the risk of CHD. The results indicated that higher maternal exposure to PM_{10} was linked to an elevated likelihood of multiple CHD (aOR 1.05, 95% CI: 1.01–1.10 for a 10 $\mu g/m^3$ increment), while higher exposure to $PM_{2.5}$ was linked to a reduced risk for patent ductus arteriosus (aOR 0.78, 95% CI: 0.68–0.91 for a 5-$\mu g/m^3$ increment), and sensitivity analyses confirmed the consistency of these results [31].

The markedly increasing association of $PM_{2.5}$ exposure during the second and third trimesters with the occurrence of CHDs was detected in a study in Suzhou, with aORs of 1.228 and 1.236 (95% CI: 1.141–1.322, 1.154–1.324 individually) for each 10 $\mu g/m^3$ increase in $PM_{2.5}$ level [16]. In a retrospective cohort study in Florida [32], exposure to elevated concentrations of $PM_{2.5}$ was linked to a higher risk of developing specific heart defects, including truncus arteriosus, coarctation of the aorta, and interrupted aortic arch. However, it is currently uncertain whether these connections have meaningful clinical relevance or can be directly attributed to exposure to air pollution. The latter findings need to be supplemented by other studies for definitive conclusions.

5.1.2. High Blood Pressure

Relevant evidence showed that air pollution exposure during pregnancy may also render offspring increasingly susceptible to high BP. A cohort study involving 1131 mother–infant pairs in Boston examined the potential correlation between systolic blood pressure (SBP) and air pollutant exposures using mixed-effects models, reporting that exposure to $PM_{2.5}$ and BC during the late pregnancy stage was associated with elevated BP among newborns (e.g., 1.0 mmHg; 95% CI: 0.1, 1.8 for a 0.32 $\mu g/m^3$ increase in mean 90 day residential BC) [33].

In another study, connections between maternal exposure to ambient $PM_{2.5}$ and elevated child BP at 3–9 years old were detected in a cohort from the USA, suggesting that reducing maternal exposure could prevent pediatric hypertension at the primary level [9]. A 5 μg/m^3 rise in $PM_{2.5}$ during the third trimester was associated with a 3.49 percent (95% CI: 0.71–6.26) elevation in child SBP or a 1.47 times (95% CI:1.17–1.85) higher hazard of elevated BP, and the connection was partially explained by the impact of $PM_{2.5}$ on fetal growth and weight during childhood, revealing novel perspectives of the mechanisms through which prenatal $PM_{2.5}$ exposure influences SBP in children.

5.2. Experimental Research

Epidemiological evidence has shown that $PM_{2.5}$ pollution during pregnancy may have a negative impact on cardiovascular system development. In fact, experimental research has corroborated the findings observed in humans.

Studies in mice revealed that $PM_{2.5}$ exposure during the in utero period may affect the development of the descendant's cardiovascular system and elevate the risk of altered BP [57–59] as well as contribute to heart failure and additional cardiovascular incidents [9,33,58]. Prominent histological changes were observed in the hearts of mature progeny mice exposed to $PM_{2.5}$ pollution during gestation [60], primarily comprising disordered cardiac cell organization, inflammation, and enlarged myocardial septum. Furthermore, male mice exhibited more severe heart damage compared with female mice in mature progeny mice. A study presented compelling evidence that exposing gravida to $PM_{2.5}$ at a concentration of 73.61 μg/m^3 substantially increased cardiac dysfunction among male descendants during their adult years [57,58], which was evidenced by changes such as remodeling and dysfunction of the left ventricle in living organisms as well as dysfunction of cardiomyocytes in a laboratory setting. Pregnant mice exposed to diesel exhaust demonstrated an enhanced vulnerability to heart failure induced by pressure overload in the offspring as they matured into adulthood [61,62]. Cardiomyocytes extracted from mice exposed to $PM_{2.5}$ during perinatal development also displayed changes in sarcomere function that were apparent at the cellular level [63].

Although these experiments were conducted solely in mice, similar observations of remarkable cardiovascular impairment caused by $PM_{2.5}$ exposure are also present in other animal species. Specifically, several studies have documented detrimental impacts on the embryonic cardiac development of zebrafish [64]. TSP and $PM_{2.5}$ exposure have been demonstrated to impair heart rate and blood flow velocity as well as affect cardiac morphology and angiogenesis [47]. Additional research substantiated that extractable organic matter (EOM) of $PM_{2.5}$ was the primary cause underlying increased cardiac malformations, such as globular chambers and pericardial edema as well as decreased heart rate [64]. Moreover, it induced DNA damage and apoptosis, inhibited cardiac differentiation, and ultimately led to heart defects in zebrafish embryos and mouse P19 embryonic cancer cells [65–67]. Current research on the impact of $PM_{2.5}$ on cardiovascular function is subject to certain limitations. Existing studies primarily focus on overall impacts while paying less attention to the specific components of $PM_{2.5}$ responsible for the related biological processes. Additionally, there are limitations in research methods and techniques, such as a lack of high-resolution molecular analysis technology and research tools at the cellular level. Therefore, it is necessary for subsequent research to employ more advanced technological approaches to enhance the understanding of the precise constituents of $PM_{2.5}$ that contribute to cardiovascular dysfunction and the related biological processes at the molecular level.

6. Neurodevelopmental Toxicity Caused by $PM_{2.5}$

6.1. Epidemiological Studies

Exposure to $PM_{2.5}$ and PM_{10} in the prenatal and early postnatal stages was found to have a detrimental impact on early childhood neurodevelopment [14,15].

6.1.1. Developmental Delay and Developmental Coordination Disorder

According to relevant studies, preschoolers exposed to higher levels of $PM_{2.5}$ exhibited higher levels of compromised neurobehavioral development, including developmental delay and DCD. Research involving the Shanghai Maternal–Child Pairs Cohort, which used the Ages and Stages Questionnaire (ASQ) to evaluate the neurological development of children at 2, 6, 12, and 24 months old, proposed that exposure to $PM_{2.5}$ during weeks 18–34 of pregnancy showed a significant correlation with ASQ scores and SDDs. $PM_{2.5}$ exposure may elevate the risk of SDDs in both sexes (RR: 1.52, 95% CI: 1.19, 2.03, per 10 $\mu g/m^3$ increase in $PM_{2.5}$ exposure), particularly in problem-solving skills among girls (RR: 2.23, 95% CI: 1.22, 4.35) [37]. Information gathered from a cohort study including 109,731 children between the ages of 3 and 5 years in China suggested that exposure to $PM_{2.5}$ during prenatal and postnatal stages was linked to diminished motor performance and greater risk of DCD [38]. The aOR was 1.06 (95% CI: 1.01, 1.10) and 1.06 (95% CI: 1.01, 1.13) for every interquartile range elevation in $PM_{2.5}$ exposure during the first 3 months and the initial 3 years, separately. The present investigation also suggested that infants who breastfed for <6 months exhibit a greater susceptibility to the effects of postnatal $PM_{2.5}$ exposure.

In a cohort study conducted within the population of Taiwan, a notable correlation was observed between gestational exposure to $PM_{2.5}$ and postponement in the development of gross motor skills, fine motor skills, and personal–social abilities [39]. Specifically, exposure during the second trimester of pregnancy was linked to an elevated probability of delayed neurodevelopment related to gross motor skills (aOR 1.09 per 10 $\mu g/m^3$ increase). The delayed development of fine motor skills was revealed to be associated with $PM_{2.5}$ exposure in the second and third trimesters (aOR 1.06), and personal–social skills were affected similarly. Nevertheless, the neurodevelopmental indicators mentioned above showed no correlation with postnatal $PM_{2.5}$ exposure. Additional research examining the consequences of $PM_{2.5}$ during pregnancy for neurodevelopment in children is essential.

6.1.2. Cognitive Impairment

Cognition is the process by which organisms perceive and acquire knowledge, while cognitive impairment refers to the presence of difficulties in higher cortical functions such as perception, attention, language, memory, and thinking [68]. There is increasing evidence stating that prenatal or postnatal $PM_{2.5}$ pollution affects the cognition of offspring. A case–control study in Utah ($n = 1032$) and a cohort study in California's agricultural Salinas Valley ($n = 568$) concluded that encountering slightly elevated outdoor $PM_{2.5}$ concentrations before delivery was indicative of greater odds of ID and small decrements in IQ in late childhood, which remained consistent across various sensitivity analyses [35,36].

According to a three-district birth cohort study carried out in Spain, the effects of $PM_{2.5}$ exposure during pregnancy on neuropsychological development were observed to be dependent on the sex of the child, with boys being more susceptible between the ages of 4 and 6 years, particularly in areas associated with memory, verbal aptitude, and overall cognitive abilities [34]. Despite the potential cognitive benefits associated with breastfeeding, this study has revealed that exposure to environmental pollutants during intrauterine development may not be mitigated by breastfeeding. A substantial correlation was observed between $PM_{2.5}$ exposure in the later stages of pregnancy (months 5–7) and the IQ of children, indicating that this specific time frame was particularly influential [36].

An interesting finding was the potential influence of the fetal sex on the $PM_{2.5}$–IQ association. Boys exhibited low verbal comprehension and working memory with average $PM_{2.5}$ exposure in utero, whereas girls exhibited a low processing speed. The connections between PM exposure during pregnancy or the early postnatal period and the neurodevelopment of offspring at 2 years of age were evaluated and compared by a study including 1331 mother–child pairs; the results indicated that exposure to $PM_{2.5}$ and PM_{10} in either of the two periods was linked to reduced scores in the mental and psychomotor developmental indices in the offspring [14]. Additionally, compared with prenatal exposure,

exposure during the early infancy phase more strongly affects neurodevelopment [14], indicating that the early postnatal phase may serve as a critical period for the impact of ambient PM on offspring development. Additional investigation is warranted to pinpoint the precise developmental timeframe when exposure to $PM_{2.5}$ pollution has the most pronounced impact.

6.1.3. Autism Spectrum Disorders

Susceptibility to ASD is determined by an interplay of genetic and environmental influences. Researchers discovered that contact with $PM_{2.5}$ during the prenatal and postnatal periods increases susceptibility of a child toward ASD [40,69].

A case–control study in Southwestern Pennsylvania revealed ~50% rise in the risk of ASD when exposed to an average cumulative level of $PM_{2.5}$ from 3 months before conception through the child's second year ($p = 0.046$) [40]. In addition, a significant association was identified between the increased risk of ASD and maternal exposure to aircraft ultrafine emission ($PM_{0.1}$) throughout pregnancy in a cohort study involving 370,723 singleton pregnancies (HR: 1.02, [95% CI: 1.01–1.03] per interquartile range [IQR] = 0.02 $\mu g/m^3$ rise) [43]. In a nested case–control study, it was observed that the relation between ASD and $PM_{2.5}$ exposure was more pronounced in the final trimester (OR = 1.42 per IQR raise in $PM_{2.5}$; 95% CI: 1.09, 1.86) when adjusting for mutual factors [41]. Yet another population-based cohort study identified that the sensitive periods of $PM_{2.5}$ exposure linked to ASD occurred early in pregnancy, demonstrating statistical significance over 1–27 weeks of gestation (cumulative HR = 1.14 [95% CI: 1.06, 1.23] per IQR [7.4 $\mu g/m^3$] increase). Furthermore, sex-stratified analysis revealed that the connections between early gestational exposure and ASD were more pronounced in boys than girls (boys HR = 1.16 [95% CI: 1.08, 1.26]; girls HR = 1.06 [95% CI: 0.89, 1.26]) [42]. While these findings contribute crucial evidence regarding the potential negative impacts of $PM_{2.5}$ exposure on the nervous system during pregnancy, the studies lack longitudinal tracking research on children's long-term neurodevelopmental outcomes. They also fail to adequately identify the critical developmental stages of $PM_{2.5}$ exposure and they overlook the moderating role of gender in its effects.

6.2. Experimental Research

6.2.1. Neural Damage and Brain Injury

$PM_{2.5}$ exposure induces neural damage and brain injury [70]. A study found gestational CAP exposure can produce neuropathological changes [71], including microglial activation and ventricular enlargement, enlarged corpus callosum, decreased hippocampal volume, aberrant white matter development, and hypomyelination [72]. Additionally, most of these effects were either exclusive to boys or more pronounced in them. Exposure to elevated levels of TSP and $PM_{2.5}$ led to the shortened length of DA neurons within the clusters of the raphe nuclei, decreased dopamine levels, and dyskinesia emergence [47]. Furthermore, exposure to $PM_{2.5}$ solely triggered intracerebral hemorrhage and disrupted the maturation of neurovascular networks. Additionally, gestational $PM_{2.5}$ exposure resulted in tau pathology in the cortical region of male descendants, which is essential for modulating neuronal maturation [73]. Previous studies have also reported that $PM_{2.5}$ triggered seasonally influenced neuronal apoptosis and synaptic impairments [74].

6.2.2. Impaired Learning and Memory

Following exposure to $PM_{2.5}$, both sexes exhibited compromised learning and short-term memory abilities accompanied by the sustained activation of glial cells within the prefrontal cortex and corpus callosum [75]. A study provided evidence that early developmental exposure to low levels of ultrafine particles can result in enduring effects on the central nervous system (CNS) functions. These consequences include enduring deficits in cognitive abilities such as learning and short-term memory, alterations in impulsive conduct and motor skills, and some persistent changes in the neurochemical processes of the brain, especially in the prefrontal cortex, the area crucial for cognitive functions [75].

Moreover, there was proof suggesting that gestational $PM_{2.5}$ exposure disrupted Hoxa5-mediated neuronal morphogenesis in male mice, resulting in impaired spatial learning and memory. Organic constituents such as PAHs exerted a more detrimental effect compared with the inorganic components [76].

6.2.3. ASD

Data from several studies have suggested that exposure to PM from traffic during pregnancy and breastfeeding contributes to the incidence of ASD and cognitive deficits [77]. Early exposure to PM was found to engender persistent behavioral impairments, which vary based on sex and may be a potential contributing factor to neurodevelopmental disorders such as ASD [78]. A study noted that mice subjected to fine PM throughout the stages of their gestational and early neonatal periods decreased social engagement in both sexes, while male descendants demonstrated more extensive repetitive impairments [78]. Mice exposed to $PM_{2.5}$ during pregnancy and the postnatal stages exhibited a more pronounced impact on the neuroinflammatory response; postnatal exposure of mice to ambient ultrafine particles reproduced numerous features consistent with ASD, such as repetitive and impulsive behaviors [79].

6.2.4. Anxiety, Depression, and Fear

Prenatal exposure plays a pivotal role in engendering anxiety-like behavior observed in adulthood [80]. A study revealed that exposing mice to $PM_{0.1}$ before mating and during gestation resulted in an increase in depressive-like reactions in male offspring [81]. Increased exposure to $PM_{2.5}$ was strongly linked with heightened fearful behaviors in boys and girls at 6 months of age, and increased prenatal exposure to PM exhibited time-dependent implications that varied across sex [82]. Overall, these studies highlighted the importance of sex differences in related toxicology studies. Additional exploration is warranted to gain a comprehensive understanding of the specific mechanisms responsible for inducing aberrant development or inflicting damage upon the neurological system during the developmental period.

7. Mechanistic Considerations of $PM_{2.5}$-Induced Developmental Toxicity

Air pollution, especially that caused by $PM_{2.5}$, has attracted considerable attention as a prominent worldwide issue over the past several years, resulting in a substantial societal burden and loss of life. Extensive evidence from human and experimental research has revealed the deleterious impacts of PM, prompting a thorough investigation into the fundamental molecular processes (Figure 1). The negative health effects observed in offspring who were exposed to fine or ultrafine PM during their formative years are believed to be influenced by three primary mechanisms: transcriptional and translational regulation, oxidative stress and inflammation responses, and epigenetic regulation (developmental toxicity responses and mechanisms of $PM_{2.5}$ are presented in Table 2). These mechanisms have offered insightful information regarding the connections between exposure to $PM_{2.5}$ and health consequences, potentially aiding in the identification of targeted interventions that may be advantageous for pregnant women who are exposed to air pollutants.

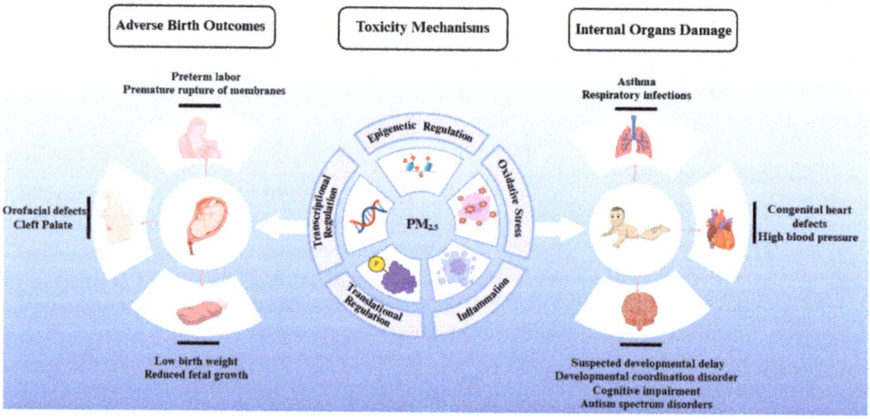

Figure 1. Schematic of biological mechanisms underlying $PM_{2.5}$-induced adverse birth outcomes and internal organ developmental injury. Image created with BioRender.com accessed on 28 March 2024. with permission.

Table 2. Summary of developmental toxicity responses and mechanisms of $PM_{2.5}$ in vivo and in vitro.

Experimental Animals/Cells	Study Design	Biological Response	Molecular Mechanism	References
Mice fetal	Pregnant mice were randomized into concentrated $PM_{2.5}$ group and FA group	Reduced fetal weight, crown–rump length, placental disorder and IUGR	AMPK/mTOR pathway	Li et al., 2022 [45]
SD rat offspring embryos	$PM_{2.5}$ was added at 6.25–200 μg/mL	Impaired embryonic growth, decreased yolk sac size, crown–rump length, head length, and somite count	ROS-MAPKs-apoptosis/cell cycle arrest pathways	Yuan et al., 2016 [83]
Zebrafish embryos/larvae	Exposed to 25, 50, 100, 200, and 400 μg/mL of $PM_{2.5}$ and TSP from 24 to 120 hpf	Elevated mortality rate, malformations, reduced development of cardiovasculature and neurovasculature	ERS and Wnt signaling	Jia et al., 2022 [47]
Male mice offspring	Pregnant mice were orally given $PM_{2.5}$ suspension (3 mg/kg/2 days) until the birth of decedents	Impaired myelin ultrastructure on PNDs 14 and 21	lncRNAs–Ctcf signaling pathway	Hou et al., 2023 [72]
Primary cortical neuron	Treated with the $PM_{2.5}$ samples at different concentration	Neuronal apoptosis and synaptic injuries	Suppression of phosphorylated ERK1/2 and CREB, activated caspase-3	Chen et al., 2017 [74]
Murine offspring	Pregnant ICR mice were exposed daily to $PM_{2.5}$ (0.4 mg/m^3) or FA, separately (for 14 consecutive days)	Locomotor hyperactivities	The excessive activity of the dopamine pathway inhibited the glycine pathway	Cui et al., 2019 [84]
Neonatal mice (14 days old)	Pregnant FVB female mice were exposed either to FA or $PM_{2.5}$ at an average concentration of 91.78 μg/m^3 for 6 h/day, 5 days/week throughout the gestation period (20 days)	Functional cardiac changes that were evident during the very early (14 days) stages of adolescence	Altered Ca^{2+} handling protein expression	Tanwar et al., 2017 [59]

Table 2. *Cont.*

Experimental Animals/Cells	Study Design	Biological Response	Molecular Mechanism	References
Pups mice PND1 and 28	Timed pregnant SD rats were treated with $PM_{2.5}$ (0.1, 0.5, 2.5, or 7.5 mg/kg) once every 3 days from day 0 to 18 of pregnancy	Significant decreases in lung volume parameters, compliance, and airflow during expiration on PND28, interstitial proliferation in lung histology	TGF-β/Smad3 pathway	Tang et al., 2017 [52]
Juvenile male rats	Gestational and early-life exposure to traffic-related PM ($PM_{2.5}$ was 200 μg/m^3) for 5 h/day, 5 days/week for 6 weeks	Decreased social behavior, increased anxiety, impaired cognition, disrupted neural integrity	Decreased levels of inflammatory and growth factors	Nephew et al., 2020 [77]
Mice offspring	Timed pregnant SD rats were treated with $PM_{2.5}$ (0.1, 0.5, 2.5, or 7.5 mg/kg) once every 3 days from day 0 to 18 of pregnancy	Fetal lung injury, lung inflammation	Promoted IL-1, IL-6, and TNF-α secretion	Tang et al., 2018 [51]
Zebrafish embryo	Exposed to EOM concentration at 5 mg/L abstracted from $PM_{2.5}$	Mitochondrial dysfunction, apoptosis and heart defects	CYP1A1 overexpression and accumulation of mtROS	Chen et al., 2023 [85]
Adult mice offspring	Male and female FVB mice were exposed to either FA or $PM_{2.5}$ at an average concentration of 38.58 μg/m^3 for 6 h/day, 5 days/week for 3 months	Cardiac dysfunction	Altered Ca^{2+} regulatory proteins, increased oxidative stress markers, inflammatory and fibrogenic mediators	Tanwar et al., 2018 [57]
Zebrafish embryos	Exposed to EOM abstracted from $PM_{2.5}$ at different concentrations at 3 hpf in the absence or presence of CH (0.5 μM) or CHIR (1 μM)	Heart defects	Activation of AHR, repressed Wnt/β-catenin signaling	Zhang et al., 2016 [64]
Zebrafish embryos	Exposed to EOM (5 mg/L) in the absence or presence of CH (0.05 μM) or NAC (0.25 μM) from 3 hpf until 72 hpf	DNA damage and apoptosis, cardiac developmental toxicity	Oxidative stress	Ren et al., 2020 [66]
Zebrafish embryos	Treated with EOM (5 mg/L) in the absence or presence of 4-PBA (5 mM), CH (0.05 mM) or NAC (0.25 mM) from 2 to 72 hpf	Apoptosis, heart defects	ER stress and Wnt signaling inhibition	Zhang et al., 2022 [67]
Mice	Exposed in the postnatal period from PNDs 4–7 and 10–13, with adult re-exposure at PNDs 57–59	Long-term impairment in learning/short-term memory, impulsivity-linked behavior and motor function	Persistent glial activation, more inflammatory cytokines including IL-6, TNF-α	Allen et al., 2014 [75]
Mice	Exposed to concentrated ambient UFP from PND 4–7 and 10–13	Repetitive and impulsive behaviors, reductions in the size of the CC and associated hypomyelination	Inflammation/microglial activation, elevated glutamate and excitatory/inhibitory imbalance, increased amygdala astrocytic activation	Allen et al., 2017 [79]

Table 2. *Cont.*

Experimental Animals/Cells	Study Design	Biological Response	Molecular Mechanism	References
Mice	Exposed to ultrafine CAPs or FA on PNDs 4–7 and 10–13	Lateral ventricle dilation	Neuroinflammatory response, alterations in cytokines and neurotransmitters	Allen et al., 2014 [86]
Zebrafish embryos	Exposed to EOM extracted from $PM_{2.5}$ (5 mg/L) in the absence or presence of FA (0.05 μM) from 3 hpf	Heart defects	Decreased SAM/SAH ratio, altered expression of genes related to DNA methylation	Jiang et al., 2019 [87]
hESCs line H1	Treated with EOM from $PM_{2.5}$ concentrations exceeding 100 μg/mL	Abnormal embryonic development, decrease in vitality	Interference with DNA methylation and mRNA expression	Wang et al., 2023 [88]
Zebrafish embryos	Treated with EOM concentrations of 5 mg/L	Apoptosis and cardiac malformations	Decreased global m^6A RNA methylation levels	Ji et al., 2023 [89]

Abbreviations: AHR, aryl-hydrocarbon receptor; CC, corpus callosum; CH, CH223191; CHIR, CHIR99021; ERS, endoplasmic reticulum stress; FA, filtered air; FVB, friend leukemia virus b; hESCs, human embryonic stem cells; hpf, hours post-fertilization; IUGR, intrauterine growth restriction; PNDs, postnatal days; UFP, ultrafine particle (<100 nm).

7.1. Transcriptional and Translational Regulation

As external pollutants can affect gene expression and alter the synthesis, activity, and function of proteins in organisms, either through direct or indirect means, transcriptional and translation regulation are considered the primary regulatory mechanisms for the negative impacts of $PM_{2.5}$. For instance, $PM_{2.5}$ interferes with embryonic development by impacting processes such as autophagy and apoptosis, leading to cellular dysfunction often associated with alterations in the relevant genetic expression. Additionally, various receptor proteins, including components of the MAPK and caspases, have been involved in mediating these developmental toxic effects. A study provided evidence that encountering $PM_{2.5}$ during gestation reduced the levels of autophagy-related proteins and suppressed autophagy flux primarily on GD15. Similarly, the activation of the AMPK/mTOR signaling pathway, which plays a crucial role in regulating autophagy, was also observed in the placenta on GD15. These findings revealed that the AMPK/mTOR pathway could be implicated in the inhibition of placental autophagy caused by $PM_{2.5}$, leading to placental dysfunction and IUGR in mice [45]. Researchers attempted to address the potential involvement of ROS–MAPK–apoptosis/cell cycle arrest pathways in the embryotoxicity triggered by $PM_{2.5}$, using whole rat embryos cultured in vitro. The results revealed that $PM_{2.5}$ treatment delayed embryonic development along with cellular apoptosis and G0/G1 phase arrest.

Additionally, ROS production and the consequent activation of JNK and ERK signaling pathways may participate in these detrimental consequences by decreasing the Bcl-2/Bax protein ratio and increasing transcription levels of $p15^{INK4B}$, $p16^{INK4A}$, and $p21^{WAF1/CIP1}$ [83,90]. Another study explored the correlation between $PM_{2.5}$ exposure and neurodegenerative effects such as neuronal apoptosis and synaptic damage. The findings demonstrated that exposure to $PM_{2.5}$ induced modifications in the expression of proteins associated with apoptosis, primarily bax and bcl-2, leading to the activation of caspase-3 and subsequent neuronal apoptosis. Moreover, $PM_{2.5}$ exposure resulted in a reduction in the expression extent of synaptic structural postsynaptic density protein 95 (PSD-95) and synaptic functional protein N-Methyl-D-Aspartate (NMDA) receptor subunit (NR2B), both crucial for synaptic integrity and function. The suppression of phosphorylated ERK1/2 and CREB accompanied these effects. One additional key finding derived from this study was that these outcomes showed a seasonal correlation, with the most pronounced alterations observed in the $PM_{2.5}$ samples obtained over the winter period [74].

The nervous system of zebrafish larvae experienced developmental toxicity due to exposure to $PM_{2.5}$, which disrupted neuronal differentiation and neurovasculogenesis processes. Exposure to elevated concentrations of $PM_{2.5}$ resulted in decreased expression levels of genes associated with dopamine regulation as well as essential neurodevelopmental genes linked to CNS development in zebrafish. This exposure also caused the loss and degeneration of dopaminergic neurons as well as decreasing the length of DA neurons in the raphe nuclei clusters [47]. This study presented empirical support for the adverse effects on cardiovascular health and neurodevelopment caused by acute exposure to TSP and $PM_{2.5}$, which were linked to abnormal gene expression. Another study also concluded from a murine model that the prenatal inhalation of $PM_{2.5}$ could potentially have detrimental consequences on the neurobehavior of offspring. This impact was linked to the overactivation of the dopamine pathway and inhibition of the glycine pathway within the brain [84].

A study examined the genetic expression profile of the cortical regions of male descendants following $PM_{2.5}$ exposure during pregnancy. This experiment revealed that prenatal $PM_{2.5}$ exposure disrupted myelin development via the lncRNAs–Ctcf signaling pathway, inducing abnormal myelin development in male offspring. The observation of reduced myelin sheath thickness in the optic nerves and a slight decline in myelin content in the corpus callosum serve as compelling evidence for this phenomenon. This study presented genomic evidence linking prenatal encounters with $PM_{2.5}$ with neurodevelopmental disorders in male descendants [72].

In addition, researchers observed that the TGF-β/Smad3 pathway served as a mediator for the increased expression of EMT, which contributed to postnatal pulmonary impairment linked to maternal contact with $PM_{2.5}$ in a rat model [52]. Additional research has demonstrated that exposure to $PM_{2.5}$ during the gestational period contributes to cardiac impairment in newborns, primarily by modifying the protein expression associated with the regulation of Ca^{2+} [59].

To summarize, the studies mentioned above have delved deeply into the mechanisms through which $PM_{2.5}$ regulates gene expression, elucidating that $PM_{2.5}$ exerts direct effects on gene expression and protein function through multiple pathways such as interfering with the binding of transcription factors to DNA, regulating RNA stability, and influencing post-translational modifications. This impact not only induces changes at the cellular level but may also trigger cascading effects in crucial biological processes such as neurodevelopment and immune regulation. These findings broadened the comprehension of a range of transcriptional and translational regulation prompted by exposure to $PM_{2.5}$, providing new insights for interventions and treatments of environmentally related diseases.

7.2. Oxidative Stress and Inflammation Response

It is widely accepted that oxidative stress and inflammation exert a crucial influence on the negative impacts of $PM_{2.5}$ on the development process of respiratory, cardiovascular, and nervous systems. There are abundant published studies describing the contribution of oxidative stress and inflammation on various body systems.

Intrauterine exposure to $PM_{2.5}$ raises susceptibility to acute infections of the bronchopulmonary system during the early developmental stage. Exposure to $PM_{2.5}$ during pregnancy leads to the onset of lung inflammation in descendants through pathways involving elevated HMGB1 expression, which in turn facilitates the secretion of IL-1, IL-6, and TNF-α [51]. Upon inhalation, on the one hand, PM directly damages cells by generating free radicals; on the other hand, it can be detected by receptors present on macrophages in the respiratory system, both of which stimulate the release of inflammatory cytokines [91,92], induce inflammatory responses, and result in newborns and young infants being more vulnerable to pulmonary infections [12]. $PM_{0.1}$ also penetrates the pulmonary endothelium and enters the bloodstream, reaching other organs [91,92]. This leads to an increase in systemic superoxide radical production due to subsequent neutrophil activation, which disrupts the integrity of endothelial cells [93]. Furthermore, a study found that higher exposure to $PM_{2.5}$ was associated with increasing concentrations of MCP-1 and IL-6 chemokines in the body as well as an increased influx of macrophages and neutrophils into multiple organs, including adipose tissue, the lungs, spleen, and thymus [94].

While the precise mechanisms remain elusive, oxidative stress and inflammation are considered to have significant implications in heart development. One study provided evidence that $PM_{2.5}$ caused abnormal heart development through oxidative stress, evidenced by altered Ca^{2+} regulatory proteins and increased levels of oxidative stress markers. Apart from oxidative stress, inflammatory response is also involved in this damage, supported by the observation that CRP expression increased nearly eightfold in offspring who were prenatally exposed to $PM_{2.5}$ [57]. Another study indicated that EOM from $PM_{2.5}$ increased mtROS production through the overexpression of CYP1A1 mediated by AHR, which aggravated the opening of the mPTP, resulting in mitochondrial dysfunction. The opening of the mPTP further caused the buildup of mtROS, ultimately leading to inherent apoptosis and heart defects. These findings indicate that mitochondria have the potential to be an attractive candidate for therapeutic targeting to prevent and treat CHDs caused by air pollution [85].

Similarly, EOM exposure triggered AHR/ROS-mediated ER stress, which subsequently intensified ROS production. Sustained ER stress upregulated CHOP, promoting DNA apoptosis and inhibiting Wnt signaling, consequently contributing to cardiac abnormalities in the embryos of the zebrafish species. This study revealed the participation of ER stress in the development of adverse cardiac defects caused by $PM_{2.5}$, indicating that targeting ER stress and inhibiting CHOP upregulation could potentially treat and prevent CHDs caused by air pollution [64,66,67].

Air pollution poses a significant threat to the brain, and $PM_{2.5}$ exposure during pregnancy might adversely impact the neurobehavior of descendants through an inflammatory response [79]. Possible mechanisms by which $PM_{2.5}$ induces neurological damage include direct neurotoxicity caused by the permeation of PM into CNS tissues, triggering a cascade of secondary neurotoxic events that include reactive microglia proliferation triggered by inflammatory signaling molecules entering the brain from the circulation. Reportedly, ultrafine PM present in the bloodstream can traverse the blood–brain barrier and the cribriform plate in the olfactory mucosa, thereby entering the cerebrum [95]. Once within the cerebrum, PM may activate reactive microgliosis and interfere with the growth of neurons even at minimal levels while inducing the death of neurons at greater doses [75,79,95,96]. Another study reported that when pregnant individuals were exposed to UFP, their offspring exhibited the enduring activation of glial cells in the corpus callosum and frontal cortex [75]. This glial activation increased the generation of inflammatory cytokines such as IL-6 and TNF-α, which perpetuated the cycle of neuroinflammation and oxidative damage [97,98]. Exaggerated microglial activation and accompanying inflammation have the potential to cause hypomyelination and ventriculomegaly by exerting toxicity on oligodendrocytes, which are responsible for myelination in the cerebrum, ultimately resulting in impaired learning and short-term memory outcomes in both sexes [79,86,99–103]. Although there is much research on the inflammation and oxidative stress caused by $PM_{2.5}$, mysteries still surround the detailed signaling pathways and interactions among various cellular factors. The relationship between the inflammatory and oxidative stress effects of different components of $PM_{2.5}$ remains unclear.

7.3. Epigenetic Regulation

Epigenetic regulation, encompassing DNA methylation, histone modification, and RNA-mediated processes, is critical in the developmental process. Epigenetic changes are responsive to external stressors and have been proposed to serve as a connection between environmental influences and genetic factors [104]. Early-life exposure to air pollutants might contribute to epigenetic dysregulation, causing developmental abnormalities, childhood and adult illnesses, and even the development of cancer later in life. To date, the molecular pathways underlying the mechanism by which $PM_{2.5}$ induces epigenetic modifications have been inadequately explored.

DNA methylation is a constituent of the extensively researched epigenetic alterations and is essential in the development of the heart. Disruptions in DNA methylation have been implicated in the occurrence of CHD [105]. Extensive research has provided insights into the aberrant DNA methylation alterations triggered by $PM_{2.5}$ exposure, which can result in disruptions of DNA methylation and mRNA expression, leading to abnormal embryonic development. Elevated prenatal exposure was correlated with an increased overall mutation rate in the placenta, which coincided with epigenetic modifications in crucial DNA repair and tumor suppressor genes, ultimately resulting in modifications in the capacity of fetal and neonatal DNA repair [106]. The transcriptome and DNA methyl group of hESCs were significantly influenced by the presence of EOM extracted from $PM_{2.5}$. The integrated examination of alterations in DNA methylation and mRNA expression revealed an increased abundance of terms associated with the VEGFR signaling pathway and extracellular matrix. These findings offered a new understanding of the molecular processes that are implicated in the detrimental impact on development triggered by $PM_{2.5}$ [88].

In addition, EOM exposure can engender significant modifications in DNA methylation either through modifying the activity of genes associated with DNA methylation or through reducing the SAM/SAH ratio. These disrupted DNA methylation patterns affect the transcription of genes implicated in cardiac development, leading to the manifestation of cardiac abnormalities in zebrafish embryos. A crucial discovery of this study is that the administration of folic acid supplements can counteract this sequence of adverse alterations induced by EOM, and the reduction in DNA methylation changes might be involved in the protective effect of folic acid against cardiac developmental toxicity [87]. m^6A RNA methylation, which is the most prevalent type of RNA modification, has been identified as a critical factor in cardiac developmental toxicity.

One study indicated that exposure to EOM derived from $PM_{2.5}$ leads to significant alterations in m^6A RNA methylation. This is achieved through the downregulation of mettl14, facilitated by the AHR. Consequently, there is an upregulation of traf4a and bbc3 genes, triggering oxidative stress and apoptosis and eventually causing irregularities in cardiac development. Fortunately, this effect can be mitigated by the use of AHR antagonists and dietary methyl donors [89]. The collected data strongly support the fact that $PM_{2.5}$ exposure leads to substantial epigenetic modifications, which may affect the activation of pivotal genes implicated in early developmental processes. These discoveries greatly enhanced the comprehension of how $PM_{2.5}$ exerts its harmful effects at the molecular level and underscore the importance of studying the components of $PM_{2.5}$.

8. Conclusions

Although there is a growing body of information regarding the effects of exposure to PM during pregnancy, the complex composition and diverse sources of $PM_{2.5}$, as well as the influence of environmental factors such as atmospheric stability and topographical features and the existence of differences in exposure levels and individual sensitivity, make it difficult to ascertain its potential health risks to humans and wildlife. Additionally, epidemiological studies may be affected by factors such as sample selection bias, information bias, or confounding, which could impact the accuracy and reliability of research results. In laboratory experiments, important factors such as species differences, exposure methods, duration, dosage, and particle composition may not be adequately discussed and considered, which could affect the scientific validity and credibility of the research conclusions. Therefore, the following aspects should be emphasized: (1) given the high adsorption capacity of $PM_{2.5}$ for various pollutants, different origins of $PM_{2.5}$ may lead to diverse negative impacts. Subsequent research should prioritize examining adducts generated by a range of contaminants, encompassing heavy metals and organic compounds while considering their combined effects and identifying the specific roles of various air toxins through the multipollutant modeling or an effect-directed analysis strategy; (2) long-term assessment, identification of critical exposure windows, and multiple influences such as mother's age, economic level, and educational attainment should be considered; (3) the role of sexes on repercussions of atmospheric contamination deserves more research. Several studies have reported that there are differences in susceptibility to $PM_{2.5}$ between sexes, and there may be a reciprocal relationship between genetic and external elements; and (4) the mechanism of PMs precrossing and postcrossing the placental barrier also needs further in-depth study, which can provide theoretical support for the treatment of PM-induced diseases.

In conclusion, there remain significant knowledge deficiencies in the comprehension of the complex signaling pathways that mediate cellular reactions to $PM_{2.5}$. Advancing our comprehension regarding the mechanisms by which $PM_{2.5}$ affects health will be instrumental in the creation of clinically relevant drugs and novel strategies to protect the public, especially children, from air pollution.

Author Contributions: Writing—original draft preparation, R.Y. and D.M.; conceptualization, Y.L., R.W. and L.F.; investigation, Q.Y., C.C. and W.W.; validation, Z.R.; writing—review and editing, T.K. and X.N.; supervision and project administration, N.S. All authors have read and agreed to the published version of the manuscript.

Funding: This research was funded by the National Key R&D Program of China (2023YFC3708305), the National Science Foundation of China (No. 22176119 and 22036005), and the Special Fund for Scientific and Technological Innovation Talent Team of Shanxi Province (No. 202204051002024).

Institutional Review Board Statement: Not applicable.

Informed Consent Statement: Not applicable.

Data Availability Statement: Not applicable.

Conflicts of Interest: The authors declare no conflicts of interest.

Abbreviations

AHR, aryl-hydrocarbon receptor; aOR, adjusted OR; ASD, autism spectrum disorders; ASQ, Ages and Stages Questionnaire; BC, black carbon; BP, blood pressure; CAP, concentrated ambient $PM_{2.5}$; CC, corpus callosum; CH, CH223191; CHDs, congenital heart diseases; CHIR, CHIR99021; CNS, Central Nervous System; CP, cleft palate alone; DCD, developmental coordination disorder; EMT, epithelial–mesenchymal transition; EOM, extractable organic matters; ERS, endoplasmic reticulum stress; FA, filtered air; FVB, friend leukemia virus b; GD, gestation day; hESCs, human embryonic stem cells; hpf, hours post-fertilization; id, intellectual disability; IQ, intelligence quotient; IUGR, intrauterine growth restriction; LBW, low birth weight; LDCDQ, Little DCD Questionnaire; MDI, Mental Developmental Index; NMDA, N-Methyl-D-Aspartate; NR2B, receptor subunit; PDI, Psychomotor Developmental Index; $PM_{0.1}$, ultrafine emission; $PM_{2.5}$, particulate matter of size $\leq$ 2.5 μm; PNDs, postnatal days; PROM, premature rupture of membranes; PSD-95, postsynaptic density protein 95; PTB, preterm birth; SBP, systolic blood pressure; SDDs, suspected developmental delay; UFP, ultrafine particle (<100 nm).

References

1. Feng, S.; Gao, D.; Liao, F.; Zhou, F.; Wang, X. The health effects of ambient $PM_{2.5}$ and potential mechanisms. *Ecotoxicol. Environ. Saf.* **2016**, *128*, 67–74. [CrossRef] [PubMed]
2. Li, R.; Zhou, R.; Zhang, J. Function of $PM_{2.5}$ in the pathogenesis of lung cancer and chronic airway inflammatory diseases. *Oncol. Lett.* **2018**, *15*, 7506–7514. [CrossRef] [PubMed]
3. Thiankhaw, K.; Chattipakorn, N.; Chattipakorn, S.C. $PM_{2.5}$ exposure in association with AD-related neuropathology and cognitive outcomes. *Environ. Pollut.* **2022**, *292*, 118320. [CrossRef] [PubMed]
4. Wang, Y.; Zhong, Y.; Liao, J.; Wang, G. $PM_{2.5}$-related cell death patterns. *Int. J. Med. Sci.* **2021**, *18*, 1024–1029. [CrossRef] [PubMed]
5. Zhu, Y.; Zhang, C.; Liu, D.; Grantz, K.L.; Wallace, M.; Mendola, P. Maternal ambient air pollution exposure preconception and during early gestation and offspring congenital orofacial defects. *Environ. Res.* **2015**, *140*, 714–720. [CrossRef] [PubMed]
6. Teng, C.; Wang, Z.; Yan, B. Fine particle-induced birth defects: Impacts of size, payload, and beyond. *Birth Defects Res. C Embryo Today* **2016**, *108*, 196–206. [CrossRef] [PubMed]
7. Goriainova, V.; Awada, C.; Opoku, F.; Zelikoff, J.T. Adverse effects of black carbon (BC) exposure during pregnancy on maternal and fetal health: A contemporary review. *Toxics* **2022**, *10*, 779. [CrossRef] [PubMed]

8. Costa, L.G.; Cole, T.B.; Dao, K.; Chang, Y.C.; Garrick, J.M. Developmental impact of air pollution on brain function. *Neurochem. Int.* **2019**, *131*, 104580. [CrossRef] [PubMed]
9. Zhang, M.; Mueller, N.T.; Wang, H.; Hong, X.; Appel, L.J.; Wang, X. Maternal exposure to ambient particulate matter $\leq$2.5 µm during pregnancy and the risk for high blood pressure in childhood. *Hypertension* **2018**, *72*, 194–201. [CrossRef] [PubMed]
10. Gouveia, N.; Bremner, S.A.; Novaes, H.M. Association between ambient air pollution and birth weight in São paulo, Brazil. *J. Epidemiol. Community Health* **2004**, *58*, 11–17. [CrossRef] [PubMed]
11. Lin, C.A.; Pereira, L.A.; Nishioka, D.C.; Conceição, G.M.; Braga, A.L.; Saldiva, P.H. Air pollution and neonatal deaths in São paulo, Brazil. *Braz. J. Med. Biol. Res.* **2004**, *37*, 765–770. [CrossRef] [PubMed]
12. Jedrychowski, W.A.; Perera, F.P.; Spengler, J.D.; Mroz, E.; Stigter, L.; Flak, E.; Majewska, R.; Klimaszewska-Rembiasz, M.; Jacek, R. Intrauterine exposure to fine particulate matter as a risk factor for increased susceptibility to acute broncho-pulmonary infections in early childhood. *Int. J. Hyg. Environ. Health* **2013**, *216*, 395–401. [CrossRef] [PubMed]
13. Korten, I.; Ramsey, K.; Latzin, P. Air pollution during pregnancy and lung development in the child. *Paediatr. Respir. Rev.* **2017**, *21*, 38–46. [CrossRef] [PubMed]
14. Wang, H.; Zhang, H.; Li, J.; Liao, J.; Liu, J.; Hu, C.; Sun, X.; Zheng, T.; Xia, W.; Xu, S.; et al. Prenatal and early postnatal exposure to ambient particulate matter and early childhood neurodevelopment: A birth cohort study. *Environ. Res.* **2022**, *210*, 112946. [CrossRef] [PubMed]
15. Li, J.; Liao, J.; Hu, C.; Bao, S.; Mahai, G.; Cao, Z.; Lin, C.; Xia, W.; Xu, S.; Li, Y. Preconceptional and the first trimester exposure to $PM_{2.5}$ and offspring neurodevelopment at 24 months of age: Examining mediation by maternal thyroid hormones in a birth cohort study. *Environ. Pollut.* **2021**, *284*, 117133. [CrossRef] [PubMed]
16. Sun, L.; Wu, Q.; Wang, H.; Liu, J.; Shao, Y.; Xu, R.; Gong, T.; Peng, X.; Zhang, B. Maternal exposure to ambient air pollution and risk of congenital heart defects in Suzhou, China. *Front. Public. Health* **2022**, *10*, 1017644. [CrossRef] [PubMed]
17. Iglesias-Vázquez, L.; Binter, A.C.; Canals, J.; Hernández-Martínez, C.; Voltas, N.; Ambròs, A.; Fernández-Barrés, S.; Pérez-Crespo, L.; Guxens, M.; Arija, V. Maternal exposure to air pollution during pregnancy and child's cognitive, language, and motor function: Eclipses study. *Environ. Res.* **2022**, *212*, 113501. [CrossRef] [PubMed]
18. Zhang, Y.; Shi, J.; Ma, Y.; Yu, N.; Zheng, P.; Chen, Z.; Wang, T.; Jia, G. Association between air pollution and lipid profiles. *Toxics* **2023**, *11*, 894. [CrossRef] [PubMed]
19. Wang, C.; Yu, G.; Menon, R.; Zhong, N.; Qiao, C.; Cai, J.; Wang, W.; Zhang, H.; Liu, M.; Sun, K.; et al. Acute and chronic maternal exposure to fine particulate matter and prelabor rupture of the fetal membranes: A nation-wide survey in China. *Environ. Int.* **2022**, *170*, 107561. [CrossRef] [PubMed]
20. DeFranco, E.; Moravec, W.; Xu, F.; Hall, E.; Hossain, M.; Haynes, E.N.; Muglia, L.; Chen, A. Exposure to airborne particulate matter during pregnancy is associated with preterm birth: A population-based cohort study. *Environ. Health* **2016**, *15*, 6. [CrossRef] [PubMed]
21. Li, Q.; Wang, Y.Y.; Guo, Y.; Zhou, H.; Wang, X.; Wang, Q.; Shen, H.; Zhang, Y.; Yan, D.; Zhang, Y.; et al. Effect of airborne particulate matter of 2.5 µm or less on preterm birth: A national birth cohort study in China. *Environ. Int.* **2018**, *121*, 1128–1136. [CrossRef] [PubMed]
22. Savitz, D.A.; Bobb, J.F.; Carr, J.L.; Clougherty, J.E.; Dominici, F.; Elston, B.; Ito, K.; Ross, Z.; Yee, M.; Matte, T.D. Ambient fine particulate matter, nitrogen dioxide, and term birth weight in New York, New York. *Am. J. Epidemiol.* **2014**, *179*, 457–466. [CrossRef] [PubMed]
23. Kirwa, K.; McConnell-Rios, R.; Manjourides, J.; Cordero, J.; Alshawabekeh, A.; Suh, H.H. Low birth weight and $PM_{2.5}$ in Puerto rico. *Environ. Epidemiol.* **2019**, *3*, e058. [CrossRef] [PubMed]
24. Rodríguez-Fernández, A.; Ramos-Castillo, N.; Ruiz-De la Fuente, M.; Parra-Flores, J.; Maury-Sintjago, E. Association of prematurity and low birth weight with gestational exposure to $PM_{2.5}$ and PM_{10} particulate matter in chileans newborns. *Int. J. Environ. Res. Public. Health* **2022**, *19*, 6133. [CrossRef] [PubMed]
25. Zhou, Y.; Gilboa, S.M.; Herdt, M.L.; Lupo, P.J.; Flanders, W.D.; Liu, Y.; Shin, M.; Canfield, M.A.; Kirby, R.S. Maternal exposure to ozone and $PM_{2.5}$ and the prevalence of orofacial clefts in four U.S. States. *Environ. Res.* **2017**, *153*, 35–40. [CrossRef] [PubMed]
26. Wu, Y.; Li, H.; Xu, D.; Li, H.; Chen, Z.; Cheng, Y.; Yin, G.; Niu, Y.; Liu, C.; Kan, H.; et al. Associations of fine particulate matter and its constituents with airway inflammation, lung function, and buccal mucosa microbiota in children. *Sci. Total Environ.* **2021**, *773*, 145619. [CrossRef] [PubMed]
27. Jung, C.R.; Chen, W.T.; Tang, Y.H.; Hwang, B.F. Fine particulate matter exposure during pregnancy and infancy and incident asthma. *J. Allergy Clin. Immunol.* **2019**, *143*, 2254–2262. [CrossRef] [PubMed]
28. Hsu, H.H.; Chiu, Y.H.; Coull, B.A.; Kloog, I.; Schwartz, J.; Lee, A.; Wright, R.O.; Wright, R.J. Prenatal particulate air pollution and asthma onset in urban children. Identifying sensitive windows and sex differences. *Am. J. Respir. Crit. Care Med.* **2015**, *192*, 1052–1059. [PubMed]
29. Hazlehurst, M.F.; Carroll, K.N.; Loftus, C.T.; Szpiro, A.A.; Moore, P.E.; Kaufman, J.D.; Kirwa, K.; LeWinn, K.Z.; Bush, N.R.; Sathyanarayana, S.; et al. Maternal exposure to $PM_{2.5}$ during pregnancy and asthma risk in early childhood: Consideration of phases of fetal lung development. *Environ. Epidemiol.* **2021**, *5*, e130. [CrossRef]
30. Chiu, Y.M.; Carroll, K.N.; Coull, B.A.; Kannan, S.; Wilson, A.; Wright, R.J. Prenatal fine particulate matter, maternal micronutrient antioxidant intake, and early childhood repeated wheeze: Effect modification by race/ethnicity and sex. *Antioxidants* **2022**, *11*, 366. [CrossRef] [PubMed]

31. Agay-Shay, K.; Friger, M.; Linn, S.; Peled, A.; Amitai, Y.; Peretz, C. Air pollution and congenital heart defects. *Environ. Res.* **2013**, *124*, 28–34. [CrossRef]
32. Tanner, J.P.; Salemi, J.L.; Stuart, A.L.; Yu, H.; Jordan, M.M.; DuClos, C.; Cavicchia, P.; Correia, J.A.; Watkins, S.M.; Kirby, R.S. Associations between exposure to ambient benzene and $PM_{2.5}$ during pregnancy and the risk of selected birth defects in offspring. *Environ. Res.* **2015**, *142*, 345–353. [CrossRef] [PubMed]
33. van Rossem, L.; Rifas-Shiman, S.L.; Melly, S.J.; Kloog, I.; Luttmann-Gibson, H.; Zanobetti, A.; Coull, B.A.; Schwartz, J.D.; Mittleman, M.A.; Oken, E.; et al. Prenatal air pollution exposure and newborn blood pressure. *Environ. Health Perspect.* **2015**, *123*, 353–359. [CrossRef] [PubMed]
34. Lertxundi, A.; Andiarena, A.; Martínez, M.D.; Ayerdi, M.; Murcia, M.; Estarlich, M.; Guxens, M.; Sunyer, J.; Julvez, J.; Ibarluzea, J. Prenatal exposure to $PM_{2.5}$ and NO_2 and sex-dependent infant cognitive and motor development. *Environ. Res.* **2019**, *174*, 114–121. [CrossRef] [PubMed]
35. Grineski, S.; Alexander, C.; Renteria, R.; Collins, T.W.; Bilder, D.; VanDerslice, J.; Bakian, A. Trimester-specific ambient $PM_{2.5}$ exposures and risk of intellectual disability in Utah. *Environ. Res.* **2023**, *218*, 115009. [CrossRef] [PubMed]
36. Holm, S.M.; Balmes, J.R.; Gunier, R.B.; Kogut, K.; Harley, K.G.; Eskenazi, B. Cognitive development and prenatal air pollution exposure in the CHAMACOS cohort. *Environ. Health Perspect.* **2023**, *131*, 37007. [CrossRef] [PubMed]
37. Wang, P.; Zhao, Y.; Li, J.; Zhou, Y.; Luo, R.; Meng, X.; Zhang, Y. Prenatal exposure to ambient fine particulate matter and early childhood neurodevelopment: A population-based birth cohort study. *Sci. Total Environ.* **2021**, *785*, 147334. [CrossRef] [PubMed]
38. Cai, J.; Shen, Y.; Meng, X.; Zhao, Y.; Niu, Y.; Chen, R.; Du, W.; Quan, G.; Barnett, A.L.; Jones, G.; et al. Association of developmental coordination disorder with early-life exposure to fine particulate matter in Chinese preschoolers. *Innovation* **2023**, *4*, 100347. [PubMed]
39. Shih, P.; Chiang, T.L.; Wu, C.D.; Shu, B.C.; Lung, F.W.; Guo, Y.L. Air pollution during the perinatal period and neurodevelopment in children: A national population study in Taiwan. *Dev. Med. Child. Neurol.* **2023**, *65*, 783–791. [CrossRef] [PubMed]
40. Talbott, E.O.; Arena, V.C.; Rager, J.R.; Clougherty, J.E.; Michanowicz, D.R.; Sharma, R.K.; Stacy, S.L. Fine particulate matter and the risk of autism spectrum disorder. *Environ. Res.* **2015**, *140*, 414–420. [CrossRef] [PubMed]
41. Raz, R.; Roberts, A.L.; Lyall, K.; Hart, J.E.; Just, A.C.; Laden, F.; Weisskopf, M.G. Autism spectrum disorder and particulate matter air pollution before, during, and after pregnancy: A nested case-control analysis within the Nurses' Health Study II cohort. *Environ. Health Perspect.* **2015**, *123*, 264–270. [CrossRef] [PubMed]
42. Rahman, M.M.; Shu, Y.H.; Chow, T.; Lurmann, F.W.; Yu, X.; Martinez, M.P.; Carter, S.A.; Eckel, S.P.; Chen, J.C.; Chen, Z.; et al. Prenatal exposure to air pollution and autism spectrum disorder: Sensitive windows of exposure and sex differences. *Environ. Health Perspect.* **2022**, *130*, 17008. [CrossRef] [PubMed]
43. Carter, S.A.; Rahman, M.M.; Lin, J.C.; Chow, T.; Yu, X.; Martinez, M.P.; Levitt, P.; Chen, Z.; Chen, J.C.; Eckel, S.P.; et al. Maternal exposure to aircraft emitted ultrafine particles during pregnancy and likelihood of ASD in children. *Environ. Int.* **2023**, *178*, 108061. [CrossRef] [PubMed]
44. Chen, M.; Wang, X.; Hu, Z.; Zhou, H.; Xu, Y.; Qiu, L.; Qin, X.; Zhang, Y.; Ying, Z. Programming of mouse obesity by maternal exposure to concentrated ambient fine particles. *Part. Fibre Toxicol.* **2017**, *14*, 20. [CrossRef] [PubMed]
45. Li, R.; Peng, J.; Zhang, W.; Wu, Y.; Hu, R.; Chen, R.; Gu, W.; Zhang, L.; Qin, L.; Zhong, M.; et al. Ambient fine particulate matter exposure disrupts placental autophagy and fetal development in gestational mice. *Ecotoxicol. Environ. Saf.* **2022**, *239*, 113680. [CrossRef] [PubMed]
46. Zhang, Y.; Li, S.; Li, J.; Han, L.; He, Q.; Wang, R.; Wang, X.; Liu, K. Developmental toxicity induced by $PM_{2.5}$ through endoplasmic reticulum stress and autophagy pathway in zebrafish embryos. *Chemosphere* **2018**, *197*, 611–621. [CrossRef] [PubMed]
47. Jia, Z.L.; Zhu, C.Y.; Rajendran, R.S.; Xia, Q.; Liu, K.C.; Zhang, Y. Impact of airborne total suspended particles (TSP) and fine particulate matter ($PM_{2.5}$)-induced developmental toxicity in zebrafish (Danio rerio) embryos. *J. Appl. Toxicol.* **2022**, *42*, 1585–1602. [CrossRef] [PubMed]
48. Jedrychowski, W.A.; Perera, F.P.; Maugeri, U.; Mroz, E.; Klimaszewska-Rembiasz, M.; Flak, E.; Edwards, S.; Spengler, J.D. Effect of prenatal exposure to fine particulate matter on ventilatory lung function of preschool children of non-smoking mothers. *Paediatr. Perinat. Epidemiol.* **2010**, *24*, 492–501. [CrossRef] [PubMed]
49. Johnson, N.M.; Hoffmann, A.R.; Behlen, J.C.; Lau, C.; Pendleton, D.; Harvey, N.; Shore, R.; Li, Y.; Chen, J.; Tian, Y.; et al. Air pollution and children's health-a review of adverse effects associated with prenatal exposure from fine to ultrafine particulate matter. *Environ. Health Prev. Med.* **2021**, *26*, 72. [CrossRef] [PubMed]
50. Kajekar, R. Environmental factors and developmental outcomes in the lung. *Pharmacol. Ther.* **2007**, *114*, 129–145. [CrossRef] [PubMed]
51. Tang, W.; Huang, S.; Du, L.; Sun, W.; Yu, Z.; Zhou, Y.; Chen, J.; Li, X.; Li, X.; Yu, B.; et al. Expression of hmgb1 in maternal exposure to fine particulate air pollution induces lung injury in rat offspring assessed with micro-CT. *Chem. Biol. Interact.* **2018**, *280*, 64–69. [CrossRef] [PubMed]
52. Tang, W.; Du, L.; Sun, W.; Yu, Z.; He, F.; Chen, J.; Li, X.; Li, X.; Yu, L.; Chen, D. Maternal exposure to fine particulate air pollution induces epithelial-to-mesenchymal transition resulting in postnatal pulmonary dysfunction mediated by transforming growth factor-β/smad3 signaling. *Toxicol. Lett.* **2017**, *267*, 11–20. [CrossRef] [PubMed]
53. Dysart, M.M.; Galvis, B.R.; Russell, A.G.; Barker, T.H. Environmental particulate ($PM_{2.5}$) augments stiffness-induced alveolar epithelial cell mechanoactivation of transforming growth factor beta. *PLoS ONE* **2014**, *9*, e106821. [CrossRef] [PubMed]

54. Yue, H.; Ji, X.; Ku, T.; Li, G.; Sang, N. Sex difference in bronchopulmonary dysplasia of offspring in response to maternal $PM_{2.5}$ exposure. *J. Hazard. Mater.* **2020**, *389*, 122033. [CrossRef] [PubMed]
55. Jin, L.; Qiu, J.; Zhang, Y.; Qiu, W.; He, X.; Wang, Y.; Sun, Q.; Li, M.; Zhao, N.; Cui, H.; et al. Ambient air pollution and congenital heart defects in Lanzhou, China. *Environ. Res. Lett.* **2015**, *10*, 074005. [CrossRef] [PubMed]
56. Padula, A.M.; Tager, I.B.; Carmichael, S.L.; Hammond, S.K.; Yang, W.; Lurmann, F.; Shaw, G.M. Ambient air pollution and traffic exposures and congenital heart defects in the San Joaquin Valley of California. *Paediatr. Perinat. Epidemiol.* **2013**, *27*, 329–339. [CrossRef] [PubMed]
57. Tanwar, V.; Adelstein, J.M.; Grimmer, J.A.; Youtz, D.J.; Katapadi, A.; Sugar, B.P.; Falvo, M.J.; Baer, L.A.; Stanford, K.I.; Wold, L.E. Preconception exposure to fine particulate matter leads to cardiac dysfunction in adult male offspring. *J. Am. Heart Assoc.* **2018**, *7*, e010797. [CrossRef] [PubMed]
58. Tanwar, V.; Gorr, M.W.; Velten, M.; Eichenseer, C.M.; Long, V.P., 3rd; Bonilla, I.M.; Shettigar, V.; Ziolo, M.T.; Davis, J.P.; Baine, S.H.; et al. In utero particulate matter exposure produces heart failure, electrical remodeling, and epigenetic changes at adulthood. *J. Am. Heart Assoc.* **2017**, *6*, e005796. [CrossRef] [PubMed]
59. Tanwar, V.; Adelstein, J.M.; Grimmer, J.A.; Youtz, D.J.; Sugar, B.P.; Wold, L.E. $PM_{2.5}$ exposure in utero contributes to neonatal cardiac dysfunction in mice. *Environ. Pollut.* **2017**, *230*, 116–124. [CrossRef] [PubMed]
60. Li, R.; Zhao, Y.; Shi, J.; Zhao, C.; Xie, P.; Huang, W.; Yong, T.; Cai, Z. Effects of $PM_{2.5}$ exposure in utero on heart injury, histone acetylation and GATA4 expression in offspring mice. *Chemosphere* **2020**, *256*, 127133. [CrossRef] [PubMed]
61. Hamanaka, R.B.; Mutlu, G.M. Particulate matter air pollution: Effects on the cardiovascular system. *Front. Endocrinol.* **2018**, *9*, 680. [CrossRef] [PubMed]
62. Weldy, C.S.; Liu, Y.; Liggitt, H.D.; Chin, M.T. In utero exposure to diesel exhaust air pollution promotes adverse intrauterine conditions, resulting in weight gain, altered blood pressure, and increased susceptibility to heart failure in adult mice. *PLoS ONE* **2014**, *9*, e88582. [CrossRef] [PubMed]
63. Gorr, M.W.; Velten, M.; Nelin, T.D.; Youtz, D.J.; Sun, Q.; Wold, L.E. Early life exposure to air pollution induces adult cardiac dysfunction. *Am. J. Physiol. Heart Circ. Physiol.* **2014**, *307*, H1353–H1360. [CrossRef] [PubMed]
64. Zhang, H.; Yao, Y.; Chen, Y.; Yue, C.; Chen, J.; Tong, J.; Jiang, Y.; Chen, T. Crosstalk between AHR and wnt/β-catenin signal pathways in the cardiac developmental toxicity of $PM_{2.5}$ in zebrafish embryos. *Toxicology* **2016**, *355–356*, 31–38. [CrossRef] [PubMed]
65. Chen, T.; Jin, H.; Wang, H.; Yao, Y.; Aniagu, S.; Tong, J.; Jiang, Y. Aryl hydrocarbon receptor mediates the cardiac developmental toxicity of EOM from $PM_{2.5}$ in P19 embryonic carcinoma cells. *Chemosphere* **2019**, *216*, 372–378. [CrossRef] [PubMed]
66. Ren, F.; Ji, C.; Huang, Y.; Aniagu, S.; Jiang, Y.; Chen, T. AHR-mediated ROS production contributes to the cardiac developmental toxicity of $PM_{2.5}$ in zebrafish embryos. *Sci. Total Environ.* **2020**, *719*, 135097. [CrossRef] [PubMed]
67. Zhang, M.; Chen, J.; Jiang, Y.; Chen, T. Fine particulate matter induces heart defects via AHR/ROS-mediated endoplasmic reticulum stress. *Chemosphere* **2022**, *307*, 135962. [CrossRef] [PubMed]
68. Meca-Lallana, V.; Gascón-Giménez, F.; Ginestal-López, R.C.; Higueras, Y.; Téllez-Lara, N.; Carreres-Polo, J.; Eichau-Madueño, S.; Romero-Imbroda, J.; Vidal-Jordana, Á.; Pérez-Miralles, F. Cognitive impairment in multiple sclerosis: Diagnosis and monitoring. *Neurol. Sci.* **2021**, *42*, 5183–5193. [CrossRef] [PubMed]
69. McGuinn, L.A.; Wiggins, L.D.; Volk, H.E.; Di, Q.; Moody, E.J.; Kasten, E.; Schwartz, J.; Wright, R.O.; Schieve, L.A.; Windham, G.C.; et al. Pre- and postnatal fine particulate matter exposure and childhood cognitive and adaptive function. *Int. J. Environ. Res. Public. Health* **2022**, *19*, 3748. [CrossRef] [PubMed]
70. Ning, X.; Li, B.; Ku, T.; Guo, L.; Li, G.; Sang, N. Comprehensive hippocampal metabolite responses to $PM_{2.5}$ in young mice. *Ecotoxicol. Environ. Saf.* **2018**, *165*, 36–43. [CrossRef] [PubMed]
71. Klocke, C.; Allen, J.L.; Sobolewski, M.; Mayer-Pröschel, M.; Blum, J.L.; Lauterstein, D.; Zelikoff, J.T.; Cory-Slechta, D.A. Neuropathological consequences of gestational exposure to concentrated ambient fine and ultrafine particles in the mouse. *Toxicol. Sci.* **2017**, *156*, 492–508. [CrossRef] [PubMed]
72. Hou, Y.; Yan, W.; Li, G.; Sang, N. Transcriptome sequencing analysis reveals a potential role of lncrna NONMMUT058932.2 and NONMMUT029203.2 in abnormal myelin development of male offspring following prenatal $PM_{2.5}$ exposure. *Sci. Total Environ.* **2023**, *895*, 165004. [CrossRef] [PubMed]
73. Hou, Y.; Wei, W.; Li, G.; Sang, N. Prenatal $PM_{2.5}$ exposure contributes to neuronal tau lesion in male offspring mice through mitochondrial dysfunction-mediated insulin resistance. *Ecotoxicol. Environ. Saf.* **2022**, *246*, 114151. [CrossRef] [PubMed]
74. Chen, M.; Li, B.; Sang, N. Particulate matter ($PM_{2.5}$) exposure season-dependently induces neuronal apoptosis and synaptic injuries. *J. Environ. Sci.* **2017**, *54*, 336–345. [CrossRef] [PubMed]
75. Allen, J.L.; Liu, X.; Weston, D.; Prince, L.; Oberdörster, G.; Finkelstein, J.N.; Johnston, C.J.; Cory-Slechta, D.A. Developmental exposure to concentrated ambient ultrafine particulate matter air pollution in mice results in persistent and sex-dependent behavioral neurotoxicity and glial activation. *Toxicol. Sci.* **2014**, *140*, 160–178. [CrossRef] [PubMed]
76. Hou, Y.; Yan, W.; Guo, L.; Li, G.; Sang, N. Prenatal $PM_{2.5}$ exposure impairs spatial learning and memory in male mice offspring: From transcriptional regulation to neuronal morphogenesis. *Part. Fibre Toxicol.* **2023**, *20*, 13. [CrossRef] [PubMed]
77. Nephew, B.C.; Nemeth, A.; Hudda, N.; Beamer, G.; Mann, P.; Petitto, J.; Cali, R.; Febo, M.; Kulkarni, P.; Poirier, G.; et al. Traffic-related particulate matter affects behavior, inflammation, and neural integrity in a developmental rodent model. *Environ. Res.* **2020**, *183*, 109242. [CrossRef] [PubMed]

78. Church, J.S.; Tijerina, P.B.; Emerson, F.J.; Coburn, M.A.; Blum, J.L.; Zelikoff, J.T.; Schwartzer, J.J. Perinatal exposure to concentrated ambient particulates results in autism-like behavioral deficits in adult mice. *Neurotoxicology* **2018**, *65*, 231–240. [CrossRef] [PubMed]
79. Allen, J.L.; Oberdorster, G.; Morris-Schaffer, K.; Wong, C.; Klocke, C.; Sobolewski, M.; Conrad, K.; Mayer-Proschel, M.; Cory-Slechta, D.A. Developmental neurotoxicity of inhaled ambient ultrafine particle air pollution: Parallels with neuropathological and behavioral features of autism and other neurodevelopmental disorders. *Neurotoxicology* **2017**, *59*, 140–154. [CrossRef] [PubMed]
80. Di Domenico, M.; Benevenuto, S.G.M.; Tomasini, P.P.; Yariwake, V.Y.; de Oliveira Alves, N.; Rahmeier, F.L.; da Cruz Fernandes, M.; Moura, D.J.; Nascimento Saldiva, P.H.; Veras, M.M. Concentrated ambient fine particulate matter ($PM_{2.5}$) exposure induce brain damage in pre and postnatal exposed mice. *Neurotoxicology* **2020**, *79*, 127–141. [CrossRef]
81. Davis, D.A.; Bortolato, M.; Godar, S.C.; Sander, T.K.; Iwata, N.; Pakbin, P.; Shih, J.C.; Berhane, K.; McConnell, R.; Sioutas, C.; et al. Prenatal exposure to urban air nanoparticles in mice causes altered neuronal differentiation and depression-like responses. *PLoS ONE* **2013**, *8*, e64128. [CrossRef] [PubMed]
82. Rahman, F.; Coull, B.A.; Carroll, K.N.; Wilson, A.; Just, A.C.; Kloog, I.; Zhang, X.; Wright, R.J.; Chiu, Y.M. Prenatal $PM_{2.5}$ exposure and infant temperament at age 6 months: Sensitive windows and sex-specific associations. *Environ. Res.* **2022**, *206*, 112583. [CrossRef] [PubMed]
83. Yuan, X.; Wang, Y.; Li, L.; Zhou, W.; Tian, D.; Lu, C.; Yu, S.; Zhao, J.; Peng, S. $PM_{2.5}$ induces embryonic growth retardation: Potential involvement of ROS-MAPKs-apoptosis and G0/G1 arrest pathways. *Environ. Toxicol.* **2016**, *31*, 2028–2044. [CrossRef] [PubMed]
84. Cui, J.; Fu, Y.; Lu, R.; Bi, Y.; Zhang, L.; Zhang, C.; Aschner, M.; Li, X.; Chen, R. Metabolomics analysis explores the rescue to neurobehavioral disorder induced by maternal $PM_{2.5}$ exposure in mice. *Ecotoxicol. Environ. Saf.* **2019**, *169*, 687–695. [CrossRef] [PubMed]
85. Chen, J.; Zhang, M.; Zou, H.; Aniagu, S.; Jiang, Y.; Chen, T. $PM_{2.5}$ induces mitochondrial dysfunction via AHR-mediated CYP1A1 overexpression during zebrafish heart development. *Toxicology* **2023**, *487*, 153466. [CrossRef] [PubMed]
86. Allen, J.L.; Liu, X.; Pelkowski, S.; Palmer, B.; Conrad, K.; Oberdörster, G.; Weston, D.; Mayer-Pröschel, M.; Cory-Slechta, D.A. Early postnatal exposure to ultrafine particulate matter air pollution: Persistent ventriculomegaly, neurochemical disruption, and glial activation preferentially in male mice. *Environ. Health Perspect.* **2014**, *122*, 939–945. [CrossRef] [PubMed]
87. Wang, J.; Liu, T.; Wang, J.; Chen, T.; Jiang, Y. Genome-wide profiling of transcriptome and DNA methylome in human embryonic stem cells exposed to extractable organic matter from $PM_{2.5}$. *Toxics* **2023**, *11*, 840. [CrossRef] [PubMed]
88. Jiang, Y.; Li, J.; Ren, F.; Ji, C.; Aniagu, S.; Chen, T. $PM_{2.5}$-induced extensive DNA methylation changes in the heart of zebrafish embryos and the protective effect of folic acid. *Environ. Pollut.* **2019**, *255*, 113331. [CrossRef] [PubMed]
89. Ji, C.; Tao, Y.; Li, X.; Wang, J.; Chen, J.; Aniagu, S.; Jiang, Y.; Chen, T. AHR-mediated m^6a RNA methylation contributes to $PM_{2.5}$-induced cardiac malformations in zebrafish larvae. *J. Hazard. Mater.* **2023**, *457*, 131749. [CrossRef] [PubMed]
90. Li, Z.; Tang, Y.; Song, X.; Lazar, L.; Li, Z.; Zhao, J. Impact of ambient $PM_{2.5}$ on adverse birth outcome and potential molecular mechanism. *Ecotoxicol. Environ. Saf.* **2019**, *169*, 248–254. [CrossRef] [PubMed]
91. MohanKumar, S.M.; Campbell, A.; Block, M.; Veronesi, B. Particulate matter, oxidative stress and neurotoxicity. *Neurotoxicology* **2008**, *29*, 479–488. [CrossRef] [PubMed]
92. Dai, J.; Sun, C.; Yao, Z.; Chen, W.; Yu, L.; Long, M. Exposure to concentrated ambient fine particulate matter disrupts vascular endothelial cell barrier function via the IL-6/HIF-1α signaling pathway. *FEBS Open Bio* **2016**, *6*, 720–728. [CrossRef] [PubMed]
93. Wang, T.; Wang, L.; Moreno-Vinasco, L.; Lang, G.D.; Siegler, J.H.; Mathew, B.; Usatyuk, P.V.; Samet, J.M.; Geyh, A.S.; Breysse, P.N.; et al. Particulate matter air pollution disrupts endothelial cell barrier via calpain-mediated tight junction protein degradation. *Part. Fibre Toxicol.* **2012**, *9*, 35. [CrossRef] [PubMed]
94. Xu, X.; Deng, F.; Guo, X.; Lv, P.; Zhong, M.; Liu, C.; Wang, A.; Tzan, K.; Jiang, S.Y.; Lippmann, M.; et al. Association of systemic inflammation with marked changes in particulate air pollution in beijing in 2008. *Toxicol. Lett* **2012**, *212*, 147–156. [CrossRef] [PubMed]
95. Maher, B.A.; Ahmed, I.A.; Karloukovski, V.; MacLaren, D.A.; Foulds, P.G.; Allsop, D.; Mann, D.M.; Torres-Jardón, R.; Calderon-Garciduenas, L. Magnetite pollution nanoparticles in the human brain. *Proc. Natl. Acad. Sci. USA* **2016**, *113*, 10797–10801. [CrossRef] [PubMed]
96. Gillespie, P.; Tajuba, J.; Lippmann, M.; Chen, L.C.; Veronesi, B. Particulate matter neurotoxicity in culture is size-dependent. *Neurotoxicology* **2013**, *36*, 112–117. [CrossRef] [PubMed]
97. Block, M.L.; Calderón-Garcidueñas, L. Air pollution: Mechanisms of neuroinflammation and CNS disease. *Trends Neurosci.* **2009**, *32*, 506–516. [CrossRef] [PubMed]
98. Wang, Y.; Xiong, L.; Tang, M. Toxicity of inhaled particulate matter on the central nervous system: Neuroinflammation, neuropsychological effects and neurodegenerative disease. *J. Appl. Toxicol.* **2017**, *37*, 644–667. [CrossRef] [PubMed]
99. Harry, G.J.; Kraft, A.D. Microglia in the developing brain: A potential target with lifetime effects. *Neurotoxicology* **2012**, *33*, 191–206. [CrossRef] [PubMed]
100. Baburamani, A.A.; Supramaniam, V.G.; Hagberg, H.; Mallard, C. Microglia toxicity in preterm brain injury. *Reprod. Toxicol.* **2014**, *48*, 106–112. [CrossRef] [PubMed]

101. Chew, L.J.; Fusar-Poli, P.; Schmitz, T. Oligodendroglial alterations and the role of microglia in white matter injury: Relevance to schizophrenia. *Dev. Neurosci.* **2013**, *35*, 102–129. [CrossRef] [PubMed]
102. El Waly, B.; Macchi, M.; Cayre, M.; Durbec, P. Oligodendrogenesis in the normal and pathological central nervous system. *Front. Neurosci.* **2014**, *8*, 145. [CrossRef] [PubMed]
103. Liu, X.B.; Shen, Y.; Plane, J.M.; Deng, W. Vulnerability of premyelinating oligodendrocytes to white-matter damage in neonatal brain injury. *Neurosci. Bull.* **2013**, *29*, 229–238. [CrossRef] [PubMed]
104. Cavalli, G.; Heard, E. Advances in epigenetics link genetics to the environment and disease. *Nature* **2019**, *571*, 489–499. [CrossRef] [PubMed]
105. Dong, W.; Matsumura, F.; Kullman, S.W. TCDD induced pericardial edema and relative COX-2 expression in medaka (Oryzias Latipes) embryos. *Toxicol. Sci.* **2010**, *118*, 213–223. [CrossRef] [PubMed]
106. Neven, K.Y.; Saenen, N.D.; Tarantini, L.; Janssen, B.G.; Lefebvre, W.; Vanpoucke, C.; Bollati, V.; Nawrot, T.S. Placental promoter methylation of DNA repair genes and prenatal exposure to particulate air pollution: An environage cohort study. *Lancet Planet. Health* **2018**, *2*, e174–e183. [CrossRef] [PubMed]

toxics

MDPI

Article

In Vitro Profiling of Toxicity Effects of Different Environmental Factors on Skin Cells

Minghui Fu [1], Yingxin Yang [1], Xiaolan Zhang [1], Bingli Lei [1,*], Tian Chen [2,3,*] and Yuanqi Chen [4]

[1] Institute of Environmental Pollution and Health, School of Environmental and Chemical Engineering, Shanghai University, Shanghai 200444, China; fmh2817@163.com (M.F.); yangyingxin2021@163.com (Y.Y.); zhangxiaolan@shu.edu.cn (X.Z.)

[2] State Environmental Protection Key Laboratory of the Assessment of Effects of Emerging Pollutants on Environmental and Human Health, Shanghai Municipal Center for Disease Control and Prevention, Shanghai 200336, China

[3] Department of Environmental Health, Shanghai Municipal Center for Disease Control and Prevention, Shanghai 200336, China

[4] Skincare Research Center of Dr. YU, Shanghai Jahwa United Co., Ltd., Shanghai 200082, China; chenyuanqi@jahwa.com

* Correspondence: leibingli@126.com (B.L.); chentian@scdc.sh.cn (T.C.)

Abstract: The skin is constantly exposed to a variety of environmental threats. Therefore, the influence of environmental factors on skin damage has always been a matter of concern. This study aimed to investigate the cytotoxic effects of different environmental factors, including cooking oil fumes (COFs), haze ($PM_{2.5}$), and cigarette smoke (CS), on epidermal HaCaT cells and dermal fibroblast (FB) cells. Cell viability, intracellular reactive oxygen species (ROS) generation, inflammatory cytokine levels, and collagen mRNA expression were used as toxicity endpoints. Additionally, the effects of ozone (O_3) on cell viability and release of inflammatory cytokines in 3D epidermal cells were also examined. The results showed that the organic extracts of CS, COFs, and $PM_{2.5}$ significantly inhibited the viability of HaCaT and FB cells at higher exposure concentrations. These extracts also increased intracellular ROS levels in FB cells. Furthermore, they significantly promoted the release of inflammatory cytokines, such as IL-1α and TNF-α, in HaCaT cells and down-regulated the mRNA expression of collagen I, III, IV, and VII in FB cells. Comparatively, SC organic extracts exhibited stronger cytotoxicity to skin cells compared to $PM_{2.5}$ and COFs. Additionally, O_3 at all test concentrations significantly inhibited the viability of 3D epidermal cells in a concentration-dependent manner and markedly increased the levels of TNF-α and IL-1α in 3D epidermal cells. These findings emphasize the potential cytotoxicity of COFs, $PM_{2.5}$, CS, and O_3 to skin cells, which may lead to skin damage; therefore, we should pay attention to these environmental factors and take appropriate measures to protect the skin from their harmful effects.

Keywords: FB cells; HaCaT cells; 3D epidermal cells; environmental factors; cytotoxicity

1. Introduction

The skin, consisting of the epidermis and dermis, is the outermost organ of the body. The outer epidermis contains keratinocytes, while the inner dermis is primarily composed of fibroblasts and connective tissues [1]. Serving as a barrier against physical and environmental factors, the skin is constantly exposed to harmful environmental stressors, which can lead to accelerated premature intrinsic skin aging and even skin carcinogenesis [2–4].

Among environmental factors, fine particulate matter ($PM_{2.5}$) in haze is a mixture of many harmful ingredients. Some of these harmful ingredients can act as catalysts for the production of reactive oxygen species (ROS) and promote skin inflammation [4,5]. Cigarette smoke (CS) aerosol is formed during smoking due to incomplete combustion [6]. The complex CS aerosol contains over 7000 harmful substances and is classified as a Group

A carcinogen by the USEPA [7]. The oxidative compounds in CS can disrupt cellular redox homeostasis, further affect the cutaneous tissue, and have a clear relationship with premature skin aging [8,9]. Oil fumes from high-temperature cooking can form aerosols through the vapor-to-particle process in a temperature gradient region [10]. Exposure to cooking oil fumes (COFs) may have carcinogenic effects on the respiratory system in humans. Epidemiological studies suggest that carcinogens produced during cooking may be one of the factors causing lung cancer in Chinese women [11,12]. Ozone (O_3) is one of the most reactive environmental oxidants that can come into contact with skin [13]. Previous studies have shown that exposure to O_3 can result in the depletion of antioxidants and the oxidation of lipids and proteins in the outermost layer of skin, the stratum corneum [14,15].

More than 90% of the urban population is exposed to contaminant concentrations above the standard limits established by the World Health Organization (WHO) [16]. In recent years, the adverse effects of environmental factors such as $PM_{2.5}$, CS, COFs, and O_3 on the respiratory system in animals and humans have attracted the attention of many researchers [17–20]. Particularly, the impact of environmental factors on the spread of COVID-19 has become a hot topic in the past two years [21–23]. Additionally, several studies have been conducted on the biological effects of some environmental factors such as PM, CS, and O_3 on skin cells. However, there is a lack of research on the effects of COFs on the epidermis and dermis of the skin. Furthermore, there is a lack of comparative studies on the cytotoxicity of different environmental factors on skin cells.

The epidermal HaCaT cells and dermal fibroblasts (FB cells) are ideal cell models for studying epidermal and dermal skin damage caused by pollutants. Fibroblasts, as one of the most important types of cells in the skin, not only synthesize and secrete collagen to provide physical support for the skin but also participate in tissue repair when the skin is damaged [24]. Increased ROS generation and decreased activity and collagen secretion of fibroblasts have been identified as important factors in wrinkle formation [24]. HaCaT cells play a role in maintaining skin barrier homeostasis [25]. Under the stimulation of environmental factors, HaCaT cells can produce a large number of cytokines, including TNF-α, IL-1α, and IL-6, which can damage the skin tissue [26]. Therefore, in this study, dermal fibroblasts (FB cells) were used to evaluate the effects of $PM_{2.5}$, COFs, and CS on ROS generation and mRNA levels of collagen genes, while HaCaT cells were used to evaluate the effects of $PM_{2.5}$, COFs, and CS on the secretion of cytokines (TNF-α and IL-1α). Additionally, 3D epidermal cells were employed to investigate the influence of O_3 on skin tissue damage. The findings of this study will highlight the hazards of different environmental factors on human skin.

2. Methods and Materials

2.1. Reagents

2′,7′-dichlorodihydrofluorescein diacetate (DCFH-DA), ter-butyl hydroperoxide (t-BHP), *tert*-butyl hydroperoxide (t-BHP), and 3-(4,5)-dimethylthiazol (-2-y1)-2,5-diphenyltetrazolium bromide (MTT) were obtained from Sigma (Saint Louis, MO, USA). The SYBR green dye and reverse-transcription kit were purchased from TOYOBO (Osaka, Japan). The ELISA kits for IL-1α and TNF-α were purchased from Mibio Co. (Shanghai, China). All the other reagents used in this study were of analytical grade, unless otherwise specified. The 3D epidermal model used in this study was obtained from Shanghai Jahwa United Co., Ltd. and is a three-dimensional cellular system of human epidermal keratinocytes (HEK).

2.2. Sample Collection and Preparation

Fine particulate matter ($PM_{2.5}$) samples were collected using a Th-150c III medium-flow atmospheric sampler with a quartz filter membrane for 24 h. The $PM_{2.5}$ samples were collected on 14 December 2019, in Shanghai, China, with an air concentration of 57 $\mu g/m^3$. For cigarette smoke (CS) collection, smoke smog was generated in a closed room by recruited volunteers who smoke and the smog was collected using an atmospheric sampler with a quartz filter membrane. Cooking oil fumes (COFs) were also collected during cooking with an atmospheric sampler with a quartz filter membrane. After collection, the samples were immediately transferred to the laboratory and stored at −20 °C until further preparation.

The $PM_{2.5}$, CS, and COFs adsorbed on the quartz filter membrane were freeze-dried. The quartz filter membranes containing these samples were then cut into pieces and extracted for 24 h using n-hexane/dichloromethane (1/1, *v*/*v*) by the microwave ultrasound method. The organic extracts were reduced to approximately 1 mL using a rotary evaporator (R-200 rotary evaporator, Büchi Labortechnik AG, Flawil, Switzerland) and further concentrated to approximately 10 μL using a gentle nitrogen flow. The solvent in the extracts was then exchanged with 200 μL dimethyl sulfoxide (DMSO). The organic extracts were stored at −20 °C until the toxicity test. Four concentration sequences were prepared by two-fold dilution from stock solutions for the toxicity test. Therefore, the concentration sequences for the $PM_{2.5}$ were 6.375, 12.75, 25.5, and 51 μg/mL, for the CS were 3, 6, 12, and 24 μg/mL, and for the COFs were 101.25, 205.5, 405, and 810 μg/mL. The final DMSO concentration used in the toxicity test was 0.1%, which was non-toxic to FB cells and HaCaT cells.

2.3. Maintenance of Skin Cells and MTT Assay

MTT is a commonly used method to detect the cell proliferation and cytotoxicity of chemicals due to its high sensitivity and ease of use. In this study, FB and HaCaT skin cells were obtained from Shanghai Jahwa United Co., Ltd. (Shanghai, China). FB and HaCaT cells were maintained in high glucose Dulbecco's modified Eagle's medium (DMEM) (Gibco, Grand Island, NY, USA) with 10% fetal bovine serum (FBS) (Gibco, Grand Island, NY, USA) and 100 units/mL penicillin/streptomycin (Invitrogen, Carlsbad, CA, USA). The cells were incubated in a 5% CO_2 incubator at 37 °C and the culture medium of the cells was refreshed every 2–3 days. The cells in their exponential growth phase were employed for the toxicity test of organic extracts. A total of 0.1% DMSO was used as the control group.

To perform the MTT assay, HaCaT and FB cells were seeded in 96-well plates with 200 μL culture medium at a density of 3×10^3 cells per well and allowed to adhere for 18–24 h. Subsequently, the cells were treated with different concentrations of organic extracts obtained from the $PM_{2.5}$, CS, and COFs for 24 h. The experiment included a control group treated with 0.1% DMSO and exposure groups with the environmental factors. Each group had six parallel samples. After exposure, the MTT assay was conducted according to the specific experimental process and the calculation method described in our previous study [27].

2.4. Reactive Oxygen Species (ROS) Detection

DCFH-DA is a fluorescent probe that has the ability to penetrate cell membrane and enter the cells. Once inside the cells, it is enzymatically hydrolyzed into DCFH (2′,7′-dichlorodihydrofluorescein). In the presence of reactive oxygen species (ROS), DCFH is oxidized and converted into highly fluorescent 2′,7′-dichlorofluorescein (DCF). Therefore, the average fluorescence intensity of cells can be used as an indicator of the instantaneous content of ROS within the cells.

To detect intracellular ROS levels, FB cells in the logarithmic growth stage were seeded in 6-well plates with a volume of 1 mL at a density of 1.5×10^5 cells per well. The cells were cultured overnight in a 5% CO_2 incubator at 37 °C to allow them to adhere. After adherence, the culture medium was discarded and fresh medium containing different concentrations of organic extracts obtained from the $PM_{2.5}$, CS, and COFs was added to treat the cells for 24 h. The specific experimental method of intracellular ROS detection can be found in our previous study [28]. Briefly, the treated cells were incubated with DCFH-DA and average fluorescence intensity was calculated using Image-pro Plus 6 software based on the fluorescence images obtained using a fluorescence microscope (Olympus BX-51; Olympus,

Tokyo, Japan). Each treatment, DMSO negative control, or t-BHP positive control, consisted of three parallel samples.

2.5. Determination of TNF-α and IL-1α Content by Sandwich ELISA

ELISA kits were employed to detect the IL-1α and TNF-α levels in the supernatant of the HaCaT cells. The HaCaT cells were seeded in 96-well plates at a density of 1×10^5 cells per well overnight. After adhesion, the cells were treated with different concentrations of the organic extracts obtained from the $PM_{2.5}$, CS, and COFs for 24 h. After treatment, conditioned media from the cell cultures were collected by centrifugation. The ELISA kits were prepared by allowing them to equilibrate for 30 min at room temperature. Then, 100 μL of standard solution and supernatant from each exposure group of environmental factors were added into the standard well and sample well, respectively, which were coated with the primary antibody. The plates were incubated for 2 h at 37 °C. After incubation, the cells were washed with D-Hanks solution and 100 μL of biotin-labeled antibody working solution was added to each well. The plates were then incubated for 1 h at 37 °C. Subsequently, the liquid in each well was discarded and 100 μL of horseradish peroxidase labeled avidin working solution was added to each well and incubated for 1 h at 37 °C. After incubation, 90 μL of substrate solution was added to each well and incubated for 10–30 min at 37 °C in the dark. Finally, 50 μL of termination solution was added to stop the reaction. The optical density (OD) values at a wavelength of 450 nm were measured and the TNF-α and IL-1α levels were calculated based on the OD values of the exposure group and the control group.

2.6. RT-qPCR

FB cells in the logarithmic growth stage were seeded at the density of 1×10^6 cells/well and exposed to different concentrations of the organic extracts obtained from the $PM_{2.5}$, CS, and COFs for 12 h. After exposure, RNA samples were collected according to the method described in our previous study [27]. The A_{260}/A_{280} ratios for all samples ranged from 1.78 to 2.25, indicating that the extracted RNA is suitable for further reverse-transcriptase polymerase chain reaction (RT-PCR).

The isolated RNA was used to perform RT-qPCR to obtain cDNA according to the instructions provided in the reverse-transcription kit manual. The cDNA was then used for second-strand synthesis and subsequent amplifications.

The PCR amplification was performed using the ABI 7500 fast system. The housekeeping gene β-actin was used as the internal reference gene for subsequent gene expression analyses. The relative expression of the target genes was calculated according to the equation: $R = 2^{-\Delta\Delta Ct}$ [29]. Specific primers for target genes, including collagen I (forward: GGACACAGAGGTTTCAGTGG; reverse: CCAGTAGCACCATCATTTCC), III (forward: TTGAAGGAGGATGTTCCCATCT; reverse: ACAGACACATATTTGGCATGGTT), IV (forward: GGGATGCTGTTGAAAGGTGAA; reverse: GGTGGTCCGGTAAATCCTGG), and VII (forward: CAGCGACGTTCTACGGATCA; reverse: TGGGAGTATCTGGTGCCTCA) were obtained from Wcgene Biotechnology Co., Ltd. (Shanghai, China).

2.7. Cell Viability and IL-1α and TNF-α Levels in 3D Epidermal Cells

The 3D epidermal cells were exposed to O_3 in a closed glove box. The O_3 was generated using O_2 through an ozone generator. The O_2 and O_3 mixtures, consisting of approximately 95% O_2 and 5% O_3, were continuously supplied to a Teflon-lined glove box at a flow rate of 70 L/min. The concentrations of O_3 in the glove box were adjusted to 500, 5000, and 50,000 mg/m^3, respectively. At the same time, 5% SDS medium and 5% PBS medium were added to separate 6-well plates as positive control and negative control, respectively. Each group, including the control groups and the O_3-exosed groups, consisted of three parallel samples.

Before O_3 exposure, the 3D epidermal cell model was washed with PBS and the residual PBS was wiped off inside and outside the model. Then, the 3D epidermal cell model was transferred to a new 6-well plate and 0.9 mL of culture solution was added to each well. The 6-well plate, containing the 3D epidermal cell model, was then exposed to different concentrations of O_3 (500, 5000, and 50,000 mg/m^3) for 1 h.

After exposure, the 3D epidermal cell model was transferred to another new 6-well plate. Then, 0.9 mL of culture solution was added to each well, and the plate was placed in an incubator for 24 h. After incubation, the supernatant was collected for the detection of IL-1α and TNF-α levels using ELISA kits. The method for detecting IL-1α and TNF-α levels is described in the previous Section (TNF-α and IL-1α levels).

The 3D epidermal cell model was transferred to a new 24-well plate to further detect cell viability. A total of 300 µL of MTT (1 mg/mL) was added and incubated for 3 h. After incubation, the MTT solution was removed from the 24-well plate, and the 3D epidermal cell model was washed three times with PBS. The surface of the model was carefully dried and the cell model was then transferred to another new 24-well plate. Next, 2 mL of isopropanol was added to each well containing the 3D epidermal cell model and the plate was covered with a sealing film to prevent evaporation. The plate was shaken at room temperature for 2 h at a speed of 120 rpm. Then, the cell model was pierced and blown three times. Subsequently, 200 µL of the purple formazan derivative was sucked out from the 24-well plate and transferred to a 96-well plate. The absorbance at 570 nm was measured.

2.8. Data Analysis

The experimental data were characterized as the mean ± standard deviation (SD). To determine the significance between the treatment group and the control group, a one-way analysis of variance (ANOVA) was performed using SPSS 19.0 (Chicago, IL, USA). A p-value of less than 0.05 was considered statistically significant.

3. Results

3.1. Effect of Different Environmental Factors on Cell Viability

We evaluated the effect of various environmental factors on cell viability. After incubation for 24 h with different concentrations of $PM_{2.5}$, we found that $PM_{2.5}$ at 6.375, 12.75, and 25.5 µg/mL had no significant cytotoxicity on HaCaT and FB cells, with cell viability maintained above 90%. However, at a concentration of 51 µg/mL, the $PM_{2.5}$ significantly inhibited the viability of HaCaT and FB cells (Figure 1A). When exposed to CS for 24 h at concentrations of 3, 6, and 12 µg/mL, there was no significant cytotoxicity on FB cells. However, at a concentration of 24 µg/mL, the CS significantly inhibited the viability of FB cells. For HaCaT cells, exposure to CS at concentrations of 6 and 24 µg/mL significantly inhibited the HaCaT cell viability (Figure 1B). At a concentration of 101.25 µg/mL, COFs had no significant effect on the viability of FB cells and HaCaT cells. However, at concentrations of 405 and 810 µg/mL, COFs significantly decreased the proliferation of FB cells, and at concentrations of 205.5–810 µg/mL, COFs significantly inhibited the viability of HaCaT cells (Figure 1C). When exposed to 810 µg/mL COFs, FB cell viability decreased by 15% and HaCaT cell viability decreased by 20%. Our results showed that lower concentrations of organic extracts from different environmental factors had no effect on the viability of FB cells and HaCaT cells, while higher concentrations attenuate their survival rates. Among the three environmental factors, CS had the strongest toxicity effects on skin cells compared to $PM_{2.5}$ and COFs, while COFs had the lowest cytotoxicity.

The highest concentrations of CS, $PM_{2.5}$, and COFs in this study significantly inhibited the viability of two skin cells. Therefore, in subsequent intracellular ROS detection in FB cells, the highest concentrations of CS, $PM_{2.5}$, and COFs were set as exposure concentrations.

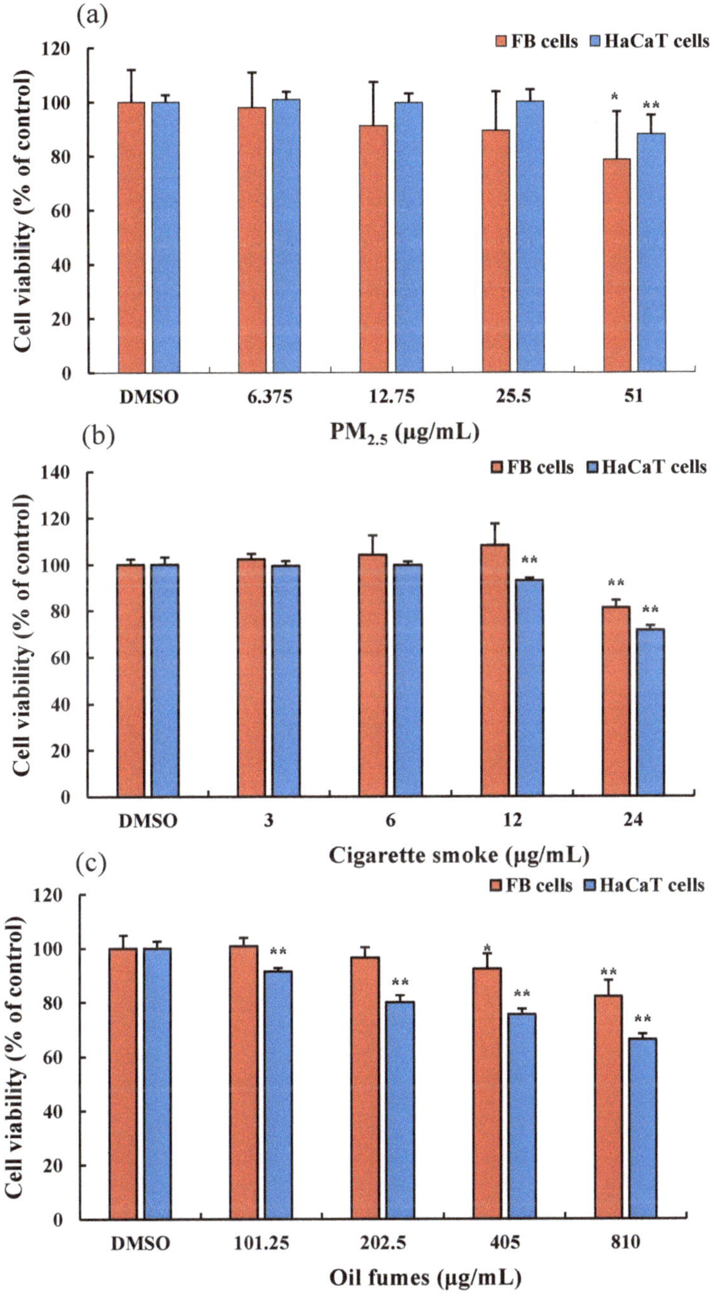

Figure 1. Effect of $PM_{2.5}$ on the viability of FB and HaCaT cells. (**a**): the organic extracts of fine particulate matter ($PM_{2.5}$); (**b**): the organic extracts of cigarette smoke (CS); and (**c**): the organic extracts of cooking oil fumes (COFs). Data are shown as the mean ± standard deviation (SD) of six parallel samples. * $p < 0.05$, ** $p < 0.01$, compared with the negative control (0.1% DMSO).

3.2. Effects of Environmental Factors on ROS Levels and the mRNA Expression of Collagen Genes in FB Cells

Based on the cell viability results, 51 μg/mL $PM_{2.5}$, 24 μg/mL CS, and 810 μg/mL COFs were selected as exposure concentrations to further investigate the effect of these three environmental factors on intracellular ROS generation in FB cells. In Figure 2a,b, we observed that t-BHP (100 μM), used as a positive control, significantly elevated intracellular ROS levels. In addition, the $PM_{2.5}$, COFs, and CS at test concentrations were found to significantly induce ROS generation in FB cells. The fluorescence images also clearly showed that various organic extracts promoted intracellular ROS generation. The levels of ROS induced by 24 μg/mL CS were similar to those induced by 54 μg/mL $PM_{2.5}$ and 810 μg/mL COFs, indicating that CS had stronger toxicity compared to the other two environmental factors.

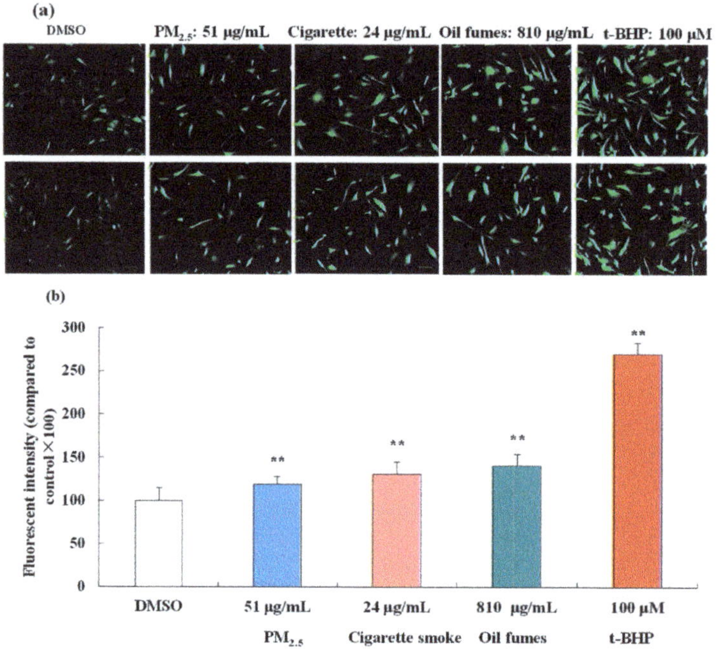

Figure 2. Effect of the $PM_{2.5}$, COFs, and CS on the levels of intracellular ROS in FB cells. (**a**): some fluorescent images of FB cells; and (**b**): ROS levels in FB cells. The scale bar is 20 μm. Data are shown as the mean ± S.D. of three parallel samples. ** $p < 0.01$, compared with negative control (0.1% DMSO).

To examine the effects of environmental factors on collagen in FB cells, collagen I, III, IV, and VII were chosen as target genes, as they are associated with skin damage and aging. The mRNA levels of these collagen genes were detected by RT-qPCR technology (Figure 3). Our results showed that exposure to $PM_{2.5}$, CS, and COFs at all test concentrations significantly decreased the mRNA levels of collagen I, III, IV, and VII. The only exception was that COFs at 202.5 μg/mL had no effect on the expression of collagen III mRNA. These findings suggest that exposure to these environmental factors can have a negative impact on the expression of collagen genes in FB cells, which may contribute to skin damage and aging.

3.3. Effects of Environmental Factors on the Levels of TNF-α and IL-1α in HaCaT Cells

To evaluate the impact of different environmental factors on the release of pro-inflammatory cytokines, ELISA kits were employed to measure the levels of TNF-α and

IL-1α in HaCaT cells. As shown in Figure 4, $PM_{2.5}$ at 51 μg/mL significantly elevated the levels of IL-1α and TNF-α. CS at concentrations of 12 and 24 μg/mL significantly increased the IL-1α levels, while at 24 μg/mL it also increased TNF-α levels. COFs at concentrations of 405 and 810 μg/mL induced significant release of TNF-α, but had no effect on the levels of IL-1α. Furthermore, the levels of IL-1α and TNF-α induced by CS were higher than those induced by $PM_{2.5}$ and COFs. These results indicate that all three environmental factors can significantly promote the release of TNF-α or IL-1α in HaCaT cells, particularly at higher exposure concentrations.

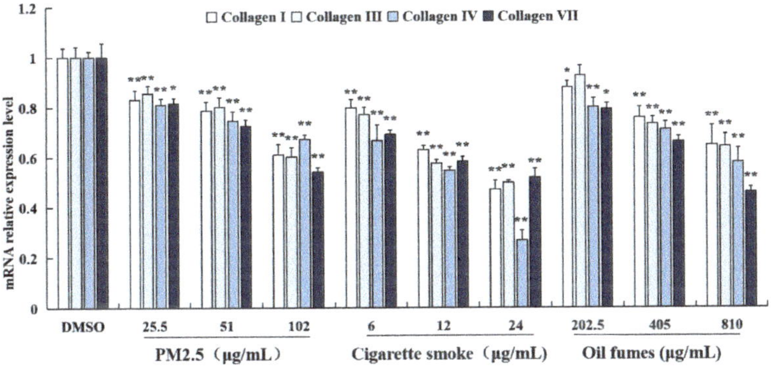

Figure 3. Effect of $PM_{2.5}$, COFs, and CS on the mRNA levels of collagen genes in FB cells. Data are characterized as the mean ± SD of four parallel samples. * $p < 0.05$, ** $p < 0.01$, compared with negative control (0.1% DMSO).

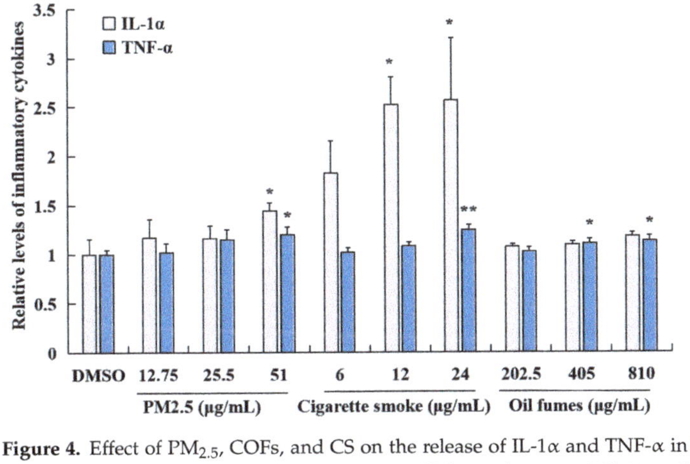

Figure 4. Effect of $PM_{2.5}$, COFs, and CS on the release of IL-1α and TNF-α in HaCaT cells. Data are characterized as the mean ± SD of three parallel samples. * $p < 0.05$, ** $p < 0.01$, compared with negative control (0.1% DMSO).

3.4. *Effect of O_3 on Cell Viability and IL-1α and TNF-α Release in 3D Epidermal Cells*

Exposure to ozone for 1 h at the test concentrations significantly inhibited the viability of 3D epidermal cells in a concentration-dependent manner (Figure 5a). In addition, ELISA analysis revealed that O_3 exposure also significantly increased the secretion of IL-1α and TNF-α by 3D epidermal cells in a concentration-dependent manner under the current environmental exposure conditions (Figure 5b).

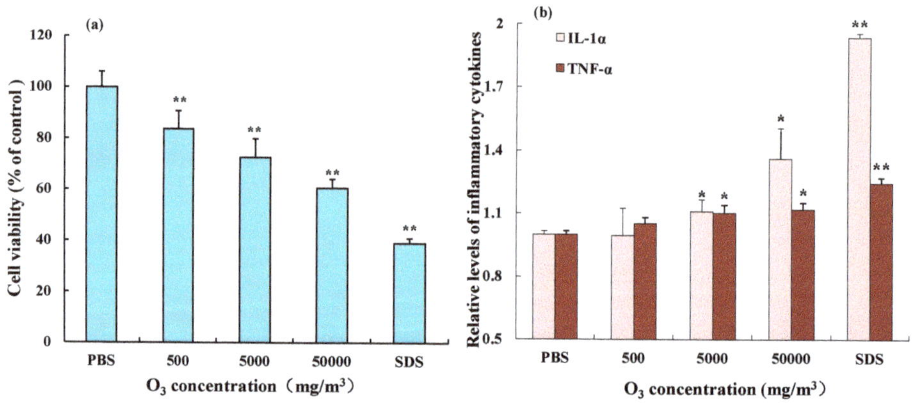

Figure 5. Effect of O_3 on the cell viability (**a**) and the IL-1α and TNF-α release (**b**) in 3D epidermal cells. Data are characterized as the mean ± SD of three parallel samples. * $p < 0.05$, ** $p < 0.01$, compared with negative control PBS.

4. Discussion

The skin serves as a crucial barrier that efficiently shields the body from the harmful effects of environmental stressors like air pollutants and ultraviolet rays [30,31]. However, excessive levels of environment stressors can result in skin damage [26,32,33]. Acute exposure to these environmental stressors can trigger the activation of various signaling pathways that coordinate adaptive stress response to maintain the homeostasis of skin cells and tissues [34].

In this study, we found that environmental stressors such as $PM_{2.5}$, COFs, and CS had a dual effect on the viability of FB and HaCaT cells. At low concentrations, these stressors promoted cell viability, while at higher concentrations, they inhibited cell viability. This may be attributed to the toxicity of pollutants present in $PM_{2.5}$, CS, and COFs. $PM_{2.5}$ is a complex mixture of harmful components, including organic pollutants, transition metals, and free radicals. CS is composed of thousands of toxic compounds such as polycyclic aromatic hydrocarbons (PAHs), tobacco-specific nitrosamines, aldehydes (formaldehyde, acrolein, and 4-hydroxynonenal), and various active free radicals [35–37]. COFs, which are commonly found in kitchen and indoor air, are considered to be the main contaminants that pose a threat to human health [38]. Therefore, it is reasonable to assume that these environmental factors can inhibit cell growth and induce cytotoxicity.

Environmental pollutants have been shown to induce the excessive production of ROS, leading to various forms of skin damage associated with oxidative stress [39,40]. ROS is directly involved in DNA oxidative damage and lipid peroxidation [41]. In the presence of hydrogen peroxide and light, redox-active metal ions, such as copper and iron, can act as catalysts for the generation of hydroxyl radicals and other ROS. These ROS can disrupt the redox balance of cells and contribute to different skin diseases [42]. In this study, we observed that $PM_{2.5}$, CS, and COFs increased the levels of intracellular ROS in FB cells. This suggests that these environmental factors can disrupt the cellular redox homeostasis, further supporting their potential to induce oxidative stress and contribute to skin damage.

In addition to disrupting the balance of cellular redox, some environmental factors can also evoke inflammation in the skin. For example, Soeur et al. [42] found that components of cigarette smoke can induce the production of pro-inflammatory mediators. They found that numerous chemicals, such as PAHs, can readily penetrate the outer layer of the skin and enter the bloodstream through the capillaries in the dermis. Once in the blood stream, they can stimulate the production of pro-inflammatory mediators, leading to adverse effects on the skin tissue. Chronic inflammatory reactions are then associated with skin disorders like atopic dermatitis and psoriasis [43]. In these conditions, the immune system is activated and releases cytokines that affect the growth and differentiation of skin cells. Several studies have shown that prolonged exposure to O_3 can increase oxidative damage and promote release of pro-inflammatory cytokines, such as interleukin-1β (IL-1β) and IL-18, leading to various inflammatory skin diseases [44,45]. Our study also observed that $PM_{2.5}$, CS, and COFs inhibited the viability of FB cells and HaCaT cells and increased the release of pro-inflammatory cytokines like TNF-α and IL-1α. In addition, O_3 inhibited the viability of 3D epidermal cells and elevated the levels of TNF-α and IL-1α in 3D epidermal cells. The findings suggest that $PM_{2.5}$, CS, COFs, and O_3 may contribute to the development of skin inflammation-related diseases.

The inflammatory changes of HaCaT cells are likely related to the levels of intracellular ROS. In the human skin, numerous contaminants can induce the excessive generation of ROS, which, in turn, causes skin inflammation and various cases of skin damage [46–48]. O_3 is known to produce active free radicals and induce inflammatory responses [49,50]. Ansary et al. [51] found that ultraviolet radiation (UVR) has also been found to cause skin inflammation through ROS. Abais et al. [41] found that exposure to air pollution exacerbates inflammatory skin diseases and ROS seems to play a key role in regulating the inflammasome activity. Environmental factors, such as $PM_{2.5}$, CS, and COFs, include a variety of pollutants. Therefore, it is reasonable to assume that environmental factors can induce inflammatory through increased ROS generation. Mokrzyński et al. [4] found that $PM_{2.5}$ can elevate ROS levels, leading to oxidative stress, inflammation, skin aging, and even skin cancer development. In addition, some studies found that ROS has been shown to induce the release of pro-inflammatory cytokines [10,16], which are important factors in skin inflammation. Therefore, excessive ROS production is considered an important initial step in cell damage, photo-aging, immune system change, and skin carcinogenesis [32].

The main indicator of skin damage is the depletion of collagen. The generation of ROS can affect the synthesis and secretion of collagen. Treatment of human dermal fibroblasts with hydrogen peroxide solution (H_2O_2) increases intracellular ROS levels, leading to the expression of matrix metalloproteinase-1 (MMP-1) and a decrease in collagen secretion [52]. Similarly, in this study, $PM_{2.5}$, CS, and COFs were found to down-regulate the mRNA expression of collagen genes and increase intracellular ROS levels in FB cells. This suggests that $PM_{2.5}$, CS, and COFs can decrease collagen secretion by increasing intracellular ROS generation, potentially leading to further skin damage. Kruk and Duchnik [53] found that oxidative stress has been shown to induce chronic inflammatory reaction, which, in turn, can lead to the collagen rupture and dysfunction of collagen fibers and skin cells. Exposure to COFs has been found to significantly increase oxidative stress biomarkers (ROS and MDA), pro-inflammatory markers (TNF-α and IL-1ß), and markers of apoptosis (NF-kappa B and Caspase-3) in rat lungs. The toxicity of COFs on the lungs can be reduced by vitamin E, suggesting that oxidative stress may be primarily responsible for the observed toxicity induced by COFs [20].

These results suggest that ROS may play an important role in the cell viability, release of pro-inflammatory cytokines, and mRNA expression of collagen I, III, IV, and VII induced by $PM_{2.5}$ and COFs. However, in comparison, CS had lower effect on ROS production, but exhibited a major effect on cytokines expression. This indicates that for CS, it is unclear whether ROS play a key role, at least in cytokines expression. Therefore, further investigation is needed to elucidate the mechanism behind these findings. For example, the use of ROS scavengers can help determine the role of ROS in these biological effects by investigating the relationship between cell viability, levels of IL-1α and TNF-α, or the mRNA expression of collagen and ROS generation.

5. Conclusions

The main biological effects of acute stressors on skin include alterations in the skin barrier, subclinical microinflammation, inflammation, immunosuppression, DNA damage, melanogenesis, and changes in sebum and sweat production. Environmental factors such as $PM_{2.5}$, CS, and COFs at the test concentrations were found to decrease the viability of FB cells and HaCaT cells. They also promoted the secretion of pro-inflammatory cytokines IL-1α and TNF-α in HaCaT cells, increased intracellular ROS levels, and down-regulated the mRNA expression of collagen I, III, IV, and VII in FB cells. In comparison, among $PM_{2.5}$, CS, and COFs, the organic extract of CS exhibited the strongest cytotoxicity, followed by $PM_{2.5}$. In addition, O_3 exposure also reduced the viability of 3D skin cells and elevated the levels of IL-1α and TNF-α. These findings are of value as they suggest that these common environmental factors can potentially damage our skin. Therefore, it is important to minimize exposure to these environmental factors to reduce skin damage. These results also offer a new perspective for the development of cosmetics. For instance, cosmetics could be designed to repair skin damage caused by these environmental factors or to provide a protective barrier against exposure to these factors.

Author Contributions: M.F.: methodology, investigation; Y.Y.: validation, data curation; X.Z.: writing—review and editing, formal analysis; B.L.: conceptualization, writing—original draft, supervision; T.C.: project administration, supervision; Y.C.: resources. All authors have read and agreed to the published version of the manuscript.

Funding: We thank the Shanghai Professional Technical Service Platform Construction Project (No. 22DZ2292100) and the Program for Changjiang Scholars and Innovative Research Team in University (No. IRT13078) for their support of this study.

Institutional Review Board Statement: This manuscript is a study on the toxicity of environmental factors to skin cells, which does not involve ethical issues.

Data Availability Statement: The datasets used and/or analyzed during the current study are available from the corresponding authors on reasonable request.

Acknowledgments: We thank Yanli Feng for providing environmental samples used in this manuscript.

Conflicts of Interest: Author Yuanqi Chen was employed by the company Skincare Research Center of Dr. YU, Shanghai Jahwa United Co., Ltd., Shanghai, China. The remaining authors declare that the research was conducted in the absence of any commercial or financial relationships that could be construed as a potential conflict of interest.

References

1. Schurer, N.Y.; Elias, P.M. The biochemistry and function of stratum corneum lipids. *Adv. Lipid Res.* **1991**, *24*, 27–56.
2. Araviiskaia, E.E.; Bieber, B.T.; Gontijo, G.; Viera, M.S.; Marrot, L.; Chubere, B.; Derno, B. The impact of airborne pollution on skin. *J. Eur. Acad. Dermatol.* **2019**, *33*, 1496–1505. [CrossRef]
3. Lee, K.J.; Park, K.H.; Hahn, J.H. Alleviation of ultraviolet-B radiation-induced photoaging by a TNFR antagonistic peptide TNFR2-SKE. *Mol. Cells* **2019**, *42*, 151–160.
4. Mokrzyrński, K.; Krzsztyńska-kuleta, O.; Zawrotniak, M.; Sarna, M. Fine particulate matter-induced oxidative stress mediated by UVA-visible light leads to keratinocyte damage. *Int. J. Mol. Sci.* **2021**, *22*, 10645. [CrossRef]
5. Magnani, N.D.; Muresan, X.M.; Belmonte, G.; Cervellati, F.; Sticozzi, C.; Pecorelli, A.; Miracco, C.; Marchini, T.; Evelson, P.; Valacchi, G. Skin damage mechanisms related to airborne particulate matter. *Exposure* **2016**, *149*, 227–236. [CrossRef]
6. Clunes, L.A.; Bridges, A.; Alexis, N.; Tarran, R. In vivo versus in vitro airway surface liquid nicotine levels following cigarette smoke exposure. *J. Anal. Toxicol.* **2008**, *32*, 201–207. [CrossRef]
7. Torres, S.; Merino, C.; Paton, B.; Correig, X.; Ramírez, N. Biomarkers of exposure to secondhand and thirdhand tobacco smoke: Recent advances and future perspectives. *Int. J. Environ. Public Health* **2018**, *15*, 2693. [CrossRef]
8. Doshi, D.N.; Hanneman, K.K.; Cooper, K.D. Smoking and skin aging in identical twins. *Arch. Dermatol.* **2007**, *143*, 1543–1546. [CrossRef]
9. Egawa, M.; Kohno, Y.; Kumano, Y. Oxidative effects of cigarette smoke on the human skin. *Int. J. Cosmet. Sci.* **1999**, *21*, 83–98. [CrossRef]
10. Liu, J.L.; Fu, M.Y.; Miao, J.Y.; Sun, Y.L.; Zhu, R.G.; Liu, C.Y.; Bi, R.C.; Wang, S.; Cao, X.Y. The toxicity of cooking oil fumes on human bronchial epithelial cells through ROS-mediated MAPK, NF-kappa B signaling pathways and NLRP3 inflammasome. *Environ. Toxicol.* **2022**, *37*, 1071–1080. [CrossRef]
11. Chen, K.C.; Tsai, S.W.; Shie, R.H.; Zeng, C.; Yang, H.Y. Indoor air pollution increases the risk of lung cancer. *Int. J. Environ. Res. Public Health* **2022**, *19*, 1164. [CrossRef] [PubMed]
12. Yang, S.C.; Jeng, S.N.; Kang, Z.C.; Lee, H. Identification of benzo[α]pyrene 7,8-diol 9, 10-epoxide N2-deoxyguanosine in human lung adenocarcinoma cells exposed to cooking oil fumes from frying fish under domestic conditions. *Chem. Res. Toxicol.* **2000**, *13*, 1046–1050. [CrossRef]

13. Kazemiparkouhi, F.; Eum, K.D.; Wang, B.; Manjourides, J.; Suh, H.H. Long-term ozone exposures and cause-specific mortality in a US Medicare cohort. *J. Expo. Sci. Environ. Epidemiol.* **2020**, *30*, 650–658. [CrossRef] [PubMed]
14. Fuks, K.B.; Hüls, A.; Sugiri, D.; Altug, H.; Vierktter, A.; Abramson, M.J.; Goebel, J.; Wagner, G.G.; Demuth, I.; Krutmann, J.; et al. Tropospheric ozone and skin aging: Results from two German cohort studies. *Environ. Int.* **2019**, *124*, 139–144. [CrossRef] [PubMed]
15. Valacchi, G.; van der Vliet, A.; Schock, B.C.; Okamoto, T.; Obermuller-Jevic, U.; Cross, C.E.; Packer, L. Ozone exposure activates oxidative stress responses in murine skin. *Toxicology* **2002**, *179*, 163–170. [CrossRef] [PubMed]
16. Ferrara, F.; Pambianchi, E.; Pecorelli, A.; Woodby, B.; Messano, N.; Therrien, J.-P.; Lila, M.A.; Valacchi, G. Redox regulation of cutaneous inflammasome by ozone exposure. *Free Radic. Biol. Med.* **2020**, *152*, 561–570. [CrossRef] [PubMed]
17. Deng, Y.T.; Li, X.M.; Liu, E.M.; Xiong, W.K.; Wang, S.; Zhu, R.; Ding, Y.B.; Zhong, Z.H. Association of early-life factors and indoor environmental exposure with asthma among children: A case-control study in Chongqing, China. *World J. Pediatr.* **2022**, *18*, 186–195. [CrossRef]
18. Gao, J.W.; Qiu, Z.W.; Cheng, W.; Gao, H.O. Children's exposure to BC and PM pollution, and respiratory tract deposits during commuting trips to school. *Ecotoxicol. Environ. Saf.* **2022**, *232*, 113253. [CrossRef]
19. Lin, H.; Long, Y.; Su, Y.J.; Song, K.; Li, C.L.; Ding, N. Air pollution and hospital admissions for critical illness in emergency department: A tertiary-center research in Changsha, China, 2016–2020. *Environ. Sci. Pollut. Res.* **2022**, *29*, 21440–21450. [CrossRef]
20. Ma, Y.S.; Deng, L.J.; Ma, P.; Wu, Y.; Yang, X.; Xiao, F.; Deng, Q.H. In vivo respiratory toxicology of cooking oil fumes: Evidence, mechanisms and prevention. *J. Hazard. Mater.* **2021**, *402*, 123455. [CrossRef]
21. Aikaterini, V.-A.; Robert, P. Environmental factors influencing the transmission of the coronavirus 2019: A review. *Environ. Chem. Lett.* **2022**, *20*, 1603–1610.
22. Mondal, S.; Chaipitakporn, C.; Kumar, V.; Wangler, B.; Gurajala, S.; Dhaniyala, S.; Sur, S. COVID-19 in New York state: Effects of demographics and air quality on infection and fatality. *Sci. Total Environ.* **2022**, *807*, 150536. [CrossRef]
23. Weaver, A.K.; Head, J.R.; Gould, C.F.; Carlton, E.J.; Remais, J.V. Environmental factors influencing COVID-19 incidence and severity. *Annu. Rev. Public Health* **2022**, *43*, 271–291. [CrossRef]
24. Kim, S.; Kim, J.; Lee, Y.I.; Jang, S.; Song, S.Y.; Lee, W.J.; Lee, J.H. Particulate matter-induced atmospheric skin aging is aggravated by UVA and inhibited by a topical L-ascorbic acid compound. *Photodermatol. Photoimmunol. Photomed.* **2022**, *38*, 123–131. [CrossRef] [PubMed]
25. Warke, M.; English, M.; De Marchi, L.; Sarkar, R.P.; Kannan, S.; Datta, R.; Rao, S. In-vitro cell culture model to determine toxic effects of soil arsenic due to direct dermal exposure. *Environ. Technol. Innov.* **2022**, *28*, 102949. [CrossRef]
26. Prieux, R.; Eeman, M.; Rothen-Rutishauser, B.; Valacchi, G. Mimicking cigarette smoke exposure to assess cutaneous toxicity. *Toxicol. In Vitro* **2020**, *62*, 104664. [CrossRef] [PubMed]
27. Lei, B.L.; Tang, Q.Q.; Sun, S.; Zhang, X.L.; Huang, Y.Y.; Xu, L.B. Insight into the mechanism of tetrachlorobisphenol A (TCBPA)-induced proliferation of breast cancer cells by GPER-mediated signaling pathways. *Environ. Pollut.* **2021**, *375*, 116636. [CrossRef] [PubMed]
28. Lei, B.L.; Sun, S.; Xu, J.; Feng, C.L.; Yu, Y.X.; Xu, G.; Wu, M.H.; Peng, W. Low-concentration BPAF- and BPF- induced cell biological effects are mediated by ROS in MCF-7 breast cancer cells. *Environ. Sci. Pollut. Res.* **2018**, *25*, 3200–3208. [CrossRef]
29. Lei, B.L.; Xu, L.B.; Huang, Y.Y.; Liu, Y.; Yu, M.J.; Tang, Q.Q. Chlorobisphenol A activated kisspeptin/GPR54-GnRH neuroendocrine signals through ERα and GPER pathway in neuronal GT1-7 cells. *Ecotoxicol. Environ. Saf.* **2022**, *233*, 113290. [CrossRef]
30. Fuyuno, Y.; Uchi, H.; Yasumatsu, M.; Morino-Koga, S.; Tanaka, Y.; Mitoma, C.; Furue, M. Perillaldehyde inhibits AHR signaling and activates NRF2 antioxidant pathway in human Keratinocytes. *Oxid. Med. Cell Longev.* **2018**, *2018*, 9524657. [CrossRef]
31. Lim, G.E.; Park, J.E.; Cho, Y.H.; Lim, D.; Kim, A.J.; Moh, S.H.; Lee, J.H.; Lee, J.S. Alpha-neoendorphin can reduce UVB-induced skin photoaging by activating cellular autophagy. *Arch. Biochem. Biophys.* **2020**, *689*, 108437. [CrossRef] [PubMed]
32. Abolhasani, R.; Araghi, F.; Tabary, M.; Aryannejad, A.; Mashinchi, B.; Robati, R.M. The impact of air pollution on skin and related disorders: A comprehensive review. *Dermatol. Ther.* **2021**, *34*, e14840. [CrossRef] [PubMed]
33. Chiang, H.M.; Chen, C.W.; Lin, T.Y.; Kuo, Y.H. N-phenetyl caffeamide and photodamage: Protecting skin by inhibiting type I procollagen degradation and stimulating collagen synthesis. *Food Chem. Toxicol.* **2014**, *72*, 154–161. [CrossRef] [PubMed]
34. Passeron, T.; Zouboulis, C.C.; Tan, J.; Andersen, M.L.; Katta, R.; Lyu, X.; Aguilar, L.; Kerob, D.; Morita, A.; Krutmann, J.; et al. Adult skin acute stress responses to short-term environmental and internal aggression from exposome factors. *J. Eur. Acad. Dermatol.* **2021**, *35*, 1963–1975. [CrossRef] [PubMed]
35. Cooke, M. The chemical components of Tobacco and Tobacco smoke. *Chromatographia* **2010**, *71*, 977. [CrossRef]
36. Ernster, V.L.; Grady, D.; Mike, R.; Black, D.; Selby, J.; Kerlikowske, K. Facial wrinkling in men and women, by smoking status. *Am. J. Public Health* **1995**, *85*, 78–82. [CrossRef]
37. Oppeltz, R.F.; Jatoi, I. Tobacco and the escalating global cancer burden. *J. Oncol.* **2011**, *2011*, 408104. [CrossRef]
38. Ding, R.; Li, J.; Zhang, Q.; Zhang, C.; Li, N.; Sun, S.; Li, C.L.; Shen, C.W.; Zhao, Q.H.; Chen, H.B.; et al. Vitamin D-3 protects intrauterine growth restriction induced by cooking oil fume derived fine particulate matters. *Ecotoxicol. Environ. Saf.* **2022**, *229*, 113103. [CrossRef]
39. Hyun, Y.J.; Piao, M.J.; Kang, K.A.; Ryu, Y.S.; Zhen, A.X.; Cho, S.J.; Kang, H.K.; Koh, Y.S.; Ahn, M.J.; Kim, T.H.; et al. 3,4-dicaffeoylquinic acid protects human keratinocytes against environmental oxidative damage. *J. Funct. Foods* **2019**, *52*, 430–441. [CrossRef]

40. Pecorelli, A.; Woodby, B.; Prieux, R.; Valacchi, G. Involvement of 4-hydroxy-2- nonenal in pollution-induced skin damage. *Biofactors* **2019**, *45*, 536–547. [CrossRef]
41. Abais, J.M.; Xia, M.; Zhang, Y.; Boini, K.M.; Li, P. Redox regulation of NLRP3 Inflammasomes: ROS as trigger or Effector. *Antioxid. Redox Sign* **2015**, *22*, 1111–1129. [CrossRef] [PubMed]
42. Soeur, J.; Belaïdi, J.-P.; Chollet, C.; Denat, L.; Dimitrov, A.; Jones, C.; Perez, P.; Zanini, M.; Zobiri, O.; Mezzache, S.; et al. Photo-pollution stress in skin: Traces of pollutants (PAH and particulate matter) impair redox homeostasis in keratinocytes exposed to UVA1. *J. Dermatol. Sci.* **2017**, *86*, 162–169. [CrossRef] [PubMed]
43. Guttman-Yassky, E.; Krueger, J.G. Atopic dermatitis and psoriasis: Two different immune diseases or one spectrum. *Curr. Opin. Immunol.* **2017**, *48*, 68–73. [CrossRef] [PubMed]
44. He, Y.; Hara, H.; Núñez, G. Mechanism and regulation of NLRP3 inflammasome activation. *Trends Biochem. Sci.* **2016**, *41*, 1012–1021. [CrossRef]
45. Latz, E.; Xiao, T.S.; Stutz, A. Activation and regulation of the inflammasomes. *Nat. Rev. Immunol.* **2013**, *13*, 397–411. [CrossRef] [PubMed]
46. Guo, M.Y.; Bi, S.Y.; Liu, J.; Xu, W.S.; Zhou, G.Q.; Liu, Y.; Chen, C.Y. C60(OH)n-loaded nanofibrous membranes protect HaCat cells from ROS-associated damage. *Chin. Chem. Lett.* **2017**, *28*, 1889–1892. [CrossRef]
47. Romani, A.; Cervellati, C.; Muresan, X.M.; Belmonte, G.; Pecorelli, A.; Cervellati, F.; Benedusi, M.; Evelson, P.; Valacchi, G. Keratinocytes oxidative damage mechanisms related to airborne particle matter exposure. *Mech. Ageing Dev.* **2018**, *172*, 86–95. [CrossRef]
48. Song, I.B.; Gu, H.; Han, H.J.; Lee, N.Y.; Cha, J.Y.; Dong, Y.K.; Kwon, J. Effects of 7-MEGATM 500 on oxidative stress, inflammation, and skin regeneration in H2O2-treated skin cells. *Toxicol. Res.* **2018**, *34*, 103–110. [CrossRef]
49. De Luca, C.; Valacchi, G. Surface lipids as multifunctional mediators of skin responses to environmental stimuli. *Mediat. Inflamm.* **2010**, *2010*, 321494. [CrossRef]
50. Valacchi, G.; Muresan, X.M.; Sticozzi, C.; Belmonte, G.; Pecorelli, A.; Cervellati, F. Ozone-induced damage in 3D-Skin Model is prevented by topical vitamin C and vitamin E compound mixtures application. *J. Dermatol. Sci.* **2016**, *82*, 209–212. [CrossRef]
51. Ansary, T.M.; Hossain, M.R.; Kamiya, K.; Komine, M.; Ohtsuki, M. Inflammatory molecules associated with ultraviolet radiation-mediated skin aging. *Int. J. Mol. Sci.* **2021**, *22*, 3974. [CrossRef] [PubMed]
52. Darawsha, A.; Trachtenberg, A.; Levy, J.; Sharoni, Y. The protective effect of carotenoids, polyphenols, and estradiol on dermal fibroblasts under oxidative stress. *Antioxidants* **2021**, *10*, 2023. [CrossRef] [PubMed]
53. Kruk, J.; Duchnik, E. Oxidative stress and skin diseases: Possible role of physical activity. *Asian Pac. J. Cancer Prev.* **2014**, *15*, 561–568. [CrossRef] [PubMed]

toxics

MDPI

Article

Comparison of Population-Weighted Exposure Estimates of Air Pollutants Based on Multiple Geostatistical Models in Beijing, China

Yinghan Wu [1], Jia Xu [1,*,†], Ziqi Liu [1,2], Bin Han [1], Wen Yang [1,*,†] and Zhipeng Bai [1,2]

[1] State Key Laboratory of Environmental Criteria and Risk Assessment, Chinese Research Academy of Environmental Sciences, Beijing 100012, China; wuyinghan21@mails.ucas.ac.cn (Y.W.); ziqi@uw.edu (Z.L.); hanbin@craes.org.cn (B.H.); baizp@craes.org.cn (Z.B.)

[2] Department of Environmental & Occupational Health Sciences, School of Public Health, University of Washington, Seattle, WA 98105, USA

* Correspondence: xu.jia@craes.org.cn (J.X.); yangwen@craes.org.cn (W.Y.)

† These authors contributed equally to this work.

Abstract: Various geostatistical models have been used in epidemiological research to evaluate ambient air pollutant exposures at a fine spatial scale. Few studies have investigated the performance of different exposure models on population-weighted exposure estimates and the resulting potential misclassification across various modeling approaches. This study developed spatial models for NO_2 and $PM_{2.5}$ and conducted exposure assessment in Beijing, China. It explored three spatial modeling approaches: variable dimension reduction, machine learning, and conventional linear regression. It compared their model performance by cross-validation (CV) and population-weighted exposure estimates. Specifically, partial least square (PLS) regression, random forests (RF), and supervised linear regression (SLR) models were developed based on an ordinary kriging (OK) framework for NO_2 and $PM_{2.5}$ in Beijing, China. The mean squared error-based R^2 (R^2_{mse}) and root mean squared error (RMSE) in leave-one site-out cross-validation (LOOCV) were used to evaluate model performance. These models were used to predict the ambient exposure levels in the urban area and to estimate the misclassification of population-weighted exposure estimates in quartiles between them. The results showed that the PLS-OK models for NO_2 and $PM_{2.5}$, with the LOOCV R^2_{mse} of 0.82 and 0.81, respectively, outperformed the other models. The population-weighted exposure to NO_2 estimated by the PLS-OK and RF-OK models exhibited the lowest misclassification in quartiles. For $PM_{2.5}$, the estimates of potential misclassification were comparable across the three models. It indicated that the exposure misclassification made by choosing different modeling approaches should be carefully considered, and the resulting bias needs to be evaluated in epidemiological studies.

Keywords: $PM_{2.5}$; NO_2; geostatistical modeling approach; exposure estimates; misclassification

1. Introduction

Long-term exposure to air pollutants has been proven to be associated with adverse health outcomes [1–3]. Current research has focused on a medium- and long-term period exposure assessment at an individual level [4], which needs accurate exposure assessment at a fine spatial scale to eliminate exposure errors [5,6]. It is a big challenge because of the sparse monitoring stations and missing coverage of specific predictors, such as satellite-based models [7].

Geostatistical models developed by the land-use regression (LUR) approach have been widely used to assess medium- and long-term exposure to air pollution in epidemiological studies [8,9]. The geostatistical models were created based on the inputs of observational and geographic data sets, in which the former was involved as outcome variables and the latter were predictor variables. The choice of model development approaches, the method for dealing with predictor variables, and the model structures can all affect model performances [10–13]. The golden standard method for model evaluation includes out-of-sample validation and hold-out cross-validation (CV) [10,14]. However, some studies laced sufficient observational data for out-of-sample model validation or hold-out CV. Also, some results for evaluating some two-step models were not easy to interpret, e.g., the predictor selection and dimension reduction methods [15,16]. In brief, evaluating the performance of exposure models developed based on limited monitoring sites was challenging, but they are still helpful for environmental health studies. In previous studies on modeling approach comparison [10,17], the model performance was evaluated by cross-validation or out-of-sample validation. Nevertheless, to further compare these models' performances, they need to be evaluated by exposure assessment in the real world, and potential exposure bias caused by different modeling algorithms needs to be assessed.

In this study, we used three modeling approaches, variable dimensionality reduction, machine learning, and variable screening, to build geostatistical models for NO_2 and $PM_{2.5}$ and to compare their model performance by estimating the misclassification of population-weighted exposure estimates in quartiles.

2. Methods

2.1. Study Area and Observations at Monitoring Sites

Beijing, China's capital city, is a mega-city with a population of 21.5 million during the research period (2015–2020) [18]. Ambient concentrations of $PM_{2.5}$ have decreased since stringent national and local environmental regulations were implemented in 2014 [19]. However, the ambient exposure level of such air pollutants is still higher than the World Health Organization (WHO) Global Air Quality Guidelines, 10 $\mu g/m^3$ for NO_2 and 5 $\mu g/m^3$ for $PM_{2.5}$ [20]. This study obtained NO_2 and $PM_{2.5}$ observational data from the Beijing air quality monitoring network (Beijing Municipal Environmental Monitoring Center). The NO_2 was measured using the ultraviolet fluorescence method, and the $PM_{2.5}$ was measured using the micro oscillating balance method at these monitoring sites [21]. A total of 35 monitoring sites were divided into 4 types, including 1 background site, 7 traffic sites, 14 urban sites, and 13 suburban sites, as shown in Figure 1. The background site is located near a reservoir in the Miyun district. The lowest NO_2 and $PM_{2.5}$ concentrations were observed at this background site. The traffic sites are close to the (A) type roads (highways and arterial roads) with a distance of less than 250 m. The other 27 monitoring sites were divided into urban and suburban sites, in which the urban sites were located inside and around the 6th-ring road, and the suburban sites were the rest of them.

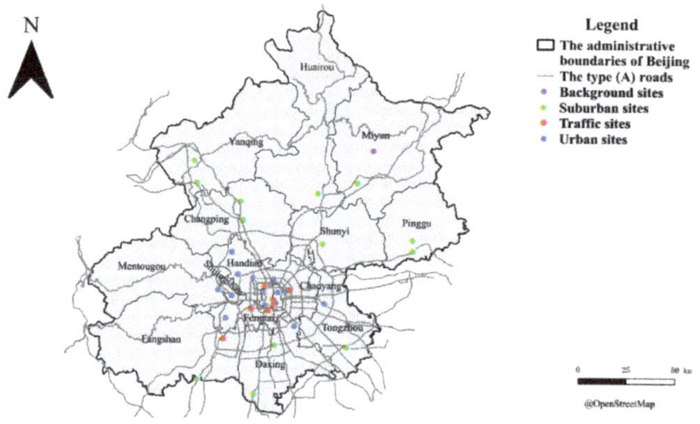

Figure 1. Map of the 35 monitoring sites in Beijing.

Annual average concentrations were obtained from the raw hourly concentrations. First, the daily averages were calculated by hourly concentration, following a criterion that 50% of the data (12 h) were available at each monitoring site. Second, these daily averages were used for calculating weekly averages, following the same criterion that 3-day data were available. Third, these weekly averages were applied for calculating annual averages, following another criterion of 25%. It allows the yearly averages to be calculated based on daily, weekly, and seasonal bases and be temporally representative. A similar temporal average strategy was used in Araki et al.'s NO_2 exposure modeling study [22]. Figure 2 depicts the calculated weekly average concentrations of NO_2 and $PM_{2.5}$, where blank spaces represent missing concentrations. The above criteria screened some of the missing data, and the rest were due to the raw data loss. Table 1 shows the statistical summary of annual average NO_2 and $PM_{2.5}$ concentrations. In 2016 and 2017, the available yearly averages were less than 35 because of the data screening criteria. After 2018, one of the 35 monitoring sites, the Beijing Botanical Garden site, was excluded from the monitoring network, as shown in Figure 1.

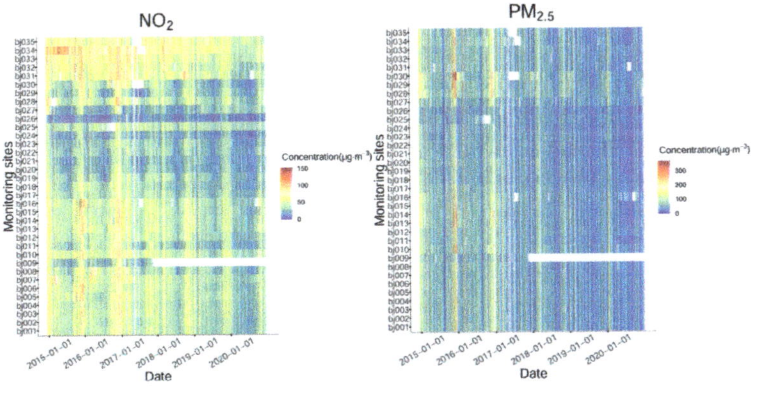

Figure 2. Weekly average concentrations of NO_2 and $PM_{2.5}$ at the 35 monitoring sites in Beijing from 2015 to 2020.

Table 1. The annual average concentrations of NO_2 and $PM_{2.5}$ from 2015 to 2020.

Pollutant	Year	No. of Sites	Missing	Annual Averages ($\mu g/m^3$)	SD ($\mu g/m^3$)
NO_2	2015	35	8.79%	49.27	15.92
	2016	34	8.79%	48.16	14.93
	2017	32	10.22%	44.09	12.57
	2018	34	3.08%	42.12	12.96
	2019	34	2.86%	37.19	10.73
	2020	34	3.62%	30.30	8.72
$PM_{2.5}$	2015	35	4.40%	82.56	13.39
	2016	35	8.79%	74.01	11.58
	2017	32	10.33%	58.60	6.59
	2018	34	3.08%	52.58	6.32
	2019	34	2.97%	43.04	5.86
	2020	34	3.85%	38.55	5.40

2.2. Geographic Variables

In this study, we collected a wide array of geographic variables, including population density, traffic network, features (e.g., airport, rail yard, railways, etc.), points of interest (POI), land-use types, Normalized Difference Vegetation Index (NDVI), topography and coordinate variables. Some of these geographic variables were related to the emission sources, such as road network, features, and POI, while others were derived from the natural characteristics in the study area, e.g., population density and elevation. The details of these geographic variables are described in Table S1 in the Supplementary Information (SI).

2.3. Algorithms for Model Development

In this study, three types of modeling approaches were applied for model development. First, we chose the partial least squares (PLS) to represent the dimension reduction modeling approach. Second, random forest (RF), an advanced and relatively simple modeling approach with relatively fewer steps, was selected as a machine learning algorithm. Third, the supervised linear regression (SLR) algorithm was chosen as a traditional modeling approach. The PLS and SLR algorithms are based on a linear regression framework [10,16]. The RF algorithm is a complex algorithm dealing with non-linear relationships between response and predictor variables and also between predictor variables [10]. The PLS and SLR models have clear and interpretable frameworks, while the RF model is less interpretable because of its hidden black box [23].

Specifically, the PLS regression algorithm reduces predictor variables to a smaller set of uncorrelated components and performs least squares regression on these components. The PLS decomposes the large geographic variable matrix into a sequence of orthogonal PLS scores computed to maximize the covariance between concentrations and their prediction. According to the experience in our previous study in Beijing [11,24], the number of PLS scores was set to be 3.

As a machine learning algorithm, RF is an ensemble learning method that combines multiple decision trees to improve the accuracy and robustness of the developed models [23]. In RF model development, potential predictor variables are forced to be partitioned into subsets, which include separate decision trees for training. The output is the average of the decision tree simulation results. The RF model provides an importance evaluation index of the variables (IncMSE) that can be used to determine the influence of predictor variables on the response variables [25]. In this study, the setting of the RF models was based on our previous experience [11]. The coefficients of the random sampling times (mtry), number of decision trees in a random forest (ntree), and a minimum number of decision tree nodes (node size) were set to be 50, 500, and 5, respectively.

The SLR model is a traditional and widely used stepwise linear regression method developed using selected geographic variables as predictors [26,27]. First, univariate linear regression is conducted to find a starting point for an SLR model, as the highest R^2 is obtained. Second, the additional predictor is added in each round to obtain the most significant increase in R^2 until the rise of the R^2 is less than 0.1. The selected variable in each round is available when its direction is plausible with the outcome pollutant. Third, the variance inflation factor (VIF) is applied to prevent multicollinearity. The selected variables with a value of VIF more than 3 were removed [28].

All the models were developed by R software (R 4.2.0, https://www.r-project.org/, accessed on 1 April 2022), using the R packages of "pls", "randomForest" and so on.

2.4. Model Structure and Validation

For LUR models, their residuals are always spatially correlated [12]. Thus, we applied a two-step model structure, a LUR model with ordinary kriging (OK), to develop a LUR-OK model. First, a LUR model was developed; second, the residuals of the LUR model were further explained by OK. The same or similar model structures were widely used in previous studies [29–31].

The developed models were evaluated by using leave-one-site-out cross-validation (LOOCV). The observed data were split into groups equal to the number of monitoring sites, in which each group included the observations from one monitoring site. One data group was used for testing (testing group), and the other remaining data groups (training group) were used to fit the model. Then, the fitted model was used to predict the testing group and repeated until predictions for all groups were generated. We used mean square error based-R-Squared (R^2_{mse}), regression-based R^2 (R^2_{reg}), and root-mean-square error

(*RMSE*) to assess the accuracy and prediction ability of the model, which was computed on observations (y_i) and predictions ($\hat{y}_i$) according to the equations below:

$$RMSE = \sqrt{\frac{1}{n}\sum_{i=1}^{n}(y_i - \hat{y}_i)} \tag{1}$$

$$R^2{}_{\mathrm{mse}} = \max\left(0, 1 - \frac{RMSE^2}{\sum_{i=1}^{n}(y_i - \overline{y})^2/n}\right) \tag{2}$$

In both equations, n is the number of observations, and $\overline{y}$ is the mean of observations. $R^2{}_{\mathrm{mse}}$ is a measure of fit to the 1:1 line and is typically lower than $R^2{}_{\mathrm{reg}}$, which is a measure of fit to the regression line. The model performance was mainly evaluated by $R^2{}_{\mathrm{mse}}$ and *RMSE*, and the $R^2{}_{\mathrm{reg}}$ was also reported for comparisons with other studies.

3. Results and Discussion

3.1. Model Development

3.1.1. PLS Models

The geographic variables were downscaled using the PLS approach. The first three PLS scores were obtained as inputs for the PLS models. The first PLS score explains most variations across the geographic data set. Thus, we evaluated correlation coefficients between the first PLS score and geographic variables to represent the influence of the geographic variables on PLS models. Figure 3 depicts these correlation coefficients for the annual NO_2 and $PM_{2.5}$ models. For NO_2 models, the correlation coefficients between the first PLS score and the geographic variables were relatively stable across the annual models. The variables of all the annual NO_2 models that were highly correlated with the first PLS score were population density, POI variables (the count of temples, restaurants, gas stations and bus stops), NDVI variables (NDVI in summer and the 75th percentile of NDVI), land-use type variables (shrubland, impervious, grassland, and forest), and the proximity variables (the distance to the type (C) road, railway, the intersection between type (A) and type (B) roads, and the intersection between type (A) roads.

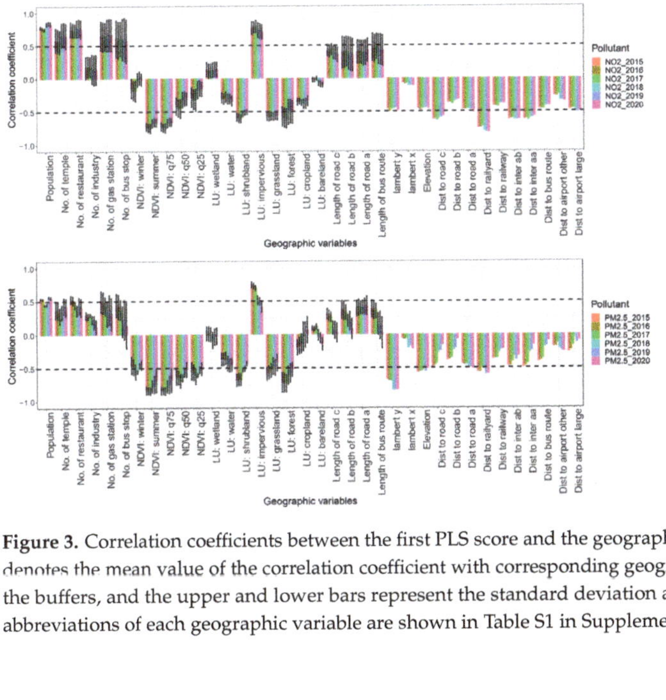

Figure 3. Correlation coefficients between the first PLS score and the geographic variables. Each box denotes the mean value of the correlation coefficient with corresponding geographic variables across the buffers, and the upper and lower bars represent the standard deviation across the buffers. The abbreviations of each geographic variable are shown in Table S1 in Supplementary Information.

Compared with the annual NO_2 models, the correlation coefficients between the first PLS score and the geographic variables varied among the annual $PM_{2.5}$ models, especially for the annual $PM_{2.5}$ models after 2017. The variables of all the annual $PM_{2.5}$ models with an absolute value of these correlation coefficients greater than 0.5 included the NDVI variables (NDVI in summer and the 75th, 50th, and 25th percentiles of NDVI), land-use type of forest, longitude (Lambert y), elevation, and distance to the railyard. The contrast of the correlation coefficients between these models presented different emission sources of NO_2 and $PM_{2.5}$. As a traffic-related primary air pollutant, the spatial distribution of NO_2 was correlated with the geographic variables of road networks. In contrast, $PM_{2.5}$ was correlated with the longitude variable because of its partially secondary species formation that originated from long-distance transportation [32].

3.1.2. RF Models

According to the IncMSE of the variables given by the RF models, the top ten variables were summarized in Figure 4. The traffic-related variables significantly influence the NO_2 models. The variables of distance to the railyard, the count of gas stations, the distance to the type (A) road, and the sum of the type (A) road length had relatively high IncMSE values in all NO_2 models. For $PM_{2.5}$, the most important variables were longitude, shrubland, and NDVI. Similar variable sensitivities were observed in the PLS models for $PM_{2.5}$, in which the longitude variable was also highlighted.

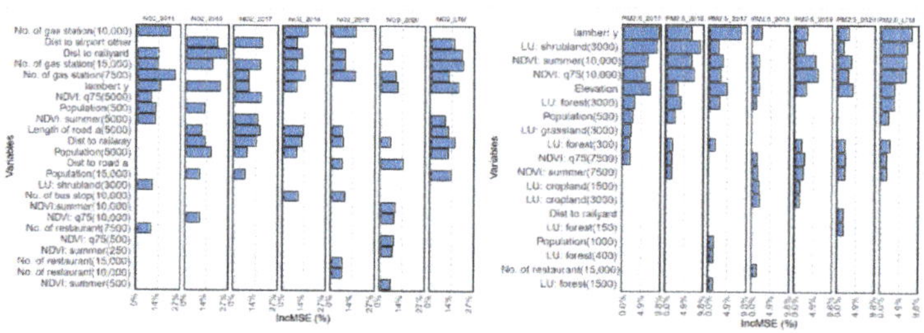

Figure 4. The geographic variables with the top ten IncMSE values in the RF model results.

3.1.3. SLR Models

Figure 5 shows the selected geographic variables by the SLR model and their regression coefficients. For NO_2 models, the traffic-related variables were involved in model development. It is consistent with the RF models. Specifically, the coefficients of the variables of the distance to the airport, railway, and railyard had relatively high values. In addition, the NDVI and land-use type of water variables were also selected. Regarding $PM_{2.5}$, the annual $PM_{2.5}$ models selected fewer variables than the NO_2 models. The variables of the distance to the airport and the distance to the type (B) road influenced the annual $PM_{2.5}$ models a lot.

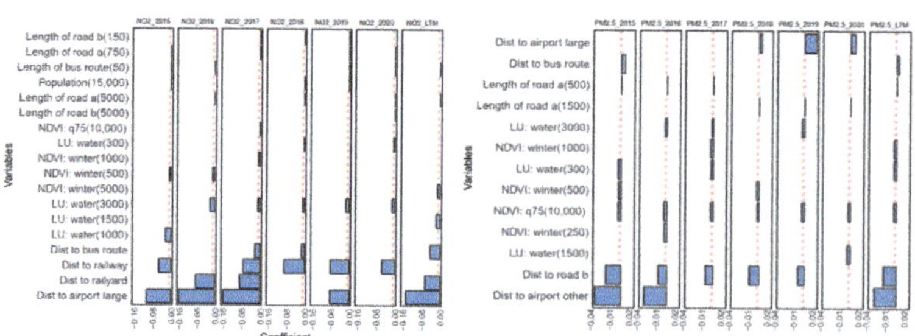

Figure 5. The coefficients of the variables selected by the SLR model.

3.1.4. Models Developed in the Urban Area

In order to compare model performance between the geostatistical models developed in the whole Beijing area and inside the 6th-ring road area that covered the total urban area. The LUR–urban (LURU) models were developed based on the monitoring sites inside and around the 6th-ring road. The coefficients of these LURU models are shown in Figures S1–S3.

For the urban model developed by the PLS approach (PLSU), some variables' correlation coefficients had significant changes, such as the variables of the count of industries (POI), water land-use type, latitude, and distance to airports for the NO_2 models and the variables of the count of industry (POI), NDVI in winter, latitude, and distance to the airports for $PM_{2.5}$ models. The predictors in the PLS and PLSU models were different. It indicated that the PLS approach could be affected when the range of the observational data was expanded as the suburban areas were included. Different model coefficients were also found when comparing RF and RFU models, SLR and SLRU models.

3.2. Model Performance

The LOOCV results of NO_2 and $PM_{2.5}$ models are shown in Tables 2 and 3, respectively. The performances of the LUR and LUR-OK models were summarized in each table. Generally, the annual PLS models performed better than others, with a higher range of R^2_{mse} for NO_2 (0.72~0.82) and $PM_{2.5}$ (0.80~0.89), which were higher than the previous studies in Beijing [33,34]. Regarding the LTM of NO_2, the PLS models had comparable good performance with the SLR models, which performed better than the RF models. Compared with the NO_2 models without an OK in the model structure, the LUR-OK models improved the model performance for PLS and SLR LTM models with a slightly higher R^2_{mse}. For annual NO_2 models, some performed worse when adding OK to the model structure. However, adding OK into the model structure worked well for RF models of $PM_{2.5}$. For annual and LTM $PM_{2.5}$, the RF-OK models improved their performance with an increase of 0.06~0.21 in R^2_{mse} compared with the RF models. In comparison, these increases in R^2_{mse} of PLS and SLR models because of adding OK were −0.17~0.01 and −0.09~0.08, respectively. For the LTM of $PM_{2.5}$, the PLS-OK model performed best among the PLS, RF, and SLR models with or without OK. A spatiotemporal covariate model was built in a previous study with an R^2_{mse} of 0.93, and its RMSE was 1.72 μg/m^3 [35]. Improved performance by adding OK in the model structure was also found in a previous study [36]. The good performance of the PLS approach on spatial modeling was concluded in the previous study [11,30]. In terms of the comparisons between the traditional SLR model and machine learning models, the SLR model underperformed in this study, which is different from the previous comparisons [10]. The controversy over machine learning approaches has existed for a long time. It may depend on the target air pollutants and the collecting method of monitoring data [13].

Different model performances were found for PLSU, RFU, and SLRU models developed in urban areas with less observational data involved in model development, as shown in Tables S2 and S3 in Supplementary Information. Compared with the models developed in the whole city area, the PLSU models had better performance for both NO_2 (LOOCV R^2_{mse}: 0.83~0.96) and $PM_{2.5}$ (LOOCV R^2_{mse}: 0.74~0.82), while RFU and SLRU models had opposite performances. The increased performance of these PLSU models might be due to overfitting. The RFU and SLRU models were sensitive to the number of observational monitoring sites. We also found worse model performances from 2018 to 2020 than those from 2015 to 2017, when observational data were missing from 2018 at the monitoring site in the western mountain area. It indicated that the monitoring sites with various observational levels were necessary for model development in the urban area [28].

Figure 6 shows the scatter plots of the long-term mean observations and LOOCV predictions of the PLS, RF, and SLR mdels for NO_2 and $PM_{2.5}$. For NO_2, the PLS (LOOCV R^2_{mse}: 0.78) and SLR (LOOCV R^2_{mse}: 0.76) models performed better than the RF models (LOOCV R^2_{mse}: 0.57). The RF model was overestimated at the background site. Similar results were found for $PM_{2.5}$ models, in which the LOOCV R^2_{mse} of PLS, RF, and SLR models were 0.80, 0.51, and 0.54, respectively. The $PM_{2.5}$ RF model performed worse at the background site than those at other types of monitoring sites.

Table 2. LOOCV results of the NO_2 models.

Year	PLS			RF			SLR		
	RMSE	R^2_{mse}	R^2_{reg}	RMSE	R^2_{mse}	R^2_{reg}	RMSE	R^2_{mse}	R^2_{reg}
2015	6.59	0.82	0.85	9.93	0.60	0.62	7.56	0.77	0.78
2016	7.64	0.73	0.78	9.90	0.55	0.57	11.46	0.39	0.44
2017	6.19	0.75	0.78	9.09	0.46	0.46	7.00	0.68	0.71
2018	6.34	0.75	0.78	8.60	0.55	0.57	7.23	0.68	0.69
2019	5.06	0.77	0.80	7.80	0.46	0.47	5.72	0.71	0.71
2020	4.55	0.72	0.77	6.79	0.37	0.38	4.81	0.69	0.70
LTM	5.66	0.78	0.81	7.93	0.57	0.59	5.97	0.76	0.76
Year	PLS-OK			RF-OK			SLR-OK		
	RMSE	R^2_{mse}	R^2_{reg}	RMSE	R^2_{mse}	R^2_{reg}	RMSE	R^2_{mse}	R^2_{reg}
2015	6.18	0.84	0.87	9.75	0.61	0.62	7.43	0.78	0.78
2016	7.74	0.72	0.78	10.23	0.52	0.55	11.42	0.40	0.46
2017	5.97	0.77	0.80	9.41	0.42	0.45	6.80	0.70	0.73
2018	5.77	0.80	0.82	8.22	0.59	0.59	7.06	0.69	0.72
2019	4.61	0.81	0.83	7.76	0.46	0.47	6.11	0.67	0.67
2020	4.53	0.72	0.77	7.67	0.20	0.29	5.38	0.61	0.64
LTM	5.16	0.82	0.84	7.92	0.57	0.58	5.73	0.78	0.78

Table 3. LOOCV results of the $PM_{2.5}$ models.

Year	PLS			RF			SLR		
	RMSE	R^2_{mse}	R^2_{reg}	RMSE	R^2_{mse}	R^2_{reg}	RMSE	R^2_{mse}	R^2_{reg}
2015	4.39	0.89	0.89	7.88	0.64	0.73	7.64	0.66	0.68
2016	4.07	0.87	0.87	6.90	0.64	0.73	7.02	0.62	0.63
2017	2.73	0.82	0.82	4.24	0.57	0.62	5.30	0.33	0.42
2018	2.33	0.86	0.86	4.80	0.41	0.47	4.17	0.55	0.56
2019	2.13	0.86	0.86	4.02	0.51	0.57	3.75	0.58	0.60
2020	2.21	0.83	0.83	4.21	0.37	0.40	3.43	0.58	0.59
LTM	3.51	0.80	0.80	5.51	0.51	0.59	5.33	0.54	0.54
Year	PLS-OK			RF-OK			SLR-OK		
	RMSE	R^2_{mse}	R^2_{reg}	RMSE	R^2_{mse}	R^2_{reg}	RMSE	R^2_{mse}	R^2_{reg}
2015	4.26	0.90	0.90	5.87	0.80	0.80	7.64	0.66	0.70
2016	4.25	0.86	0.87	5.51	0.77	0.77	7.05	0.62	0.67
2017	2.64	0.83	0.84	3.03	0.78	0.78	5.64	0.24	0.43
2018	3.45	0.69	0.72	3.99	0.59	0.59	3.90	0.61	0.62
2019	2.10	0.87	0.87	3.37	0.66	0.67	3.38	0.66	0.69
2020	2.31	0.81	0.82	4.00	0.43	0.45	3.29	0.62	0.63
LTM	3.38	0.81	0.82	4.42	0.68	0.69	5.11	0.58	0.60

3.3. Prediction in the Urban Area

A square covering the 6th ring road in Beijing was picked to show the predictions around urban areas. It was divided into 3301 grids at a 1 km spatial scale. These grids are categorized according to the quartile distributions of model predictions, as shown in Figure 7. For NO_2, the grids with high predictions were clustered in the central urban area. In addition, the hotspots of the PLS and SLR model predictions were highlighted across the road network, while the grids with high RF predictions were aggregated (Figure 7). Regarding $PM_{2.5}$, noticeable spatial differences were found across the three model predictions. The hotspots of the PLS model predictions were sparsely distributed, while the RF predictions were highlighted in the southern part of Beijing. In comparison, the SLR model predictions were shown with clear spatial clusters. The contrast among the three $PM_{2.5}$ model predictions arises from the difference in the selection of geographical variables as primary predictors and the variations in the significance of predictors during model development. Figures S4 and S5 in Supplementary Information show the correlation coefficient between the three models. For LTM, the correlation coefficients of NO_2 models among the three approaches were 0.72~0.83, and it was 0.81~0.85 in $PM_{2.5}$ models. The correlation coefficient between PLS and SLR was the lowest regardless of whether in either NO_2 models or $PM_{2.5}$ models. The lower correlation coefficients of SLR with the other two models may be related to the fact that the variables were screened in SLR while the other two modeling methods were not.

Since the LUR-OK model performed better than the LUR models in LTM predictions, we focused on using the LUR-OK model to make predictions for population-weighted exposure estimates. Figure 8 depicts the box plots of the spatial predictions at a 1 km spatial scale (shown as grids in Figure 7) for NO_2 and $PM_{2.5}$ in the urban area. Regarding the annual predictions, a noticeable decline was found for $PM_{2.5}$ year by year. It is expected that the air quality level in Beijing has become better in recent years [37]. Meanwhile, regarding NO_2, the decline in annual mean concentrations was almost flat from 2015 to 2017, especially for PLS-OK and RF-OK predictions. Comparing the predictions among different models, the PLS-OK and RF-OK models had comparable median predictions. In contrast, SLR had relatively low median predictions, especially for annual mean NO_2 prediction in 2017 (34.98 $\mu g/m^3$) and NO_2 and $PM_{2.5}$ LTM predictions (NO_2: 37.58 $\mu g/m^3$; $PM_{2.5}$: 71.43 $\mu g/m^3$). The NO_2 predictions obtained a more considerable divergence across the three models with the coefficient of variation (COV) of 11.85~19.41 for three NO_2 models, compared with the $PM_{2.5}$ predictions among the three models with the COV of 7.57 ~11.88. It indicated that the NO_2 models were more sensitive to the predictors derived from the geographic variables than the $PM_{2.5}$ models.

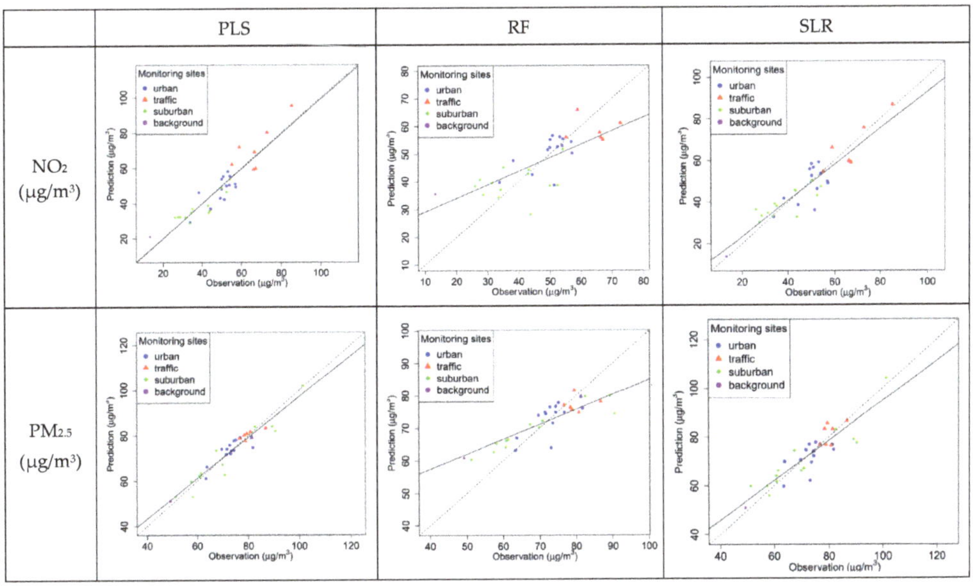

Figure 6. The average observations and LOOCV predictions of the three models for NO_2 and $PM_{2.5}$ from 2015 to 2020. Dashed lines denote the 1:1 line, and solid lines represent linear regression lines.

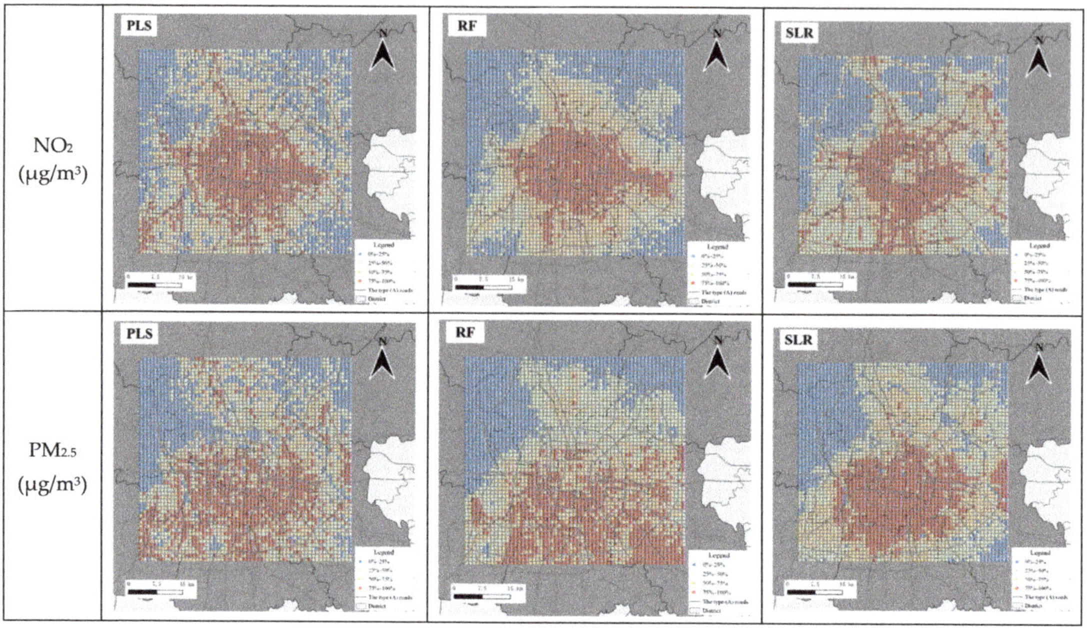

Figure 7. Maps of the long-term mean NO_2 and $PM_{2.5}$ predictions from 2015 to 2020.

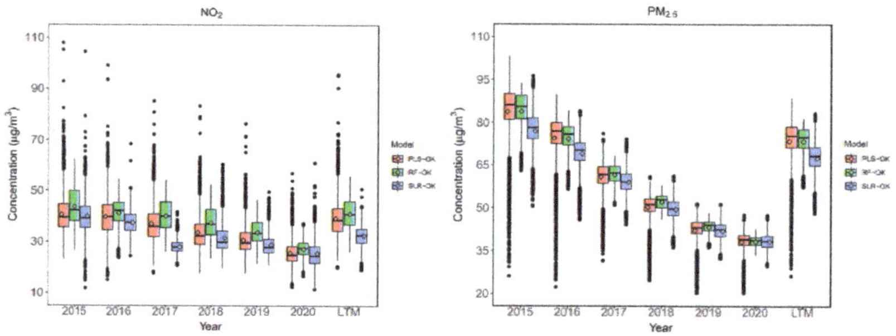

Figure 8. Distributions of annual averages and long-term means (LTM) from 2015 to 2020 of NO_2 and $PM_{2.5}$ predicted by three models. Each box's upper, middle, and lower lines denote 75%, 50%, and 25% of the concentration. The dots represent the predictions that are higher or lower than 1.5 times the IQR from the median. The point in the box represents the means of the predictions.

3.4. Population-Weighted Exposure Estimates

The population-weighted exposure estimates (PEE) in urban areas from 2015 to 2020 were predicted using the PLS-OK, RF-OK, and SLR-OK models. The long-term mean values of PEE in the urban area from 2015 to 2020 were calculated based on the model predictions and population density across the 1 km grids [38]. The total population in the prediction area was 15.94 million, accounting for about 76% of the entire population in Beijing, ranging from 211 to 32,097 persons/km^2 across the grids in the urban area. The misclassification of PEE in quartiles between the three models was estimated personally.

Figure 9 depicts the misclassification of PEE in quartiles between the PLS-OK, RF-OK, and SLR-OK models. Tables S4 and S5 in Supplementary Information summarizes the percentage of misclassification in quartiles for NO_2 and $PM_{2.5}$. For NO_2, the total misclassification of particular PEE between the PLS-OK and RF-OK models was 37.87%,

49.27% between PLS-OK and RF-OK models, and 50.49% between RF-OK and SLR-OK models. The contrast between PLS-OK and RF-OK models was smaller than the other two pairs. Compared with the PEE predicted by the PLS-OK model, 19.16% of them indicated by the RF-OK model were overestimated, and 18.72% were underestimated. Overestimation and underestimation between the PEE predicted using the PLS-OK and SLR-OK models were 23.25% and 26.03%, respectively. Most of the misclassifications happened across the adjacent quartiles. For comparison between the PLS-OK and RF-OK models, only 4.74% of the PEE was misclassified into the upper or lower quartiles that were not adjacent. This number was about 10% for other pairs of comparisons. It indicated that the PEE of NO_2 predicted by PLS-OK and RF-OK models obtained similar results, which resulted in the least misclassifications of the PEE in quartiles across the three models. Regarding the PEE of $PM_{2.5}$, the misclassification in quartiles was comparable between the three models.

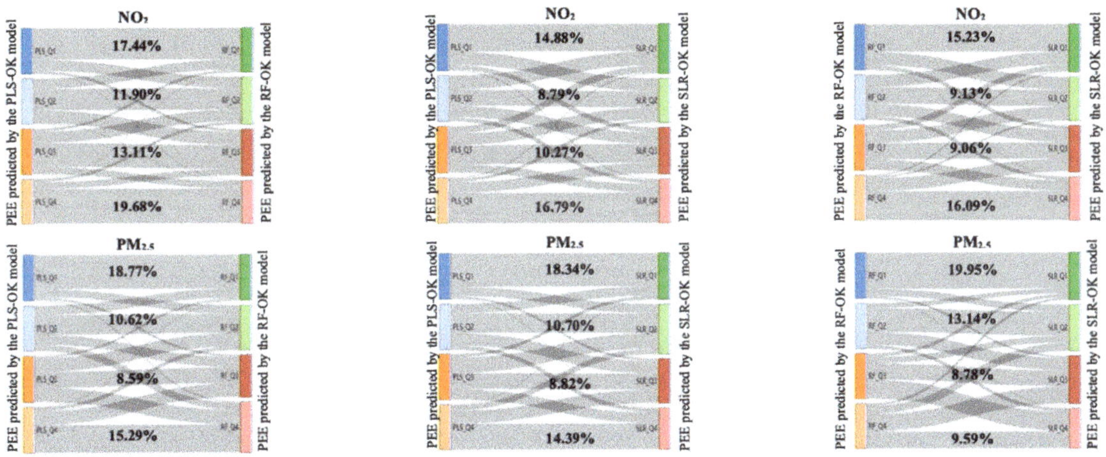

Figure 9. The misclassification of the PEE in quartiles between the PLS-OK, RF-OK, and SLR-OK models for NO_2 and $PM_{2.5}$. The four classifications from top to bottom denote the ranges of 0~25%, 25~50%, 50~75%, and 75~100% of PEE. The numbers indicate the non-misclassified percentage in quartiles.

3.5. Strengths and Limitations

This study compared three geostatistical model performances in an air pollutant exposure assessment study in a metropolitan city in China. The findings have a broad implication for environmental studies. First, the three approaches chosen for model development represent a variety of advanced and traditional, complicated, and simple geostatistical modeling methods. The usage of each modeling approach is distinctive. The SLR models outperformed the RF models. However, compared with the PLS model predictions, the RF model predictions had fewer misclassifications than the SLR predictions. Second, this study focused on spatial model comparisons, which may provide a reference for spatiotemporal modeling studies. For primary pollutants, like NO_2, the spatial distribution of air pollutants highly relies on local features related to emission sources. A comprehensive array of geographic variables could influence the model performance at a fine spatial scale. The PLS approach has such potential for exposure assessment on directly emitted air pollutants [39]. Third, the interpretability of machine learning models is challenging. Although its usage is potentially limited because of its black box instinct, it possesses the capability for utilization in an urban area abundant with spatially dense observational data on the basis of RF model performance in this study.

There were also some limitations in this study. First, there is a lack of additional data for model development and out-of-sample validation. In this study, the observational data used for model development was derived from the national and regional monitoring network. Increasing the abundance of spatial data would enhance the accuracy and stability of the model [40]. Second, the spatial models might be overestimated as less spatially rich observational data were involved in model development. To make use of the limited spatial information from these relatively sparse monitoring sites, an out-of-sample CV was not used in this study. To address these limitations, we plan to conduct mobile monitoring in the next step of our study. In addition, the inclusion of health outcomes for analyzing the impact of exposure bias caused by choosing different exposure models will be considered.

4. Conclusions

Using three geostatistical modeling approaches, we developed spatial models for NO_2 and $PM_{2.5}$ in Beijing. After evaluating the model performances with LOOCV, we found that the PLS model exhibited the best performance among the three models. A hybrid model framework, which used OK to further explain the residuals, could improve the model performance. We compared the model performance by making predictions at a 1 km spatial scale in the urban area. The misclassification of population-weighted exposure estimates in quartiles caused by using a different modeling approach was also conducted. For NO_2, both the PLS-OK and RF-OK models showed the least misclassification in the comparisons. The $PM_{2.5}$ models obtained more misclassification than the NO_2 models.

Supplementary Materials: The following supporting information can be downloaded at: https://www.mdpi.com/article/10.3390/toxics12030197/s1, Figure S1: Correlation coefficients between the first PLS score and the corresponding geographic variables in PLSU; Figure S2: The geographic variables with the top ten IncMSE values in RFU results; Figure S3: The coefficients of the variables selected by the SLRU; Figure S4: The correlation coefficients of NO_2 models among the three approaches; Figure S5: The correlation coefficients of $PM_{2.5}$ models among the three approaches; Table S1: Details of the geographic variables; Table S2: LOOCV results of the NO_2 LURU models; Table S3: LOOCV results of the $PM_{2.5}$ LURU models; Table S4: The NO_2 misclassification between LUR models; Table S5: Quartile distribution of the $PM_{2.5}$ misclassification between LUR models.

Author Contributions: Conceptualization, J.X. and W.Y.; methodology, J.X.; software, Y.W., J.X. and Z.L.; formal analysis, Y.W., J.X. and Z.L.; investigation, J.X., W.Y., B.H. and Z.B.; resources, W.Y., B.H. and Z.B.; data curation, Y.W. and J.X.; writing—original draft preparation, Y.W.; writing—review and editing, Y.W. and J.X.; visualization, Y.W.; supervision, J.X. and W.Y.; project administration, J.X.; funding acquisition, Z.B. All authors have read and agreed to the published version of the manuscript.

Funding: This research was funded by the National Key Research and Development Program funded by the Ministry of Science and Technology of the People's Republic of China, Grant number 2019YFE0115100.

Institutional Review Board Statement: Not applicable.

Informed Consent Statement: Not applicable.

Data Availability Statement: In this study, the observational data of air pollutants are available online. Most of the GIS features were obtained from open sources. The geographic variables are unavailable due to privacy or ethical restrictions.

Conflicts of Interest: The authors declare no conflicts of interest.

References

1. Hoek, G.; Beelen, R.; de Hoogh, K.; Vienneau, D.; Gulliver, J.; Fischer, P.; Briggs, D. A review of land-use regression models to assess spatial variation of outdoor air pollution. *Atmos. Environ.* **2008**, *42*, 7561–7578. [CrossRef]
2. Brauer, M.; Lencar, C.; Tamburic, L.; Koehoorn, M.; Demers, P.; Karr, C. A cohort study of traffic-related air pollution impacts on birth outcomes. *Environ. Health Perspect.* **2008**, *116*, 680–686. [CrossRef]
3. Miller, K.A.; Sullivan, J.H. Long-Term Exposure to Air Pollution and Incidence of Cardiovascular Events in Women. *N. Engl. J. Med.* **2007**, *356*, 447–458. [CrossRef] [PubMed]
4. Shaffer, R.M.; Blanco, M.N.; Li, G.; Adar, S.D.; Carone, M.; Szpiro, A.A.; Kaufman, J.D.; Larson, T.V.; Larson, E.B.; Crane, P.K. Fine particulate matter and dementia incidence in the adult changes in thought study. *Environ. Health Perspect.* **2021**, *129*, 087001. [CrossRef] [PubMed]
5. Batterman, S.; Chambliss, S.; Isakov, V. Spatial resolution requirements for traffic-related air pollutant exposure evaluations. *Atmos. Environ.* **2014**, *94*, 518–528. [CrossRef] [PubMed]

6. Steinle, S.; Reis, S.; Sabel, C.E. Quantifying human exposure to air pollution—Moving from static monitoring to spatio-temporally resolved personal exposure assessment. *Sci. Total Environ.* **2013**, *443*, 184–193. [CrossRef] [PubMed]
7. Xiao, Q.Y.; Wang, Y.J.; Chang, H.H.; Meng, X.; Geng, G.N.; Lyapustin, A.; Liu, Y. Full-coverage high-resolution daily PM2.5 estimation using MAIAC AOD in the Yangtze River Delta of China. *Remote Sens. Environ.* **2017**, *199*, 437–446. [CrossRef]
8. Kaufman, J.D.; Adar, S.D.; Barr, R.G.; Budoff, M.; Burke, G.L.; Curl, C.L.; Daviglus, M.L.; Roux, A.V.D.; Gassett, A.J.; Jacobs, D.R., Jr.; et al. Association between air pollution and coronary artery calcification within six metropolitan areas in the USA (the Multi-Ethnic Study of Atherosclerosis and Air Pollution): A longitudinal cohort study. *Lancet* **2016**, *388*, 696–704. [CrossRef] [PubMed]
9. Raaschou-Nielsen, O.; Andersen, Z.J.; Beelen, R.; Samoli, E.; Stafoggia, M.; Weinmayr, G.; Hoffmann, B.; Fischer, P.; Nieuwenhuijsen, M.J.; Brunekreef, B.; et al. Air pollution and lung cancer incidence in 17 European cohorts: Prospective analyses from the European Study of Cohorts for Air Pollution Effects (ESCAPE). *Lancet Oncol.* **2013**, *14*, 813–822. [CrossRef]
10. Chen, J.; de Hoogh, K.; Gulliver, J.; Hoffmann, B.; Hertel, O.; Ketzel, M.; Bauwelinck, M.; van Donkelaar, A.; Hvidtfeldt, U.A.; Katsouyanni, K.; et al. A comparison of linear regression, regularization, and machine learning algorithms to develop Europe-wide spatial models of fine particles and nitrogen dioxide. *Environ. Int.* **2019**, *130*, 104934. [CrossRef]
11. Xu, J.; Yang, W.; Bai, Z.; Zhang, R.; Zheng, J.; Wang, M.; Zhu, T. Modeling spatial variation of gaseous air pollutants and particulate matters in a Metropolitan area using mobile monitoring data. *Environ. Res.* **2022**, *210*, 112858. [CrossRef]
12. Mercer, L.D.; Szpiro, A.A.; Sheppard, L.; Lindstroem, J.; Adar, S.D.; Allen, R.W.; Avol, E.L.; Oron, A.P.; Larson, T.; Liu, L.J.S.; et al. Comparing universal kriging and land-use regression for predicting concentrations of gaseous oxides of nitrogen (NOx) for the Multi-Ethnic Study of Atherosclerosis and Air Pollution (MESA Air). *Atmos. Environ.* **2011**, *45*, 4412–4420. [CrossRef]
13. Kerckhoffs, J.; Hoek, G.; Portengen, L.; Brunekreef, B.; Vermeulen, R.C.H. Performance of Prediction Algorithms for Modeling Outdoor Air Pollution Spatial Surfaces. *Environ. Sci. Technol.* **2019**, *53*, 1413–1421. [CrossRef]
14. Wang, M.; Brunekreef, B.; Gehring, U.; Szpiro, A.; Hoek, G.; Beelen, R. A New Technique for Evaluating Land-use Regression Models and Their Impact on Health Effect Estimates. *Epidemiology* **2016**, *27*, 51–56. [CrossRef] [PubMed]
15. Xu, J.; Yang, Z.; Han, B.; Yang, W.; Duan, Y.; Fu, Q.; Bai, Z. A unified empirical modeling approach for particulate matter and NO_2 in a coastal city in China. *Chemosphere* **2022**, *299*, 134384. [CrossRef] [PubMed]
16. Keller, J.P.; Olives, C.; Kim, S.Y.; Sheppard, L.; Sampson, P.D.; Szpiro, A.A.; Oron, A.P.; Lindstrom, J.; Vedal, S.; Kaufman, J.D. A Unified Spatiotemporal Modeling Approach for Predicting Concentrations of Multiple Air Pollutants in the Multi-Ethnic Study of Atherosclerosis and Air Pollution. *Environ. Health Perspect.* **2015**, *123*, 301–309. [CrossRef]
17. de Hoogh, K.; Korek, M.; Vienneau, D.; Keuken, M.; Kukkonen, J.; Nieuwenhuijsen, M.J.; Badaloni, C.; Beelen, R.; Bolignano, A.; Cesaroni, G. Comparing land use regression and dispersion modelling to assess residential exposure to ambient air pollution for epidemiological studies. *Environ. Int.* **2014**, *73*, 382–392. [CrossRef] [PubMed]
18. The People's Government of Beijing Municipality. Available online: https://www.beijing.gov.cn (accessed on 1 October 2023).
19. Feng, L.; Liao, W. Legislation, plans, and policies for prevention and control of air pollution in China: Achievements, challenges, and improvements. *J. Clean. Prod.* **2016**, *112*, 1549–1558. [CrossRef]
20. WHO. *WHO Global Air Quality Guidelines: Particulate Matter (PM2.5 and PM10), Ozone, Nitrogen Dioxide, Sulfur Dioxide and Carbon Monoxide*; World Health Organization: Geneva, Switzerland, 2021.
21. Zhao, S.; Yu, Y.; Yin, D.; He, J.; Liu, N.; Qu, J.; Xiao, J. Annual and diurnal variations of gaseous and particulate pollutants in 31 provincial capital cities based on in situ air quality monitoring data from China National Environmental Monitoring Center. *Environ. Int.* **2016**, *86*, 92–106. [CrossRef]
22. Araki, S.; Shima, M.; Yamamoto, K. Spatiotemporal land use random forest model for estimating metropolitan NO_2 exposure in Japan. *Sci. Total Environ.* **2018**, *634*, 1269–1277. [CrossRef]
23. Wu, C.; Fang, C.; Wu, X.; Zhu, G. Health-Risk Assessment of Arsenic and Groundwater Quality Classification Using Random Forest in the Yanchi Region of Northwest China. *Expo. Health* **2019**, *12*, 761–774. [CrossRef]
24. Xu, J.; Yang, W.; Han, B.; Wang, M.; Wang, Z.; Zhao, Z.; Bai, Z.; Vedal, S. An advanced spatio-temporal model for particulate matter and gaseous pollutants in Beijing, China. *Atmos. Environ.* **2019**, *211*, 120–127. [CrossRef]
25. Genuer, R.; Poggi, J.M.; Tuleau-Malot, C. Variable selection using Random Forests. *Pattern Recognit. Lett.* **2010**, *31*, 2225–2236. [CrossRef]
26. Beelen, R.; Hoek, G.; Vienneau, D.; Eeftens, M.; Dimakopoulou, K.; Pedeli, X.; Tsai, M.Y.; Kunzli, N.; Schikowski, T.; Marcon, A.; et al. Development of NO_2 and NO_x land use regression models for estimating air pollution exposure in 36 study areas in Europe—The ESCAPE project. *Atmos. Environ.* **2013**, *72*, 10–23. [CrossRef]
27. de Hoogh, K.; Gulliver, J.; van Donkelaar, A.; Martin, R.V.; Marshall, J.D.; Bechle, M.J.; Cesaroni, G.; Cirach Pradas, M.; Dedele, A.; Eeftens, M.; et al. Development of West-European $PM_{2.5}$ and NO_2 land use regression models incorporating satellite-derived and chemical transport modelling data. *Environ. Res.* **2016**, *151*, 1–10. [CrossRef]
28. Eeftens, M.; Tsai, M.Y.; Ampe, C.; Anwander, B.; Beelen, R.; Bellander, T.; Cesaroni, G.; Cirach, M.; Cyrys, J.; de Hoogh, K.; et al. Spatial variation of $PM_{2.5}$, PM_{10}, $PM_{2.5}$ absorbance and PM coarse concentrations between and within 20 European study areas and the relationship with NO_2—Results of the ESCAPE project. *Atmos. Environ.* **2012**, *62*, 303–317. [CrossRef]
29. Lu, T.; Marshall, J.D.; Zhang, W.; Hystad, P.; Kim, S.-Y.; Bechle, M.J.; Demuzere, M.; Hankey, S. National Empirical Models of Air Pollution Using Microscale Measures of the Urban Environment. *Environ. Sci. Technol.* **2021**, *55*, 15519–15530. [CrossRef] [PubMed]

30. Sampson, P.D.; Richards, M.; Szpiro, A.A.; Bergen, S.; Sheppard, L.; Larson, T.V.; Kaufman, J.D. A regionalized national universal kriging model using Partial Least Squares regression for estimating annual $PM_{2.5}$ concentrations in epidemiology. *Atmos. Environ.* **2013**, *75*, 383–392. [CrossRef] [PubMed]
31. Kim, S.-Y.; Bechle, M.; Hankey, S.; Sheppard, L.; Szpiro, A.A.; Marshall, J.D. Concentrations of criteria pollutants in the contiguous U.S., 1979–2015: Role of prediction model parsimony in integrated empirical geographic regression. *PLoS ONE* **2020**, *15*, e0228535. [CrossRef] [PubMed]
32. Wang, L.; Liu, Z.; Sun, Y.; Ji, D.; Wang, Y. Long-range transport and regional sources of $PM_{2.5}$ in Beijing based on long-term observations from 2005 to 2010. *Atmos. Res.* **2015**, *157*, 37–48. [CrossRef]
33. Zhang, L.; Tian, X.; Zhao, Y.; Liu, L.; Li, Z.; Tao, L.; Wang, X.; Guo, X.; Luo, Y. Application of nonlinear land use regression models for ambient air pollutants and air quality index. *Atmos. Pollut. Res.* **2021**, *12*, 101186. [CrossRef]
34. Dong, J.; Cai, X.; Tian, L.; Chen, F.; Xu, Q.; Li, T.; Chen, X. Satellite-based estimates of daily NO_2 exposure in urban agglomerations of China and application to spatio-temporal characteristics of hotspots. *Atmos. Environ.* **2023**, *293*, 119453. [CrossRef]
35. Lyu, Y.; Kirwa, K.; Young, M.; Liu, Y.; Liu, J.; Hao, S.; Li, R.; Xu, D.; Kaufman, J.D. A high-resolution computationally-efficient spatiotemporal model for estimating daily $PM_{2.5}$ concentrations in Beijing, China. *Atmos. Environ.* **2022**, *290*, 119349. [CrossRef]
36. Shi, T.; Dirienzo, N.; Requia, W.J.; Hatzopoulou, M.; Adams, M.D. Neighbourhood scale nitrogen dioxide land use regression modelling with regression kriging in an urban transportation corridor. *Atmos. Environ.* **2020**, *223*, 117218. [CrossRef]
37. Xu, J.; Zhang, Z.; Zhao, X.; Cheng, S. Downward trend of NO_2 in the urban areas of Beijing-Tianjin-Hebei region from 2014 to 2020: Comparison of satellite retrievals, ground observations, and emission inventories. *Atmos. Environ.* **2023**, *295*, 119531. [CrossRef]
38. National Bureau of Statistics. Available online: https://www.stats.gov.cn/english/ (accessed on 27 November 2023).
39. Ma, X.; Zou, B.; Deng, J.; Gao, J.; Longley, I.; Xiao, S.; Guo, B.; Wu, Y.; Xu, T.; Xu, X.; et al. A Comprehensive Review of the Development of Land Use Regression Approaches for Modeling Spatiotemporal Variations of Ambient Air Pollution: A Perspective from 2011 to 2023. *Environ. Int.* **2024**, *183*, 108430. [CrossRef]
40. Basagana, X.; Rivera, M.; Aguilera, I.; Agis, D.; Bouso, L.; Elosua, R.; Foraster, M.; de Nazelle, A.; Nieuwenhuijsen, M.; Vila, J.; et al. Effect of the number of measurement sites on land use regression models in estimating local air pollution. *Atmos. Environ.* **2012**, *54*, 634–642. [CrossRef]

toxics

MDPI

Article

The Impact of Atmospheric Cadmium Exposure on Colon Cancer and the Invasiveness of Intestinal Stents in the Cancerous Colon

Shuai Zhang [1], Ruikang Li [2,*], Jing Xu [1,*], Yan Liu [2] and Yanjie Zhang [3]

1 Department of General Surgery, Tianjin Union Medical Center, No. 190 Jieyuan Road, Hongqiao District, Tianjin 300121, China; gelinbarlitony@126.com
2 Tianjin Key Laboratory of Urban Transport Emission Research & State Environmental Protection Key Laboratory of Urban Ambient Air Particulate Matter Pollution Prevention and Control, College of Environmental Science and Engineering, Nankai University, Tianjin 300071, China; liuyanwork@nankai.edu.cn
3 Tianjin Youmei Environment Technology, Ltd., Tianjin 300300, China; yiying5120@126.com
* Correspondence: nklrkstudy@163.com (R.L.); xujingdoc@126.com (J.X.)

Abstract: Background: Inhalation exposure to carcinogenic metals such as cadmium (Cd) is a significant global health concern linked to various cancers. However, the precise carcinogenic mechanism underlying inhalation exposure remains elusive. Methods: In this study, CT26 mouse colon cancer (CC) cells were implanted into BALB/c mice to establish CC mouse models. Some of the CC mice were implanted with intestinal stents. The mice were exposed to atomized oxygen and nitrogen (O_2/N_2) gas containing Cd. Results: Atmospheric Cd intensified inflammation in CC cells and heightened Nicotinamide Adenine Dinucleotide Phosphate (NADPH) Oxidase 1 (NOX1) activity, which is an indirect measurement of increased reactive oxygen species (ROS) production. This escalated ROS production triggered abnormal Wnt protein secretion, activated the Wnt/β-catenin signaling pathway, and stimulated CC cell proliferation. No discernible body weight effect was seen in the CC mice, possibly due to the later-stage tumor weight gain, which masked the changes in body weight. Cd facilitated colon tumor restructuring and cell migration at the later stage. The implantation of intestinal stents inhibited the expression of Superoxide Dismutase 1 (SOD1) in the colon tumors of the CC mice, with no evident effects on the expression levels of NOX1, SOD2, and Catalase (CAT) enzymes. Elevated ROS levels, indirectly reflected by enzyme activity, did not substantially impact the Wnt/β-catenin signaling pathway and even contributed to slowing its imbalance. Stent implantation eased the inflammation occurring in colon tumors by reducing CC cell proliferation but it induced discomfort in the mice, leading to a reduction in food intake and weight. Conclusions: Cd partially fosters CC tumorigenesis via the ROS-mediated Wnt/β-catenin signaling pathway. The effect of Cd on the invasive effect of intestinal stents in the cancerous colon is not significant.

Keywords: cadmium; tumor; colon cancer; reactive oxygen species; Wnt/β-catenin pathway

1. Introduction

In recent years, attention has increasingly turned towards the issue of air pollution, which is paralleled by a growing body of research into the impact of air pollution on colon cancer (CC). CC stands as the second leading cause of cancer-related deaths globally [1]. The risk factors linked to CC are primarily categorized into modifiable elements (such as smoking, obesity, and diet) and non-modifiable factors (like family history, age, and sex). Recent studies have illustrated that exposure to environmental pollutants, notably heavy metals, could elevate the risk of CC. Among some common heavy metal pollutants are cadmium, arsenic, lead, mercury, and chromium [2–4].

Cadmium (Cd), a hazardous metal that is prevalent in the environment and commonly used in industrial processes, is classified as a human carcinogen by the International

Agency for Research on Cancer (IARC) [5,6]. Mounting evidence indicates that the presence of Cd in aquatic environments can induce various adverse health outcomes in humans, including cancers [7,8], cardiovascular diseases [9,10], and inflammatory conditions [11,12]. Nevertheless, the impact of Cd in the atmosphere on human health, particularly concerning CC, remains elusive. Recent investigations have revealed a notable increase in plasma Cd levels among CC patients compared to healthy individuals [13]. Additionally, studies have demonstrated that Cd can prompt cellular transformation and carcinogenesis in human colon cell line CRL-1807 models [14]. There are speculations that these cellular responses are correlated with specific molecular mechanisms triggered by Cd exposure, such as the induction of oxidative stress, β-catenin mutation, the upregulation of cyclooxygenase-2 (COX-2), and the initiation of proinflammatory responses. However, further research is needed to comprehensively elucidate the intricate connections between Cd exposure and the molecular pathways involved in CC development. While the molecular mechanisms behind Cd-induced carcinogenesis necessitate further investigation, there is a consensus that Reactive Oxygen Species (ROS) play a pivotal role in cellular damage triggered by Cd, which subsequently culminates in cancer development. The Nicotinamide Adenine Dinucleotide Phosphate (NADPH) Oxidase (NOX) complex stands as a critical physiological system for ROS generation. Studies have revealed that Cd has the capability to activate NOX to produce ROS, which disrupts the integrity of the outer mitochondrial membrane, thereby engendering the production of superoxide radicals, hydroxyl radicals, and hydrogen peroxide, and thus causing cell damage [15]. In the context of CC cells, the Wnt/β-catenin pathway, which is controlled by ROS generated via NOX, regulates the proliferation of CC cells [16]. Wnt ligands constitute a diverse and highly conserved group of secreted proteins [17]. Their influence extends across various cellular processes, encompassing cell proliferation, stem cell self-renewal, the determination of cell fate, the establishment of cell polarity, and the orchestration of convergent extension behavior during cell migration [18–20]. Each of these orchestrated consequences, steered by Wnt signaling, is crucial for maintaining normal intestinal development. This pathway often exhibits differential regulation between normal and cancerous tissues, particularly in cancers such as hepatocellular carcinoma, prostate cancer, and CC [21]. Within healthy cells (Figure S1), in the absence of Wnt signaling, β-catenin is bound and regulated by a multi-subunit complex consisting of recombinant axis inhibition protein (Axin), Adenomatous Polyposis Coli (APC), Casein Kinase 1α (CK1α), and Glycogen Synthase Kinase 3β (GSK3β). This complex promotes β-catenin phosphorylation, facilitating its interaction with β-Transducin Repeat-Containing Proteins (β-TRCPs) and leading to subsequent ubiquitination and degradation, thus maintaining low β-catenin expression levels. Conversely, in cancer cells where Wnt signaling is active (Figure S2), Wnt signaling engages specific receptors like frizzled proteins, leading to low-density Lipoprotein Receptor-related Protein (LRP) phosphorylation. This culminates in the formation of the Wnt–Frizzled-LRP complex, triggering disheveled (DVL) activation and conglomerate aggregation toward the receptor. DVL activation intensifies GSK3β phosphorylation, thereby impeding β-catenin degradation [22]. Consequently, β-catenin accumulates in the nucleus, interacts with coactivators like T-Cell Factor and Lymphoid Enhancer Factor (TCF/LEF), and stimulates downstream Wnt target gene transcription, thus fostering cancer cell proliferation. Additionally, heightened ROS production incites an inflammatory cascade. The COX-2 pathway emerges as a pivotal inflammatory pathway implicated in CC [23]. Substantial data highlight the significantly elevated COX-2 gene expression in cancerous colon mucosa compared to healthy tissues [24–26]. The primary contributor to the carcinogenic effect of COX-2 is believed to be its chief metabolite, prostaglandin E2 (PGE2), which exerts its biological function by binding to its target receptor, prostaglandin receptor 4 (EP4) [27]. In addition, Iba1 is a macrophage/microglia-specific calcium-binding protein whose level can also reflect the degree of cellular inflammatory response [28]. However, the precise molecular mechanism by which Cd in the atmospheric milieu induces CC remains an area to be fully elucidated.

Advancements in medical devices and technologies have led to the gradual adoption of intestinal stents as the primary treatment for colon tract decompression. Evidence-based medicine has validated the short-term safety and efficacy of this approach [29–31]. Nevertheless, significant concerns persist regarding long-term tumor prognosis in CC patients who have undergone bowel stenting as a form of conversion therapy. Studies have indicated that the preoperative placement of bowel stents in CC patients disrupts tumor prognosis and potentially triggers tumor cell dissemination during the stent insertion process [32]. Further studies are, therefore, needed to verify the effect of intestinal stents on colon tumors. By studying the impact of intestinal stents on the CC pathology and Matrix Metalloproteinase-2 (MMP-2), MMP-9, and 8-hydroxy-2′-deoxyguanosine (8-OHdG) expression levels, the impact of intestinal stents on long-term tumor prognosis will be explained from a molecular perspective. Among these enzymes, MMP-2 primarily participates in tissue remodeling, cellular migration, and angiogenesis [33]. MMP-9 primarily participates in the activation and migration of inflammatory cells [34]. 8-OHdG serves as a commonly utilized biomarker to detect oxidative DNA damage resulting from oxidative stress [35]. However, the impact of atmospheric Cd on the invasiveness of stents in the cancerous colon remains largely unexplored.

Hence, this study employed CT26WT CC mouse models with implanted stents. These mouse models were subjected to atomized air containing Cd via inhalation to mimic atmospheric exposure, aiming to investigate the influence of Cd in the environment on CC patients with implanted intestinal stents. The hypothesis posited here is that Cd in the atmosphere fosters the proliferation and dissemination of CC cells through a mechanism reliant on the NOX-ROS-COX-2-Wnt/β-catenin pathways. A preliminary verification of this hypothesis is illustrated in Figure 1.

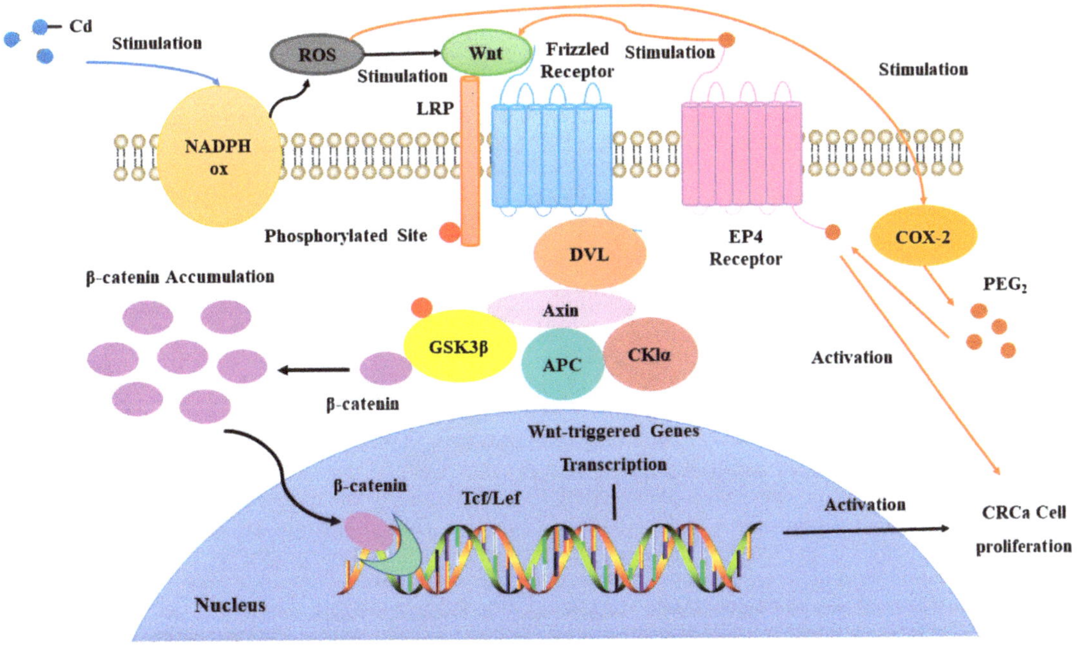

Figure 1. Hypotheses for the mechanism of Cd-induced proliferation of CC cells in atmospheric environments.

2. Materials and Methods

2.1. Animal and Experimental Design

CT26 mouse CC cells, along with the culture medium, were procured from Wuhan Pricella Life Technology Co., Ltd. (Wuhan, Hubei Province, China) These CC cells were nurtured in 1640 complete medium containing 10% Fetal Bovine Serum (FBS) and 1% bis-antibodies in a 5% carbon dioxide (CO_2) incubator at 37 °C. Forty-five 6-week-old female BALB/c mice were acquired from Beijing Sipeifu Biotechnology Co., Ltd. (Beijing, China) and were housed in accordance with the institutional animal care guidelines. To facilitate acclimation, the mice were allowed a week in the new environment before utilization. The mice were housed in plastic cages (5 mice/cage) under the following conditions: a relative humidity of 50 ± 10%, a 12/12 h light/dark cycle, and a temperature of 23 ± 2 °C.

For the implantation of CC cells, 1×10^7/mL of cells (200 μL/piece) was cultured on the mucosa of the posterior colon wall in the mice, and tumor formation was observed over a 2-week period utilizing a small-animal live imaging device (InVivo Smart-LF, VISQUE, Seoul, Republic of Korea). The BALB/c mice were then randomly divided into 9 groups based on body weight; the healthy groups included a blank group (H-Blank), a control group (H-Control), and a Cd group (H-Cd). The groups with CC cells but without an intestinal stent included a blank group (C-Blank), a control group (C-Control), and a Cd group (C-Cd). The groups with CC cells and an intestinal stent included a blank group (C-S-Blank), a control group (C-S-Control), and a Cd group (C-S-Cd). The mice in the intestinal stent groups were implanted with metal spring coils (length of 5 mm, inner diameter of 2 mm, outer diameter of 3 mm, and wire diameter of 0.2 mm) through the anus and cultured for 2 weeks. The Cd groups were exposed to a simulated environment of oxygen and nitrogen (O_2/N_2) mixed with atomized gas containing Cd for the subsequent 4 weeks. The blank groups were exposed to the actual environment without gas introduction, while the control groups were exposed to a simulated environment with the introduction of O_2/N_2 mixed with atomized gas. Throughout the experiment, the mice were weighed twice weekly, and any signs of weight loss were closely monitored. At 27 weeks of age, all mice were euthanized using CO_2 asphyxiation, and whole-colon intestinal tissues were collected. The tissue samples were promptly fixed in 10% formalin or frozen in liquid nitrogen for further analysis.

A corresponding preliminary experiment was conducted before the formal experiment in this study. The experimental design was tested for validity and efficacy. Groups of 5 mice were verified to have ≥80% power on the primary endpoint, and it was confirmed that the number of rats in each group was the minimum necessary to ensure that the experiment was able to detect the intended effect. All experiments were conducted in accordance with the biomedical research guidelines stipulated by the Experimental Biology Society of Tianjin People's Hospital and were approved by the Animal Use Experimental Ethics Committee of Tianjin Union Medical Center.

2.2. Establishment of the Simulation Environment

The reference was drawn from the average concentration of Cd in the atmospheric environment spanning from January 2016 to February 2017, specifically under heavy pollution weather conditions (AQI > 200), in Heping District, Tianjin. During this period, the average concentration was recorded at 4.33 ng/m^3. As demonstrated in Formula (1), the estimated quantity of Cd inhaled by humans in such an atmospheric environment amounted to 46.76 ng per day, whereas the estimated intake for BALB/c mice in this atmospheric environment was 0.13 ng per day. The formula is as follows:

$$E = C \times B \times t \quad (1)$$

where E is the respiratory exposure to Cd in the atmospheric environment, in ng; C is the average concentration of Cd in the atmospheric environment, in ng/m^3; and B is the respiratory rate, in m^3/d. The respiratory rate of BALB/c mice is 19.16 mL/min [36], which is 0.03 m^3/d, and the respiratory rate of humans is 10.8 m^3/d [37]; *t* is the exposure time, in d. The Cd solution used in the experiment to simulate a polluted atmospheric environment was a solution derived from the Cd inductively coupled plasma (ICP) standard solution obtained from O2si, USA. To align with the inhalation volume for both humans and BALB/c mice, the Cd ICP standard solution was prepared at a concentration of 0.23 μg/mL. The compressed air inlet of the medical nebulizer was connected to a fresh air cylinder (21% O_2/79% N_2) to generate dispersion nebulization gas. The actual concentration of cadmium in the atomized environment was 4.1~4.5 ng/m^3.

2.3. *In Vivo Imaging*

The mice were anesthetized with gas. The mice were intraperitoneally injected with D-luciferin sodium salt physiological saline solution (10 mg/mL) at a dose of 150 mg/kg. Fifteen minutes after injection, the anesthetized mice were placed in an in vivo imaging device for observation and imaging.

2.4. *Histopathology*

All tumor and mucosa specimens underwent hematoxylin and eosin (H&E) staining for histopathological assessment. The samples were fixed with paraformaldehyde and then decalcified in a decalcifying solution. The dehydration of the samples was performed by using alcohol, and the removal of the tissues from the paraffin was carried out using a xylene solution. The tissue samples underwent embedding by being dipped in a melted wax solution and placed in an embedding frame. After being positioned appropriately according to the embedding surface requirements, the samples were cooled on a −20 °C freezing platform until the wax solidified. After solidification, the wax block was removed from the embedding frame, trimmed, and placed on a paraffin microtome for slicing. The resulting slices were floated on 40 °C warm water in a spreading machine to flatten the tissue. Subsequently, the tissue was picked up with a glass slide and placed in a 60 °C oven for baking. Following baking, the slices were dewaxed in xylene twice and dehydrated using absolute ethanol. Hydration of the sample sections was performed using a series of ethanol concentrations (95%, 80%, and 70%) and distilled water. Subsequent staining involved hematoxylin staining solution application, followed by differentiation. The samples underwent dehydration, transparency treatment, and sealing. Observation and imaging were conducted using a fluorescence microscope (ECLIPSE Ci, Nikon, Tokyo, Japan) to analyze the stained tissue sections.

2.5. *Immunohistochemistry*

To achieve cell permeability and block endogenous peroxidase, the sample sections underwent immersion in a blocking/permeabilization solution (at room temperature and shielded from light). To uncover the antigen-determining area for antigen retrieval, the slices were submerged in 0.01 M sodium citrate buffer (pH = 6.0) and heated in a microwave oven until boiling, with the regular replenishment of the solution to prevent desiccation. To obstruct the influence of non-specific proteins, the surrounding tissue was outlined using a histochemical pen, followed by the application of 5% sheep serum within the outlined area. The diluted primary antibody was directly added and allowed to incubate overnight at 4 °C. Following this, the diluted secondary antibody was applied, and the sections were placed in a constant-temperature oven at 37 °C. The subsequent steps involved the addition of streptavidin peroxidase (SP) conjugates, placement in a 37 °C oven, and the introduction of diaminobenzidine (DAB). Staining progression was observed under a fluorescence microscope while controlling the duration based on the color observed. Subsequently, a hematoxylin staining solution was applied to stain nuclear proteins, followed by the use of phosphate-buffered saline (PBS) to restore their blue coloration. The samples underwent dehydration, transparency treatment, and sealing. Observation and imaging were conducted using a fluorescence microscope to analyze the stained tissue sections.

2.6. Western Blot Analysis

Western blot analysis was conducted utilizing specific antibodies targeting β-catenin (1:1000, BIOSS), phospho-GSK3β (1:1000, BIOSS), actin (1:3000, Affinity), SOD1 (1:1000, Affinity), SOD2 (1:1000, Affinity), CAT (1:1000, BIOSS), and NOX1 (1:1000, Affinity).

2.7. Statistical Analysis

Differences between treatment groups were assessed through analysis of variance (ANOVA). Statistical significance was determined at $p < 0.05$. For cases where significant differences were observed, specific post hoc comparisons between treatment groups were conducted using the Student–Newman–Keuls test. All statistical analyses were conducted using SPSS software (version 27.0, SPSS Inc., Chicago, IL, USA). The data were assessed for normality and homoskedasticity before performing the ANOVA (analysis of variance) and the Student–Newman–Keuls test. Normality was tested using the Shapiro–Wilk test, and the results showed that the data conformed to a normal distribution ($p > 0.05$). Homoscedasticity was assessed using Levene's test, and the results showed that each group of data had similar variance ($p > 0.05$). These results showed that the data of this study met the basic assumptions of ANOVA and the Student–Newman–Keuls test, thus providing a reliable basis for subsequent statistical analysis.

3. Results

3.1. Colon Tumor Invasion and Metastasis Capabilities

The mice lost weight within 4 days after the CC cells were implanted, as shown in Figure 2D,I. With tumor progression, a gradual adaptation was apparent. However, upon the implantation of intestinal stents on day 23, the mice with CC cells experienced weight loss, as indicated in Figure 2G,I. Interestingly, the injection of O_2/N_2 atomized gas and Cd-O_2/N_2 atomized gas exhibited no notable impact on the mice's body weight compared to the control groups.

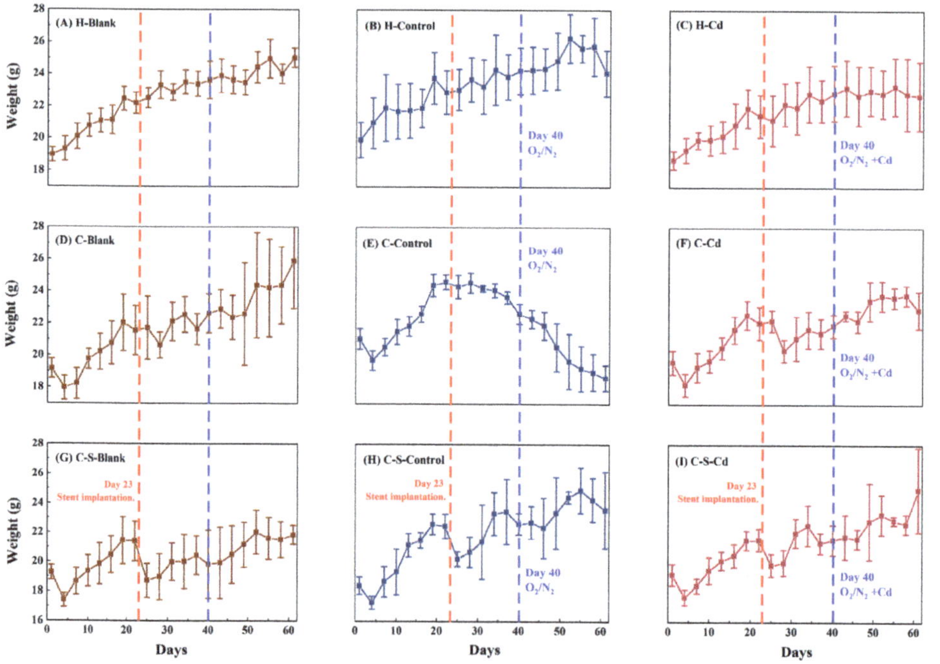

Figure 2. Changes in body weight of mice (g). Data were means ± SEM.

As illustrated in Figure 3, there was extensive proliferation of the CC cells from the third to the eighth week, resulting in an enhancement of fluorescence signals within the colon tumor tissues. Notably, compared to the blank and control groups, the injection of Cd-O_2/N_2 atomized gas further significantly intensified the proliferation of CC cells (C-Blank: $p < 0.01$; C-Control: $p < 0.001$). However, upon the implantation of intestinal stents, the proliferative capacity of CC cells showed a statistically significant decrease (C-Blank: $p < 0.01$; C-Cd: $p < 0.001$).

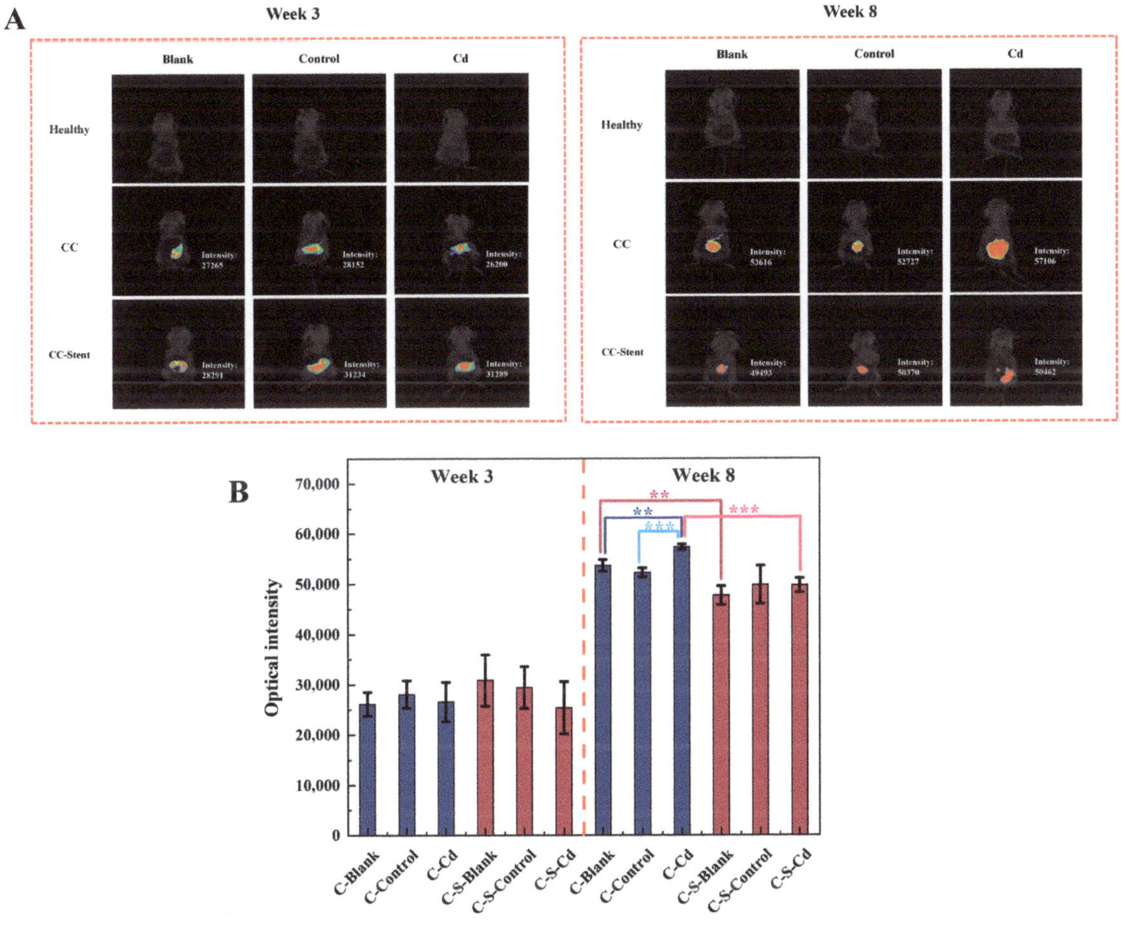

Figure 3. In vivo imaging was performed at the 3rd and 8th weeks after the start of the experiment (before sampling) to observe the (**A**) in situ tumor formation of the colon and (**B**) the changes in fluorescence intensity. (**B**) Data were means ± SEM of 5 mice. ** $p < 0.01$, *** $p < 0.001$. Among them, if there is no asterisk between the two columns, it means there is no statistical significance.

In comparison to the healthy mice, statistically significantly elevated expression levels were observed for β-catenin (H-Blank and H-Control: $p < 0.05$; H-Cd: $p < 0.001$) and phospho-GSK3β (H-Cd: $p < 0.001$) within the colon tumors of the CC mice, as depicted in Figure 4. The injection of Cd-O_2/N_2 atomized gas further significantly augmented the expression levels of β-catenin (C-Blank and C-Control: $p < 0.001$; C-S-Control: $p < 0.05$) and phospho-GSK3β (C-Blank: $p < 0.01$; C-Control, C-S-Blank and C-S-Control: $p < 0.05$). Conversely, the implantation of intestinal stents statistically significantly suppressed the expression of phospho-GSK3β (C-Cd: $p < 0.05$). However, its effect on the expression level of β-catenin was not significant. In addition, the implantation of intestinal stents had no statistically significant effect on the expression levels of β-catenin and phospho-GSK3β in the colon tumors of the CC mice in the blank and control groups.

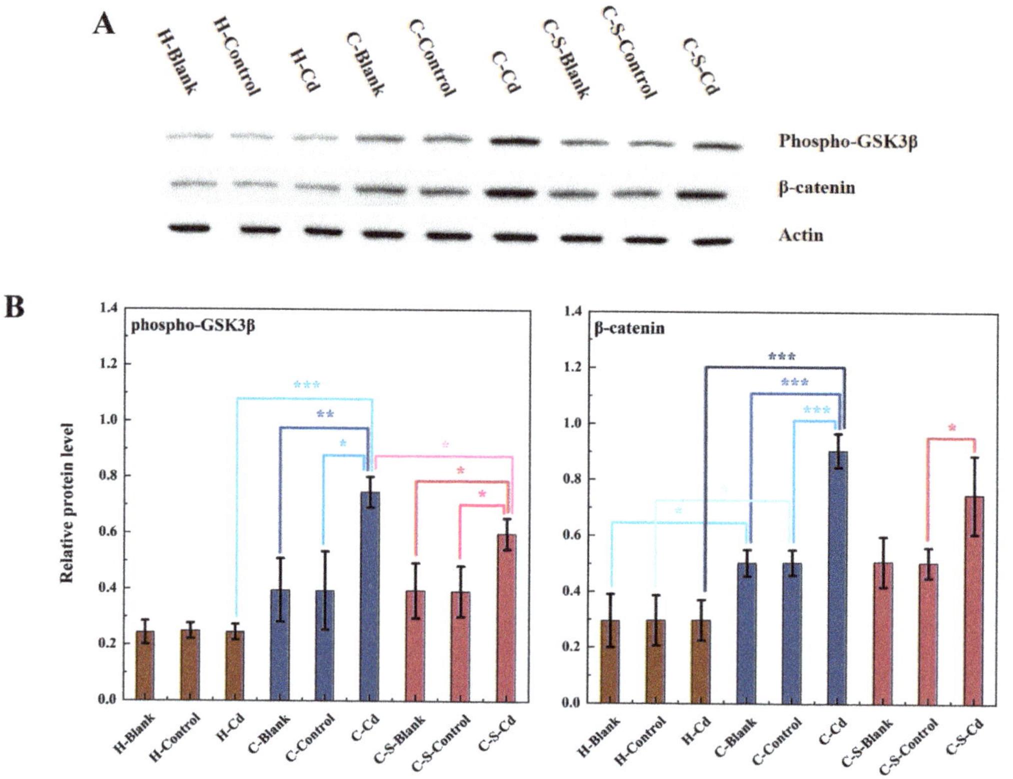

Figure 4. The expression of phospho-GSK3β and β-catenin in colon tumors of mice in each group was detected. (**A**) Expression of phospho-GSK3β and β-catenin in colon tumors was determined by immunoblotting. Expression of actin served as an internal control. (**B**) Relative levels of β-catenin and phospho-GSK3β in colon tumors. Data were means ± SEM of 5 mice. * $p < 0.05$, ** $p < 0.01$, *** $p < 0.001$. Among them, if there is no asterisk between the two columns, it means there is no statistical significance.

The assessment of colon tumor invasion and metastatic potential involved the examination and analysis of MMP-2 expression. In comparison to the healthy mice, statistically significantly heightened MMP-2 expression was observed in the colon mucosa of the CC mice (H-Blank and H-Cd: $p < 0.01$), as depicted in Figure 5. Notably, the injection of Cd-O_2/N_2 atomized gas statistically significantly amplified MMP-2 expression in the colon tumors of the CC mice relative to the blank and control groups (C-Control, C-S-Blank, and C-S-Control: $p < 0.05$). The impact of intestinal stent implantation on MMP-2 expression level was not statistically significant.

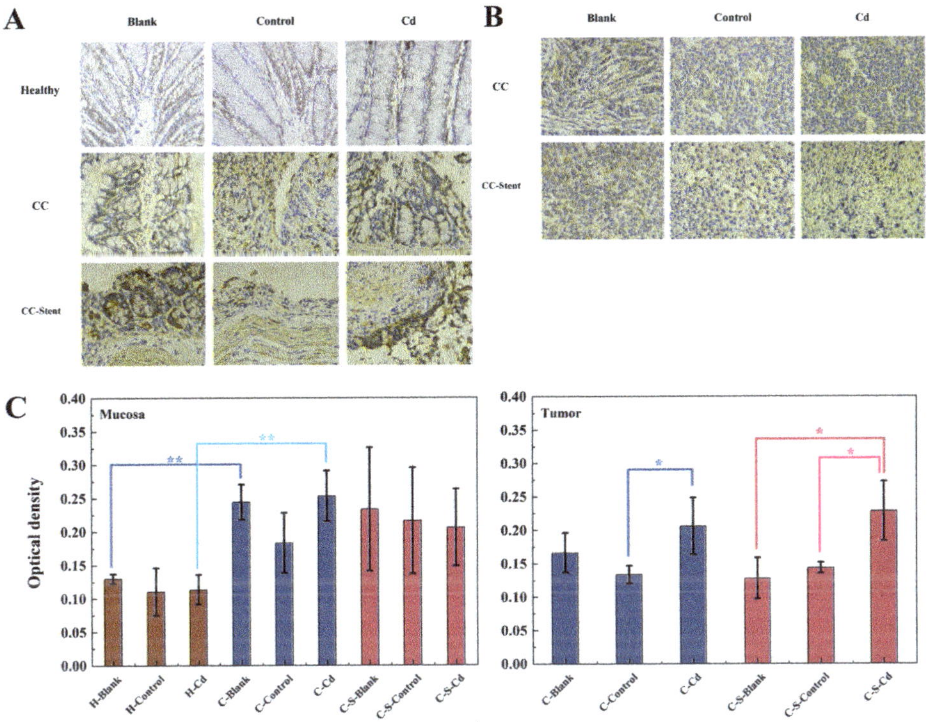

Figure 5. The expression of MMP-2 in colon tumors and mucosa of mice in each group was detected. (**A**) Immunohistochemical staining of MMP-2 in colonic mucosa in indicated treatments. Magnification was 400×. (**B**) Immunohistochemical staining of MMP-2 in colonic tumors in indicated treatments. Magnification was 400×. (**C**) Optical density was used to represent the expression of MMP-2 in colon mucosa and tumors. Data were means ± SEM of 5 mice. * $p < 0.05$, ** $p < 0.01$. Among them, if there is no asterisk between the two columns, it means there is no statistical significance.

3.2. Oxidative Stress

Carcinogenic metals are renowned for their capacity to induce ROS [38]. Due to resource limitations that hindered the ability to conduct direct ROS measurements, this study instead measured the activities of NOX1, SOD1, SOD2, and CAT enzymes, which are key players in the cellular anti-oxidant defense system and in oxidative stress, to indirectly illustrate changes in the production of ROS [39–41]. As depicted in Figure 6, NOX1 expression levels were statistically significantly increased in the colon tumors of the CC mice when compared to their healthy counterparts (H-Cd: $p < 0.05$). Notably, the alterations in the expression levels of NOX1, β-catenin, and phospho-GSK3β followed a similar pattern. Additionally, statistically significantly decreased expression levels were observed for SOD1 (H-Blank: $p < 0.05$; H-Cd: $p < 0.001$), SOD2 (H-Cd: $p < 0.01$), and CAT (H-Blank: $p < 0.01$; H-Control and H-Cd: $p < 0.001$) in these tumors. The effect on the expression levels of NOX1 and SOD2 after the transplantation of CC cells into the mice in the blank and control groups was not statistically significant. The injection of Cd-O_2/N_2 atomized gas further significantly suppressed the expression of SOD1 (C-Blank and C-Control: $p < 0.001$; C-S-Blank: $p < 0.05$), SOD2 (C-Control: $p < 0.05$), and CAT (C-Blank and C-Control: $p < 0.01$) in the colon tumors of the CC mice. The effect of Cd-O_2/N_2 atomized gas on the expression levels of NOX1, SOD2, and CAT in the colon tumors of the CC mice with intestinal stents implanted in them was not statistically significant. Conversely, the implantation of intestinal stents statistically significantly inhibited SOD1 expression in the colon tumors of the CC mice (C-Blank: $p < 0.01$). However, the effect on the expression of NOX1, SOD2, and CAT was not statistically significant. In addition, the implantation of intestinal stents had no statistically significant effect on the expression of NOX1, SOD1, SOD2, and CAT in the colon tumors of the CC mice exposed to a Cd-O_2/N_2 atomized gas environment.

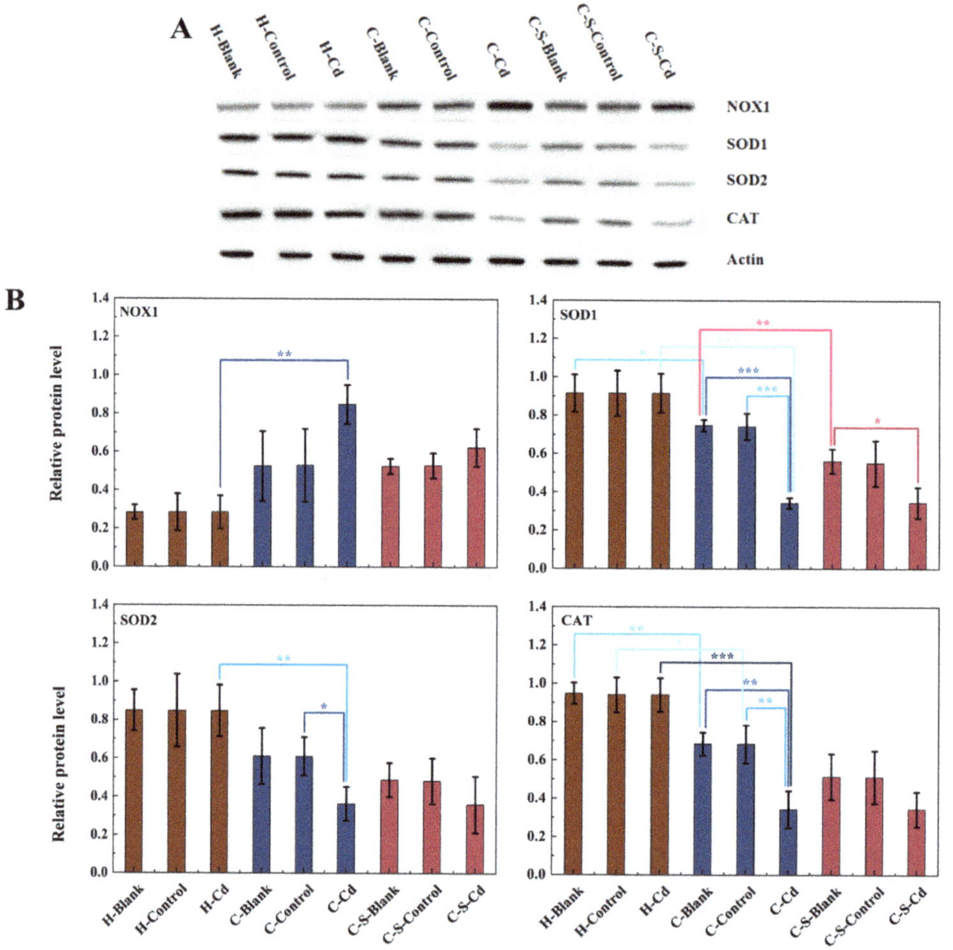

Figure 6. The expression of NOX1, SOD1, SOD2, and CAT in colon tumors of mice in each group was detected. (**A**) Expression of NOX1, SOD1, SOD2, and CAT in colon tumors was determined by immunoblotting. Expression of actin served as an internal control. (**B**) Relative levels of NOX1, SOD1, SOD2, and CAT in colon tumors. Data are means ± SEM of 5 mice. * $p < 0.05$, ** $p < 0.01$, *** $p < 0.001$. Among them, if there is no asterisk between the two columns, it means there is no statistical significance.

Relative to the healthy mice, statistically significantly elevated expression levels of 8-OHdG were observed within the colon mucosa of the CC-afflicted mice (H-Control and H-Cd: $p < 0.01$), as illustrated in Figure 7. The injection of Cd-O_2/N_2 atomized gas further significantly amplified the expression of 8-OHdG in the colon mucosa (C-Blank: $p < 0.05$). The implantation of intestinal stents had no significant effect on the expression of 8-OHdG in the colon mucosa of the CC mice.

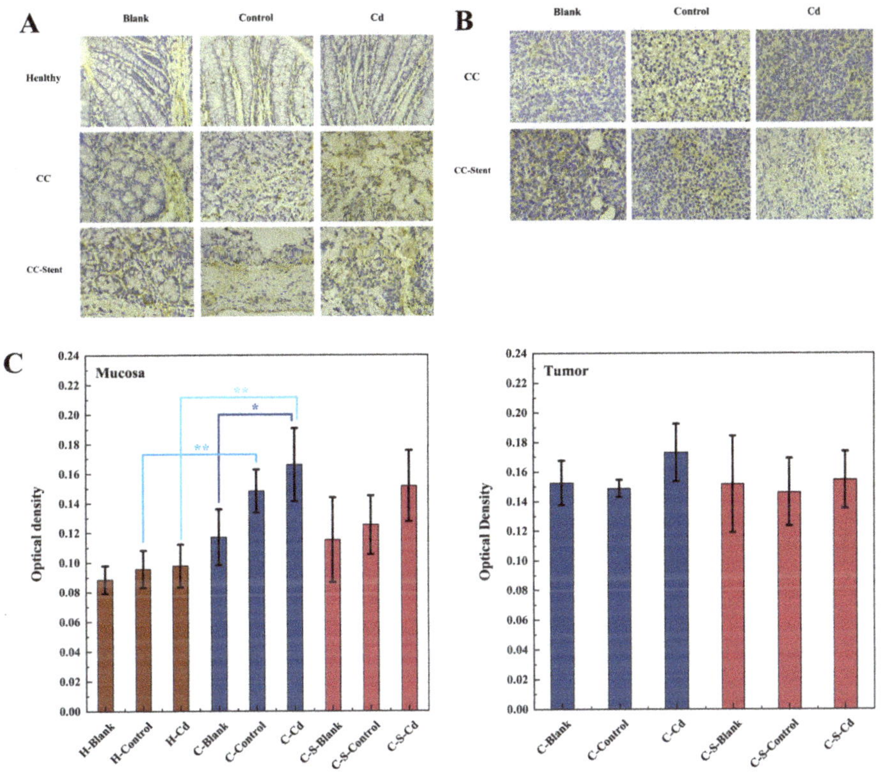

Figure 7. The expression of 8-OHdG in colon tumor and mucosa of mice in each group was detected. (**A**) Immunohistochemical staining of 8-OHdG in colonic mucosa in indicated treatments. Magnification was 100×. (**B**) Immunohistochemical staining of 8-OHdG in colonic tumor in indicated treatments. Magnification was 100×. (**C**) Optical density was used to represent the expression of 8-OHdG in colon mucosa and tumor. Data are means ± SEM of 5 mice. * $p < 0.05$, ** $p < 0.01$. Among them, if there is no asterisk between the two columns, it means there is no statistical significance.

3.3. Inflammation

As depicted in Figure 8, the colon mucosa of the healthy mice exhibited a well-maintained structure characterized by neatly arranged glands and an absence of inflammatory cell infiltration. Conversely, the colon mucosa of the CC mice displayed evident damage, with disordered glandular arrangement and noticeable infiltration of inflammatory cells. Remarkably, the mucosa of the CC mice implanted with intestinal stents exhibited severe damage, featuring disorganized glands and pronounced inflammatory cell infiltration. Notably, the tumors observed across in all groups of mice exhibited irregular nuclear morphology and variable sizes. Cell arrangement appeared disordered, lacked a distinct tissue structure, and showcased irregular intercellular spaces.

Relative to the healthy mice, statistically significantly heightened MMP-9 expression was observed within the colon mucosa of the CC mice (H-Cd: $p < 0.05$), as depicted in Figure 9. The implantation of CC cells had no statistically significant effect on the expression levels of MMP-9 in the colon mucosa of the CC mice in the blank and control groups. The injection of Cd-O_2/N_2 atomized gas statistically significantly suppressed the expression of MMP-9 in the colon tumors of the CC mice (C-Blank: $p < 0.05$). However, the effect on MMP-9 expression in the colon mucosa of the CC mice that had been implanted with intestinal stents was not significant. Similarly, the implantation of intestinal stents statistically significantly suppressed MMP-9 expression in the colon tumors of the CC mice (C-Control: $p < 0.01$; C-Cd: $p < 0.05$). Variations in MMP-9 expression were noted in the colon tumors of the CC mice in the blank and control groups ($p < 0.05$).

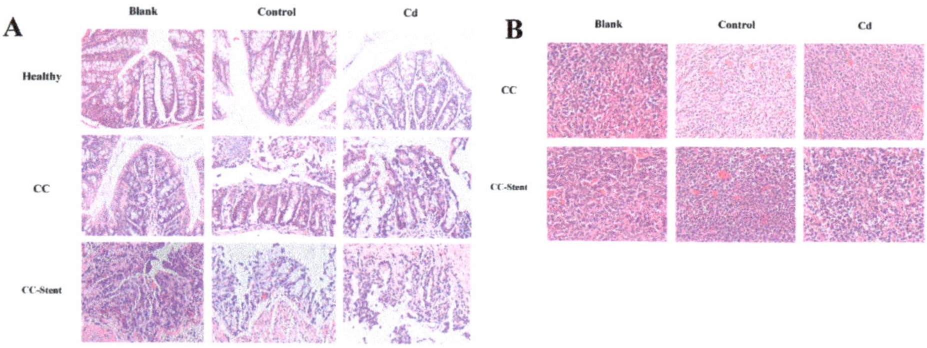

Figure 8. The pathology of colon tumor and mucosa of mice in each group was observed. (**A**) Representative H&E staining demonstrating mucosa from indicated treatments (red arrow indicates inflammatory cell infiltration). Magnification was 100×. (**B**) Representative H&E staining demonstrating tumors from indicated treatments. Magnification was 100×.

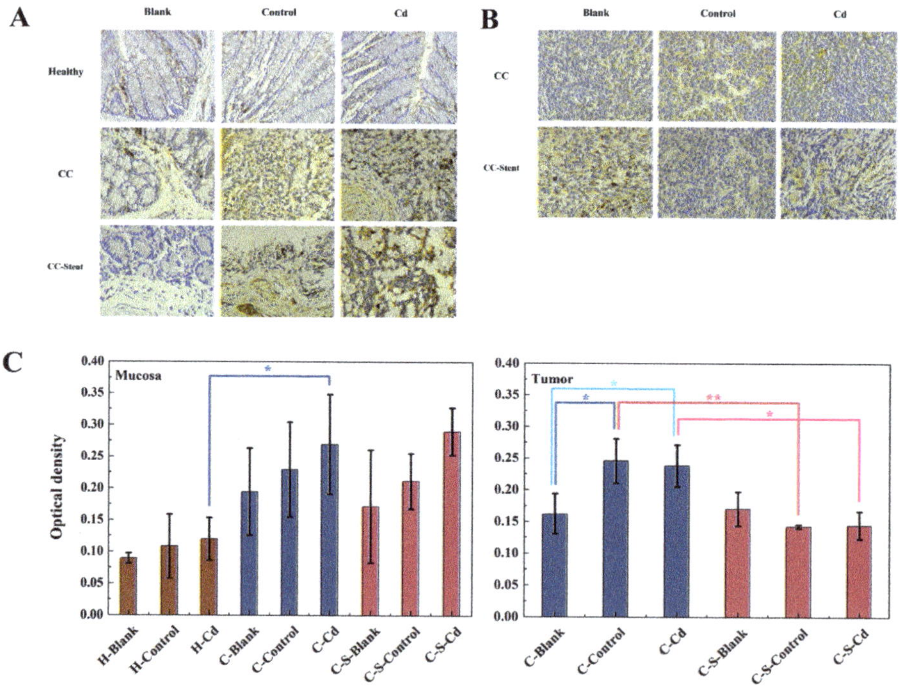

Figure 9. The expression of MMP-9 in colon tumors and mucosa of mice in each group was detected. (**A**) Immunohistochemical staining of MMP-9 in colonic mucosa in indicated treatments. Magnification was 400×. (**B**) Immunohistochemical staining of MMP-9 in colonic tumors in indicated treatments. Magnification was 400×. (**C**) Optical density was used to represent the expression of MMP-9 in colon mucosa and tumors. Data are means ± SEM of 5 mice. * $p < 0.05$, ** $p < 0.01$. If there is no asterisk between the two columns, it means there is no statistical significance.

As depicted in Figure 10, the expression of COX-2 was notably suppressed in the colon tumors of the CC mice compared to their healthy counterparts (H-Cd: $p < 0.01$). The implantation of CC cells had no statistically significant effect on the expression levels of COX-2 in the colon mucosa of the CC mice in the blank and control groups. The injection of Cd-O_2/N_2 atomized gas further significantly inhibited COX-2 expression within these colon tumors (C-Blank: $p < 0.01$; C-Control: $p < 0.05$), but the effect on COX-2 expression in the colon mucosa of the CC mice that had been implanted with intestinal stents was not significant.

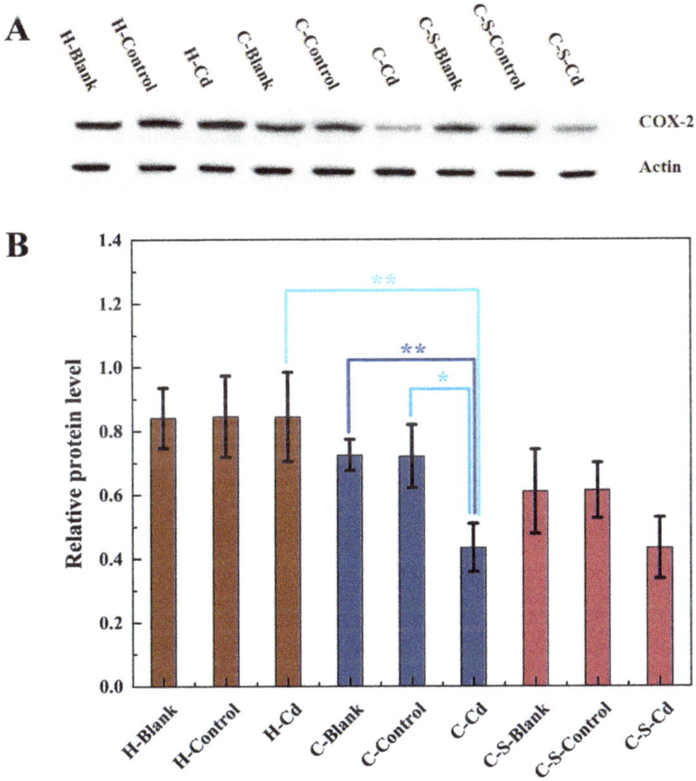

Figure 10. The expression of COX-2 in colon tumor of mice in each group was detected. (**A**) Expression of COX-2 in colon tumors was determined by immunoblotting. Expression of actin served as an internal control. (**B**) Relative levels of COX-2 in colon tumors. Data are means ± SEM of 5 mice. * $p < 0.05$, ** $p < 0.01$. If there is no asterisk between the two columns, it means there is no statistical significance.

The implantation of CC cells had no significant effect on Iba1 expression. Notably, the injection of Cd-O_2/N_2 atomized gas led to a statistically significant reduction in Iba1 expression in the colon mucosa (C-Control: $p < 0.05$) and tumors (C-Control: $p < 0.01$; C-S-Blank: $p < 0.05$; C-S-Control: $p < 0.01$), as depicted in Figure 11. Significant variation in the expression of Iba1 was observed in the colon mucosa of the blank and control groups following stent implantation.

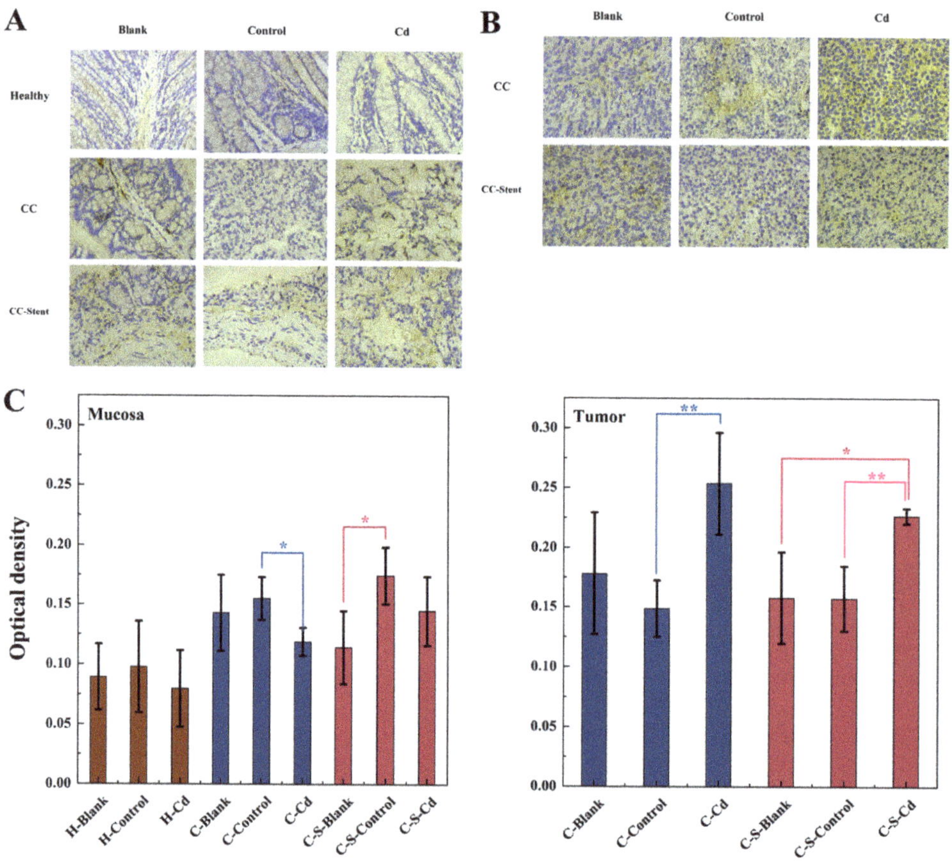

Figure 11. The expression of Iba1 in colon tumors and mucosa of mice in each group was detected. (**A**) Immunohistochemical staining of Iba1 in colonic mucosa in indicated treatments. Magnification was 400×. (**B**) Immunohistochemical staining of Iba1 in colonic tumors in indicated treatments. Magnification was 400×. (**C**) Optical density was used to represent the expression of Iba1 in colon mucosa and tumors. Data are means ± SEM of 5 mice. * $p < 0.05$, ** $p < 0.01$. If there is no asterisk between the two columns, it means there is no statistical significance among them.

4. Discussion

In this study, mouse models of CC were employed to investigate the implications of exposure to the heavy metal Cd in the atmospheric environment on CC progression and its impact on the invasiveness of intestinal stents within the cancerous colon. An abnormal secretion of Wnt protein within CC cells triggered an unconventional activation of the Wnt/β-catenin signaling pathway, culminating in the phosphorylation of GSK3β. Consequently, this cascade hindered the ubiquitination process of β-catenin, resulting in its intracellular accumulation and the subsequent promotion of CC cell proliferation [42]. The proliferation demands imposed on CC cells led to increased energy consumption, contributing to an initial decline in body weight among the CC mice [43]. Subsequently, in the later stages of the trial, an observable rise in tissue protein degradation within the colon mucosa of the CC mice significantly contributed to the invasive nature of colon tumors. Additionally, Cd amplified CC cell proliferation by further stimulating GSK3β phosphorylation and leading to subsequent intracellular β-catenin accumulation. This finding aligns with the observations made by Wei [44], who noted the role of Cd in advancing malignant tumors by inhibiting GSK3β activity while concurrently enhancing β-catenin expression. Similarly, Chakraborty [45] suggested that Cd-induced alterations in cancerous conditions plausibly occur through the Wnt signaling pathways. This enhancement did not produce statistically significant changes in the body weight of the CC mice compared to the healthy mice, likely due to the overshadowing effect of increased tumor tissue weight in the later stages of the experiment. Additionally, in the latter phase of the study, Cd notably facilitated colon tumor remodeling and instigated tumor cell migration. This corroborates with Wang's [46] findings, wherein Cd exposure induced MMP-2 mRNA expression and consequently fostered the migration and invasion capabilities of human breast cancer cells. The implantation of intestinal stents alleviated GSK3β phosphorylation and reduced intracellular β-catenin accumulation, thereby slowing down CC cell proliferation. A stent takes up part of the intestinal space and prevents colon tumors from expanding. Additionally, intestinal stents can reduce the blood supply to colon tumors. Colon tumor growth requires large amounts of oxygen and nutrients, and if the blood supply is reduced, the reproductive capacity of CC cells will be inhibited [47]. This aligns with Matsuda's [48] observations, suggesting that the mechanical compression induced by intestinal stents could hinder cancer cell proliferation in cases of malignant large bowel obstruction. However, the implantation of intestinal stents induced gastrointestinal discomfort in the CC mice, resulting in reduced food intake and weight loss. Furthermore, their implantation easily triggered inflammation and infection, compelling the body to expend additional energy to manage the immune response [49].

ROS generated by oxidative stress in the colon mucosa of the CC mice, indirectly reflected by enzyme activity, induced oxidative DNA damage, significantly contributing to the proliferation and spread of CC cells. This aligns with the conclusions drawn by Nilsson [50]. Additionally, NOX1 activity was heightened within CC cells; this is an indirect indicator of increased ROS, and increased ROS levels abnormally activate the Wnt/β-catenin signaling pathway by disrupting Wnt protein secretion. Consequently, this abnormal activation fosters the uncontrolled proliferation of CC cells [51–53]. Cd exacerbates ROS production by further amplifying NOX1 activity in CC cells, a phenomenon also observed by Tyagi [54] and Lian [55]. The implantation of intestinal stents inhibited the expression of SOD1 in the colon tumors of the CC mice. However, the impact on NOX1, SOD2, and CAT enzyme activities was not evident. SOD, which is categorized into three groups (SOD1, SOD2, and SOD3), plays a crucial role in maintaining intracellular ROS homeostasis [56]. Specifically, SOD1 facilitates the dismutation of O^{2-} into H_2O_2, a stable ROS messenger that is pivotal for regulating oxidative stress and supporting oncogene-driven cancer cell proliferation [57]. SOD2 scavenges superoxide radicals formed in the respiratory electron transport chain, thereby impacting cell cycle signaling and cancer progression [58]. CAT acts as an enzymatic scavenger by catalyzing the breakdown of H_2O_2 into oxygen and water, shielding cells from H_2O_2 toxicity and serving as a key element in the biological defense system [59]. Consequently, it was indirectly demonstrated via measurements of enzyme activity that there was no substantial increase in intracellular ROS after intestinal stent implantation, suggesting a less pronounced impact on the Wnt/β-catenin signaling pathway. This effect even contributes to the slowing down of the dysregulation of the Wnt/β-catenin signaling pathway.

The CC mice exhibited colon mucosal damage, disordered glandular arrangement, and infiltration of the inflammatory cells. However, upon the implantation of intestinal stents, severe damage to the colon mucosa and a noticeable infiltration of inflammatory cells were observed. Cd exhibited a dual impact on the immune response within the colon mucosa of the CC mice. It inhibited the expression of Iba1, likely due to its induction of oxidative stress, thus triggering the generation of oxygen free radicals in colon cells. This unfavorable effect on immune cells resulted in the a reduced production of inflammatory cytokines, thereby mitigating the inflammatory response [60]. Conversely, Cd promoted the expression of Iba1 in the colon tumors of the CC mice. This indicated that Cd heightened the inflammatory response in CC cells, consequently fostering the proliferation of colon tumor cells. It stimulated the activity of certain immune cells, notably macrophages, thereby triggering inflammatory reactions and elevating the expression levels of immune markers such as Iba1. A similar study by Yang [61] also reported increased gliosis, as indicated by a rise in the number of Iba1-positive cells, following Cd poisoning. Moreover, intestinal stents inhibited the expression of MMP-9 and COX-2 in colon tumors. This inhibition is linked to the ability of intestinal stents to suppress the activity of inflammation-related cells, possibly including those responsible for producing MMP-9 and COX-2 in colon tumors. However, this speculation necessitates further validation and investigation.

There are several points in this study that require further investigation. First, there was a difference in the expression of MMP-9 between the C-Blank and C-Control groups, but there was no difference between the C-S-Blank and C-S-Control groups. This might be due to the control group being exposed to O_2/N_2 atomized gas, which increased the proportion of oxygen and nitrogen in the atmospheric environment under which the mice lived, which, in turn, might lead to oxidative reactions in CC cells and promote the expression of MMP-9 in the tumors of the CC mice. The implantation of intestinal stents may inhibit this reaction. However, there is currently a lack of research in this area. Therefore, more research is needed to verify this speculation. Moreover, the expression of Iba1 was opposite to that of MMP-9. This difference might occur due to the reaction of the metal stent with substances in the actual atmospheric environment. Second, compared to the C-control and C-Cd mice, the mice in the C-S-Control and C-S-Cd groups exhibited significantly lower MMP-9 expression levels, but the mice in the C-S-Blank group showed a significantly lower expression level than the C-Blank mice. There was no significant change in the expression level of MMP-9 across the groups. This might be due to the difference in gas composition in the actual and simulated atmospheric environments. This study did not research the interaction of substances in the actual atmospheric environment and gas components with cadmium, intestinal stents, and colon cancer cells. Thus, further research is needed in the future.

5. Conclusions

The presence of the heavy metal Cd in an atmospheric milieu acts as a catalyst in the progression of tumorigenesis within murine models of CC. The implementation of intestinal stents demonstrates a mitigating effect on tumor incidence within these CC murine models. Significantly, an aberrant activation of the ROS-mediated Wnt/β-catenin signaling pathway emerges as a pivotal mechanism contributing to the facilitation of this tumorigenic promotion. Cd partially fosters CC tumorigenesis via the ROS-mediated Wnt/β-catenin signaling pathway. The effect of Cd on the invasive effect of intestinal stents in the cancerous colon is not significant.

Supplementary Materials: The following supporting information can be downloaded at: https://www.mdpi.com/article/10.3390/toxics12030215/s1, Figure S1: Basic conditions in healthy cells.; Figure S2: Cumulative mutations of β-catenin in cancer cells.

Author Contributions: S.Z.: Conceptualization, Validation, Investigation, Resources, Supervision, Project administration. R.L.: Methodology, Software, Validation, Formal analysis, Investigation, Data curation, Writing—original draft, Writing—review and editing, Visualization, Supervision. J.X.: Resources, Project administration. Y.L.: Resources, Supervision. Y.Z.: Resources, Supervision. All authors have read and agreed to the published version of the manuscript.

Funding: This work was supported by Tianjin People's Hospital (2020YJ001), Tianjin Municipal Health Commission, Key Research of Integrated Traditional Chinese and Western Medicine (2023056), Tianjin Medical Key Discipline (Specialty) Construction Project (TJYXZDXK-058B), Natural Science Foundation of Tianjin (21JCYBJC01070), Scientific Research Project of Tianjin Union Medical Center (2020YJ003), Beijing Science and Technology Innovation Medical Development Foundation (KC2021-JX-0186-93).

Institutional Review Board Statement: The animal study protocol was conducted in accordance with the Declaration of Helsinki and approved by the Ethics Committee of Tianjin People's Hospital, 2024-B06, 27 January 2024.

Informed Consent Statement: Not applicable.

Data Availability Statement: The original data presented in the study are included in the article/Supplementary Materials; further inquiries can be directed to the corresponding authors.

Conflicts of Interest: Author Yanjie Zhang was employed by the company Tianjin Youmei Environment Technology, Ltd. The remaining authors declare that the research was conducted in the absence of any commercial or financial relationships that could be construed as a potential conflict of interest.

References

1. Tian, R.; Chen, J.; Niu, R. The development of low-molecular weight hydrogels for applications in cancer therapy. *Nanoscale* **2022**, *6*, 3474–3482. [CrossRef]
2. Lin, X.; Peng, L.; Xu, X.; Chen, Y.; Zhang, Y.; Huo, X. Connecting gastrointestinal cancer risk to cadmium and lead exposure in the Chaoshan population of Southeast China. *Environ. Sci. Pollut. Res.* **2018**, *25*, 17611–17619. [CrossRef]
3. Rinaldi, L.; Barabino, G.; Klein, J.P.; Bitounis, D.; Pourchez, J.; Forest, V.; Boudard, D.; Leclerc, L.; Sarry, G.; Roblin, X.; et al. Metals distribution in colorectal biopsies: New insight on the elemental fingerprint of tumour tissue. *Digest. Liver Dis.* **2015**, *47*, 602–607. [CrossRef]
4. Sarkar, S.; Mukherjee, S.K.; Roy, K.; Ghosh, P. Evaluation of Role of Heavy Metals in Causation of Colorectal Cancer. *J. Evol. Med. Dent. Sci.* **2020**, *9*, 1036–1039. [CrossRef]
5. Briffa, J.; Sinagra, E.; Blundell, R. Heavy metal pollution in the environment and their toxicological effects on humans. *Heliyon* **2020**, *6*, e04691. [CrossRef]
6. Rahman, Z.; Singh, V.P. The relative impact of toxic heavy metals (THMs) (arsenic (As), cadmium (Cd), chromium (Cr)(VI), mercury (Hg), and lead (Pb)) on the total environment: An overview. *Environ. Monit Assess.* **2019**, *191*, 419. [CrossRef]
7. Nawrot, T.S.; Martens, D.S.; Hara, A.; Plusquin, M.; Vangronsveld, J.; Roels, H.A.; Staessen, J.A. Association of total cancer and lung cancer with environmental exposure to cadmium: The meta-analytical evidence. *Cancer Cause Control* **2015**, *26*, 1281–1288. [CrossRef] [PubMed]
8. Nishijo, M.; Nakagawa, H.; Suwazono, Y.; Nogawa, K.; Sakurai, M.; Ishizaki, M.; Kido, T. Cancer mortality in residents of the cadmium-polluted Jinzu River basin in Toyama, Japan. *Toxics* **2018**, *6*, 23. [CrossRef]
9. Lin, H.C.; Hao, W.M.; Chu, P.H. Cadmium and cardiovascular disease: An overview of pathophysiology, epidemiology, therapy, and predictive value. *Rev. Port. Cardiol.* **2021**, *40*, 611–617. [CrossRef]
10. Tellez-Plaza, M.; Jones, M.R.; Dominguez-Lucas, A.; Guallar, E.; Navas-Acien, A. Cadmium exposure and clinical cardiovascular disease: A systematic review topical collection on nutrition. *Curr. Atheroscler. Rep.* **2013**, *15*, 356. [CrossRef] [PubMed]
11. Salama, S.A.; Mohamadin, A.M.; Abdel-Bakky, M.S. Arctigenin alleviates cadmium-induced nephrotoxicity: Targeting endoplasmic reticulum stress, Nrf2 signaling, and the associated inflammatory response. *Life Sci.* **2021**, *287*, 120121. [CrossRef]
12. Taş, İ.; Zhou, R.; Park, S.Y.; Yang, Y.; Gamage, C.D.B.; Son, Y.J.; Paik, M.J.; Kim, H. Inflammatory and tumorigenic effects of environmental pollutants found in particulate matter on lung epithelial cells. *Toxicol. In Vitro* **2019**, *59*, 300–311. [CrossRef]
13. Mahmood, M.H.R.; Qayyum, M.A.; Yaseen, F.; Farooq, T.; Farooq, Z.; Yaseen, M.; Irfan, A.; Muddassir, K.; Zafar, M.N.; Qamar, M.T.; et al. Multivariate Investigation of Toxic and Essential Metals in the Serum from Various Types and Stages of Colorectal Cancer Patients. *Biol. Trace Elem. Res.* **2022**, *200*, 31–48. [CrossRef]
14. Lu, J.; Zhou, Z.; Zheng, J.; Zhang, Z.; Lu, R.; Liu, H.; Shi, H.; Tu, Z. 2D-DIGE and MALDI TOF/TOF MS analysis reveal that small GTPase signaling pathways may play an important role in cadmium-induced colon cell malignant transformation. *Toxicol. Appl. Pharm.* **2015**, *288*, 106–113. [CrossRef] [PubMed]
15. Chou, W.C.; Jie, C.; Kenedy, A.A.; Jones, R.J.; Trush, M.A.; Dang, C.V. Role of NADPH oxidase in arsenic-induced reactive oxygen species formation and cytotoxicity in myeloid leukemia cells. *Proc. Natl. Acad. Sci. USA* **2004**, *101*, 4578–4583. [CrossRef]
16. Coant, N.; Ben Mkaddem, S.; Pedruzzi, E.; Guichard, C.; Tréton, X.; Ducroc, R.; Freund, J.-N.; Cazals-Hatem, D.; Bouhnik, Y.; Woerther, P.-L.; et al. NADPH Oxidase 1 Modulates WNT and NOTCH1 Signaling To Control the Fate of Proliferative Progenitor Cells in the Colon. *Mol. Cell. Biol.* **2010**, *30*, 2636–2650. [CrossRef] [PubMed]
17. Yu, M.; Qin, K.; Fan, J.; Zhao, G.; Zhao, P.; Zeng, W.; Chen, C.; Wang, A.; Wang, Y.; Zhong, J.; et al. The evolving roles of Wnt signaling in stem cell proliferation and differentiation, the development of human diseases, and therapeutic opportunities. *Genes Dis.* **2023**, *11*, 101026. [CrossRef] [PubMed]
18. Braunschweig, L.; Meyer, A.K.; Wagenführ, L.; Storch, A. Oxygen regulates proliferation of neural stem cells through Wnt/β-catenin signalling. *Mol. Cell. Neurosci.* **2015**, *67*, 84–92. [CrossRef] [PubMed]
19. Qiu, W.; Chen, L.; Kassem, M. Activation of non-canonical Wnt/JNK pathway by Wnt3a is associated with differentiation fate determination of human bone marrow stromal (mesenchymal) stem cells. *Biochem. Biophys. Res. Commun.* **2011**, *413*, 98–104. [CrossRef] [PubMed]

20. Yadav, R.P.; Baranwal, S. Kindlin-2 regulates colonic cancer stem-like cells survival and self-renewal via Wnt/β-catenin mediated pathway. *Cell. Signal.* **2024**, *113*, 110953. [CrossRef]
21. Jung, Y.S.; Park, J.I. Wnt signaling in cancer: Therapeutic targeting of Wnt signaling beyond β-catenin and the destruction complex. *Exp. Mol. Med.* **2020**, *52*, 183–191. [CrossRef] [PubMed]
22. Li, Y.; Bavarva, J.H.; Wang, Z.; Guo, J.; Qian, C.; Thibodeau, S.N.; Golemis, E.A.; Liu, W. HEF1, a novel target of Wnt signaling, promotes colonic cell migration and cancer progression. *Oncogene* **2011**, *30*, 2633–2643. [CrossRef]
23. Naji, S.; Issa, K.; Eid, A.; Iratni, R.; Eid, A.H. Cadmium induces migration of colon cancer cells: Roles of reactive oxygen species, p38 and cyclooxygenase-2. *Cell. Physiol. Biochem.* **2019**, *52*, 1517–1534. [CrossRef] [PubMed]
24. Mahmoud, A.S.; Umair, A.; Azzeghaiby, S.N.; Hussain, F.; Hanouneh, S.; Tarakji, B. Expression of Cyclooxygenase-2 (COX-2) in Colorectal Adenocarcinoma: An Immunohistochemical and Histopathological Study. *Asian Pac. J. Cancer Prev.* **2014**, *15*, 6787–6790. [CrossRef]
25. Peng, L.; Zhou, Y.; Wang, Y.; Mou, H.; Zhao, Q. Prognostic Significance of COX-2 Immunohistochemical Expression in Colorectal Cancer: A Meta-Analysis of the Literature. *PLoS ONE* **2013**, *8*, e58891. [CrossRef]
26. Tatsuguchi, A.; Kishida, T.; Fujimori, S.; Tanaka, S.; Gudis, K.; Shinji, S.; Furukawa, K.; Tajiri, T.; Sugisaki, Y.; Fukuda, Y.; et al. Differential expression of cyclo-oxygenase-2 and nuclear β-catenin in colorectal cancer tissue. *Aliment. Pharm. Ther. Symp. Ser.* **2006**, *2*, 153–159. [CrossRef]
27. Breyer, R.M.; Bagdassarian, C.K.; Myers, S.A.; Breyer, M.D. Prostanoid Receptors: Subtypes and Signaling. *Annu. Rev. Pharmacol. Toxicol.* **2001**, *41*, 661–690. [CrossRef] [PubMed]
28. Waller, R.; Narramore, R.; Simpson, J.E.; Heath, P.R.; Verma, N.; Tinsley, M.; Barnes, J.R.; Haris, H.T.; Henderson, F.E.; Matthews, F.E.; et al. Heterogeneity of cellular inflammatory responses in ageing white matter and relationship to Alzheimer's and small vessel disease pathologies. *Brain Pathol.* **2021**, *31*, e12928. [CrossRef]
29. Shigeta, K.; Baba, H.; Yamafuji, K.; Kaneda, H.; Katsura, H.; Kubochi, K. Outcomes for Patients with Obstructing Colorectal Cancers Treated with One-Stage Surgery Using Transanal Drainage Tubes. *J. Gastrointest. Surg.* **2014**, *18*, 1507–1513. [CrossRef]
30. Shingu, Y.; Hasegawa, H.; Sakamoto, E.; Komatsu, S.; Kurumiya, Y.; Norimizu, S.; Taguchi, Y. Clinical and oncologic safety of laparoscopic surgery for obstructive left colorectal cancer following transanal endoscopic tube decompression. *Surg. Endosc.* **2013**, *27*, 3359–3363. [CrossRef]
31. Yoshida, S.; Watabe, H.; Isayama, H.; Kogure, H.; Nakai, Y.; Yamamoto, N.; Sasaki, T.; Kawakubo, K.; Hamada, T.; Ito, Y.; et al. Feasibility of a new self-expandable metallic stent for patients with malignant colorectal obstruction. *Digest. Endosc.* **2013**, *25*, 160–166. [CrossRef]
32. Maruthachalam, K.; Lash, G.E.; Shenton, B.K.; Horgan, A.F. Tumour cell dissemination following endoscopic stent insertion. *Brit. J. Surg.* **2007**, *94*, 1151–1154. [CrossRef]
33. Santos, A.; Lopes, C.; Frias, C.; Amorim, I.; Vicente, C.; Gärtner, F.; Matos, A. Immunohistochemical evaluation of MMP-2 and TIMP-2 in canine mammary tumours: A survival study. *Vet. J.* **2021**, *190*, 396–402. [CrossRef] [PubMed]
34. Lee, T.H.; Chen, J.L.; Liu, P.S.; Tsai, M.M.; Tsai, M.M.; Wang, S.J.; Hsieh, H.L.; Hsieh, H.L. Rottlerin, a natural polyphenol compound, inhibits upregulation of matrix metalloproteinase-9 and brain astrocytic migration by reducing PKC-δ-dependent ROS signal. *J. Neuroinflamm.* **2020**, *17*, 177. [CrossRef]
35. Bláhová, L.; Janoš, T.; Mustieles, V.; Rodríguez-Carrillo, A.; Fernández, M.F.; Bláha, L. Rapid extraction and analysis of oxidative stress and DNA damage biomarker 8-hydroxy-2′-deoxyguanosine (8-OHdG) in urine: Application to a study with pregnant women. *Int. J. Hyg. Environ. Health* **2023**, *250*, 114175. [CrossRef] [PubMed]
36. Xie, J.X.; Xi, Y.; Zhang, Q.L.; Lai, K.F.; Zhong, N.S. Impact of short term forced oral breathing induced by nasal occlusion on respiratory function in mice. *Respir. Physiol. Neurobiol.* **2015**, *205*, 37–41. [CrossRef] [PubMed]
37. Jaques, P.A.; Kim, C.S. Measurement of total lung deposition of inhaled ultrafine particles in healthy men and women. *Inhal. Toxicol.* **2000**, *12*, 715–731. [CrossRef] [PubMed]
38. Wang, L.; Wise, J.T.F.; Zhang, Z.; Shi, X. Progress and Prospects of Reactive Oxygen Species in Metal Carcinogenesis. *Curr. Pharm. Rep.* **2016**, *2*, 178–186. [CrossRef] [PubMed]
39. Chocry, M.; Leloup, L.; Kovacic, H. Progress and Prospects of Reversion of resistance to oxaliplatin by inhibition of p38 MAPK in colorectal cancer cell lines: Involvement of the calpain/Nox1 pathway. *Oncotarget* **2017**, *8*, 103710–103730. [CrossRef] [PubMed]
40. Skrzycki, M.; Czeczot, H.; Chrzanowska, A.; Otto-Ślusarczyk, D. The level of superoxide dismutase expression in primary and metastatic colorectal cancer cells in hypoxia and tissue normoxia. *Pol. Merkur. Lek.* **2015**, *39*, 281–286.
41. Tang, Z.; Meng, S.Y.; Yang, X.X.; Xiao, Y.; Wang, W.T.; Liu, Y.H.; Wu, K.F.; Zhang, X.C.; Guo, H.; Zhu, Y.Z.; et al. Neutrophil-Mimetic, ROS Responsive, and Oxygen Generating Nanovesicles for Targeted Interventions of Refractory Rheumatoid Arthritis. *Small* **2023**, 2307379. [CrossRef]
42. Zhang, X.; Li, C.; Wu, Y.; Cui, P. The research progress of Wnt/β-catenin signaling pathway in colorectal cancer. *Clin. Res. Hepatol. Gastroenterol.* **2023**, *47*, 102086. [CrossRef] [PubMed]
43. DU, J. Association between shortage of energy supply and nuclear gene mutations leading to carcinomatous transformation. *Mol. Clin. Oncol.* **2016**, *4*, 11–12. [CrossRef] [PubMed]
44. Wei, Z.; Shaikh, Z.A. Cadmium stimulates metastasis-associated phenotype in triple-negative breast cancer cells through integrin and β-catenin signaling. *Toxicol. Appl. Pharm.* **2017**, *328*, 70–80. [CrossRef] [PubMed]

45. Chakraborty, P.K.; Scharner, B.; Jurasovic, J.; Messner, B.; Bernhard, D.; Thévenod, F. Chronic cadmium exposure induces transcriptional activation of the Wnt pathway and upregulation of epithelial-to-mesenchymal transition markers in mouse kidney. *Toxicol. Lett.* **2010**, *198*, 69–76. [CrossRef] [PubMed]
46. Wang, Y.; Shi, L.; Li, J.; Li, L.; Wang, H.; Yang, H. Long-term cadmium exposure promoted breast cancer cell migration and invasion by up-regulating TGIF. *Ecotoxicol. Environ. Saf.* **2019**, *175*, 110–117. [CrossRef]
47. Feng, Y.; Chen, Y.; Chen, Y.; He, X.; Khan, Y.; Hu, H.; Lan, P.; Li, Y.; Wang, X.; Li, G.; et al. Intestinal stents: Structure, functionalization and advanced engineering innovation. *Biomater. Adv.* **2022**, *137*, 212810. [CrossRef]
48. Matsuda, A.; Miyashita, M.; Matsumoto, S.; Sakurazawa, N.; Kawano, Y.; Yamahatsu, K.; Sekiguchi, K.; Yamada, M.; Hatori, T.; Yoshida, H. Colonic stent-induced mechanical compression may suppress cancer cell proliferation in malignant large bowel obstruction. *Surg. Endosc.* **2019**, *33*, 1290–1297. [CrossRef]
49. Choi, S.J.; Min, J.W.; Yun, J.M.; Ahn, H.S.; Han, D.J.; Lee, H.J.; Kim, Y.O. Portal vein thrombosis with sepsis caused by inflammation at colonic stent insertion site. *Korean J. Gastroenterol.* **2015**, *65*, 316–320. [CrossRef]
50. Nilsson, R.; Liu, N.A. Nuclear DNA damages generated by reactive oxygen molecules (ROS) under oxidative stress and their relevance to human cancers, including ionizing radiation-induced neoplasia part I: Physical, chemical and molecular biology aspects. *Radiat. Med. Prot.* **2020**, *1*, 140–152. [CrossRef]
51. Kajla, S.; Mondol, A.S.; Nagasawa, A.; Zhang, Y.; Kato, M.; Matsuno, K.; Yabe-Nishimura, C.; Kamata, T. A crucial role for Nox 1 in redox-dependent regulation of Wnt-β-catenin signaling. *FASEB J.* **2012**, *26*, 2049–2059. [CrossRef]
52. Wang, X.; Mandal, A.K.; Saito, H.; Pulliam, J.F.; Lee, E.Y.; Ke, Z.J.; Lu, J.; Ding, S.; Li, L.; Shelton, B.J.; et al. Arsenic and chromium in drinking water promote tumorigenesis in a mouse colitis-associated colorectal cancer model and the potential mechanism is ROS-mediated Wnt/β-catenin signaling pathway. *Toxicol. Appl. Pharm.* **2012**, *262*, 11–21. [CrossRef]
53. Zhang, Z.; Wang, X.; Cheng, S.; Sun, L.; Son, Y.O.; Yao, H.; Li, W.; Budhraja, A.; Li, L.; Shelton, B.J.; et al. Reactive oxygen species mediate arsenic induced cell transformation and tumorigenesis through Wnt/β-catenin pathway in human colorectal adenocarcinoma DLD1 cells. *Toxicol. Appl. Pharm.* **2011**, *256*, 114–121. [CrossRef]
54. Tyagi, A.; Chandrasekaran, B.; Navin, A.K.; Shukla, V.; Baby, B.V.; Ankem, M.K.; Damodaran, C. Molecular interplay between NOX1 and autophagy in cadmium-induced prostate carcinogenesis. *Free Radical. Biol. Med.* **2023**, *199*, 44–55. [CrossRef]
55. Lian, S.; Xia, Y.; Khoi, P.N.; Ung, T.T.; Yoon, H.J.; Kim, N.H.; Kim, K.K.; Jung, Y.D. Cadmium induces matrix metalloproteinase-9 expression via ROS-dependent EGFR, NF-κB, and AP-1 pathways in human endothelial cells. *Toxicology* **2015**, *338*, 104–116. [CrossRef]
56. Zelko, I.N.; Mariani, T.J.; Folz, R.J. Superoxide dismutase multigene family: A comparison of the CuZn-SOD (SOD1), Mn-SOD (SOD2), and EC-SOD (SOD3) gene structures, evolution, and expression. *Free Radical. Biol. Med.* **2002**, *33*, 337–349. [CrossRef]
57. Picazo, C.; Padilla, C.A.; McDonagh, B.; Matallana, E.; Bárcena, J.A.; Aranda, A. Regulation of metabolism, stress response, and sod1 activity by cytosolic thioredoxins in yeast depends on growth phase. *Adv. Redox. Res.* **2023**, *9*, 100081. [CrossRef]
58. Miar, A.; Hevia, D.; Muñoz-Cimadevilla, H.; Astudillo, A.; Velasco, J.; Sainz, R.M.; Mayo, J.C. Manganese superoxide dismutase (SOD2/MnSOD)/catalase and SOD2/GPx1 ratios as biomarkers for tumor progression and metastasis in prostate, colon, and lung cancer. *Free Radical. Biol. Med.* **2015**, *85*, 45–55. [CrossRef]
59. Ighodaro, O.M.; Akinloye, O.A. First line defence antioxidants-superoxide dismutase (SOD), catalase (CAT) and glutathione peroxidase (GPX): Their fundamental role in the entire antioxidant defence grid. *Alex. J. Med.* **2018**, *54*, 287–293. [CrossRef]
60. Shah, R.; Ibis, B.; Kashyap, M.; Boussiotis, V.A. The role of ROS in tumor infiltrating immune cells and cancer immunotherapy. *Metabolism* **2024**, *151*, 155747. [CrossRef]
61. Yang, J.Y.; Wang, J.; Hu, Y.; Shen, D.Y.; Xiao, G.L.; Qin, X.Y.; Lan, R.F. Paeoniflorin improves cognitive dysfunction, restores glutamate receptors, attenuates gliosis and maintains synaptic plasticity in cadmiumintoxicated mice. *Arab. J. Chem.* **2023**, *16*, 104406. [CrossRef]

toxics MDPI

Article

Investigation of the Association between Air Pollution and Non-Alcoholic Fatty Liver Disease in the European Population: A Mendelian Randomization Study

Jing Yang [1,†], Yaqi Zhang [1,†], Yin Yuan [1,2,†], Zhongyang Xie [1] and Lanjuan Li [1,*]

[1] State Key Laboratory for Diagnosis and Treatment of Infectious Diseases, National Clinical Research Center for Infectious Diseases, National Medical Center for Infectious Diseases, Collaborative Innovation Center for Diagnosis and Treatment of Infectious Diseases, The First Affiliated Hospital, Zhejiang University School of Medicine, 79 Qingchun Rd., Hangzhou 310003, China; 11818049@zju.edu.cn (J.Y.); 12118240@zju.edu.cn (Y.Z.); yuanyin@zju.edu.cn (Y.Y.); zyxie@zju.edu.cn (Z.X.)

[2] Department of Biology, The David H. Koch Institute for Integrative Cancer Research at MIT, Massachusetts Institute of Technology, Cambridge, MA 02139, USA

[*] Correspondence: ljli@zju.edu.cn

[†] These authors contributed equally to this work.

Abstract: Non-alcoholic fatty liver disease (NAFLD) is currently the most prevalent chronic liver disease worldwide. At the same time, the relationship between air pollution and the likelihood of developing NAFLD has been a subject of debate due to conflicting findings in previous observational research. Our objective was to examine the potential correlation between air pollutant levels and the risk of NAFLD in the European population by employing a two-sample Mendelian randomization (MR) analysis. The UK Biobank Consortium provided the summary statistics for various air pollution indicators ($PM_{2.5}$, $PM_{2.5}$ absorbance, $PM_{2.5-10}$, PM_{10}, NO_2, and NO_x). Additionally, information on NAFLD was obtained from three studies, including one derivation set and two validation sets. Heterogeneity, pleiotropy, and sensitivity analyses were performed under different MR frameworks, and instrumental variables associated with confounders (such as education, smoking, alcohol, and BMI) were detected by tools. In the derivation set, causal relationships between $PM_{2.5}$, NO_2, and NAFLD were observed in univariable Mendelian randomization (UVMR) (Odds Ratio (OR) = 1.99, 95% confidence interval (95% CI) = [1.22–3.22], $p = 0.005$; OR = 2.08, 95% CI = [1.27–3.40], $p = 0.004$, respectively). After adjustment for air pollutants or alcohol intake frequency in multivariable Mendelian randomization (MVMR), the above genetic correlations disappeared. In validation sets, the null associations remained in UVMR. Our findings from MR analysis using genetic data did not provide evidence for a causal association between air pollution and NAFLD in the European population. The associations observed in epidemiological studies could be partly attributed to confounders.

Keywords: air pollution; NAFLD; UK Biobank; Finngen; Mendelian randomization

1. Introduction

The escalating prevalence of non-alcoholic fatty liver disease (NAFLD) has made it a major global health issue. The estimated worldwide incidence rate of NAFLD stands at approximately 24% [1]. Notably, dietary patterns and lifestyle choices have been recognized as crucial elements linked to the emergence of NAFLD, with countries exhibiting a higher consumption of high-calorie diets experiencing a greater incidence of the disease. Furthermore, NAFLD independently contributes to the likelihood of various comorbidities, including hypertension, type 2 diabetes (T2D), and cardiovascular diseases (CVDs) [2–4]. Although metabolic disorders have been established as the primary risk factor for NAFLD, increasing evidence supports the view that exposure to certain environmental factors may have a profound impact on liver disease, including NAFLD.

A matter of concern is the detrimental impact of air pollution on human health, as over 80% of city dwellers are exposed to air pollutants whose levels exceed the thresholds set by the World Health Organization (WHO) [5]. Air pollutants typically encompass particulate matter (PM) and specific chemical gases. PM can be categorized based on its physical diameter: particulate matter with aerodynamic diameters $\leq$ 2.5 μm ($PM_{2.5}$); particulate matter with diameters $\leq$ 10 μm and >2.5 μm ($PM_{2.5\text{–}10}$); particulate matter with diameters > 10 μm (PM_{10}). The chemical substances include gases such as nitrogen dioxide (NO_2), nitrogen oxides (NO_x), sulfur dioxide (SO_2), ozone (O_3), and so on. $PM_{2.5}$, originating from vehicle exhaust emissions, industrial emissions, and combustion processes, is the pollutant most commonly detected among them. Air pollutants have been officially classified by the International Agency for Research on Cancer (IARC) as the main category of substances that cause cancer in humans. A number of studies have consistently demonstrated correlations between air pollution and various forms of cancer, including lung cancer [6], gastrointestinal cancer [7], ovarian cancer [8], and others [9]. As a kind of well-established and extensively widespread industrial contaminant, $PM_{2.5}$ possesses the capacity to deeply infiltrate the respiratory system, disturb the exchange of gases, and infiltrate the bloodstream, consequently presenting a substantial risk in relation to respiratory ailments, cardiovascular conditions, and mental well-being. In the year 2015, surrounding $PM_{2.5}$ became the fifth leading cause of death, accounting for 4.2 million fatalities and 103.1 million disability-adjusted life-years (DALYs). The aforementioned statistics represented 7.6% of all deaths worldwide and 4.2% of global DALYs, with a noteworthy majority (59%) concentrated in the eastern and southern Asian regions [10].

It is crucial to acknowledge that the emergence of numerous illnesses is an intricate consequence arising from the interaction among various genetic factors, lifestyle choices, and environmental elements. Previous research has indicated that genetic polymorphism plays a vital part in investigating the effects of contaminants on different physiological and immune functions in the human body. For instance, a study rooted in genetics has demonstrated that women with the *GPX4*-rs376102 AC/CC genotype exhibit heightened vulnerability to atmospheric pollutants, consequently increasing the likelihood of preterm births [11]. Similarly, elderly individuals with *PARP4* G-C-G and *ERCC1* T-C are prone to increased levels of fasting blood sugar when exposed to $PM_{2.5}$, $PM_{2.5\text{–}10}$, and PM_{10} [12]. Moreover, the presence of indoor $PM_{2.5}$ and environmental tobacco smoke during pregnancy greatly increases the occurrence of lower respiratory tract infections in newborns who possess the *GSTM1* null, *GSTP1*-rs1695 AG/GG, or *Nrf2*-rs6726395 GG genotypes [13].

While several observational studies have suggested a correlation between air pollution and NAFLD, it is crucial to obtain further evidence to establish a more robust causal relationship. This requirement stems from the potential influence of confounding factors, misclassification, and the inherent difficulties associated with reverse causality that are prevalent in observational study designs. MR research is usually likened to a natural randomized controlled trial (RCT), as it relies on the random assignment of genetic variations/alleles from parents during meiosis in pregnancy. Conceptually, MR research shares similarities with a RCT, wherein participants are randomly placed in different experimental groups. This implies that there is no discernible association between individuals possessing a specific genetic variation and exposure factors, thus rendering it a natural random allocation. Moreover, due to the inherent stability of the human genome once established, confounding biases that are arduous to regulate (e.g., lifestyle, economic status) are significantly diminished, thereby yielding more dependable causal evidence. At the pragmatic level of implementation, MR studies employ genetic variations (single nucleotide polymorphisms, SNPs) as instrumental variables to deduce a causal relationship between exposures and outcomes. Additionally, genome-wide association studies (GWASs) furnish an extensive repertoire of genetic variation analysis data related to human diseases by testing the correlation between millions of genetic variations and disease outcomes. To establish the causal connection between air pollution and NAFLD, a two-sample MR (TSMR) analysis was performed.

2. Materials and Methods

2.1. Study Design

The genetic variations employed in this analysis are required to adhere to the three assumptions of Mendelian randomization (MR) [14], as presented in Figure 1. Firstly, the genetic instrumental variables (IVs) related to air pollution, such as $PM_{2.5}$, $PM_{2.5}$ absorbance, $PM_{2.5–10}$, PM_{10}, NO_2, and NO_x exposure levels, exhibit significant associations. Secondly, the relationship between these genetic IVs and NAFLD remains unaffected by confounding factors. Lastly, the genetic IVs solely influence the risk of NAFLD through exposure.

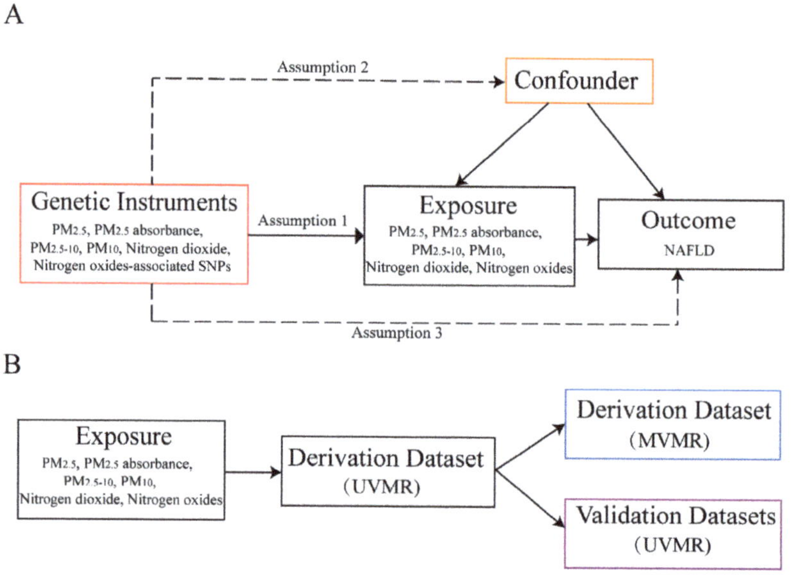

Figure 1. MR assumptions and the design flow chart of this study. (**A**) MR assumptions: assumptions 1, 2, and 3. The solid line represents direct putative causal effects that air pollution genetic instrumental variants are reliably associated with air pollutant levels and influence the risk of NAFLD through the exposures in assumption 1. The dotted line represents that genetic instrumental variants are not associated with any measured or unmeasured confounders and do not influence the risk of NAFLD through other pathways in assumptions 2 and 3, respectively. (**B**) The flow chart of the study design. MR, Mendelian randomization; PM, particulate matter; NAFLD, non-alcoholic fatty liver disease; UVMR, univariable Mendelian randomization; MVMR, multivariable Mendelian randomization.

The study design depicted in Figure 1 provides an overview of the research methodology. The objective of this MR study was to examine the possible causal connection between the atmospheric contaminants ($PM_{2.5}$, $PM_{2.5}$ absorbance, $PM_{2.5–10}$, PM_{10}, NO_2, and NO_x) and NAFLD. Firstly, a derivation outcome set was obtained from the same source as the previous observational study [15], and a univariate Mendelian randomization (UVMR) study model was employed for discovery purposes. Subsequently, exposures with positive UVMR results and the confounding factors identified in the aforementioned observational study were included for multivariate Mendelian randomization (MVMR) analysis. Additionally, validation outcome sets from two distinct populations were employed to improve the overall dependability of this research. It is important to mention that this research followed the reporting recommendations specified in Strengthening observational studies using Mendelian randomization (STROBE-MR) [16]. The Supplementary Materials contain the STROBE-MR checklist for reference.

2.2. Data Sources

The summary datasets for the air pollution GWASs in Europe were obtained from the MRC-IEU, a unit of the Medical Research Council that has streamlined its process to perform GWASs on the imputed genetic dataset of the entire UK Biobank population of 500,000 individuals with efficiency, effectiveness, and uniformity. Land use regression (LUR) models were used to measure the relevant indicators for air pollution in Europe, which include $PM_{2.5}$, $PM_{2.5}$ absorbance, $PM_{2.5–10}$, PM_{10}, NO_2, and NO_x [17]. Other datasets could also be found in the IEU open GWAS project, including the alcohol-intake frequency dataset. The NAFLD GWAS summary datasets were derived from three studies that exclusively included individuals of European descent (GWAS ID: ebi-a-GCST90054782 [18], ebi-a-GCST90091033 [19], finn-b-NAFLD [20]). Considering the distinct sources of the queues and different sample overlap ratios of these datasets, we employed the first dataset as the derivation dataset and the other two datasets as the validation datasets. Consisting of 10 centers in the United States, the eMERGE Network is a substantial genetic research establishment. With a population of around 200,000 Estonian adults, the Estonian Biobank is an organized biobank established by the Estonian Genome Center of the University of Tartu (EGCUT). FinnGen is an extensive research project that integrates inherent gene data obtained from recently gathered and existing samples from 400,000 participants in the Finnish biobank. It also incorporates digital health registers to offer innovative understandings of the genetics of human disorders [20].

The specific information of the datasets, such as cohort sources, diagnostic codes, and data adjustment methods, is listed in Tables 1 and S1. All documents in this undertaking originated from the project website and were accessible to the general public. In the respective original studies, all participants provided informed consent. Therefore, there is no requirement for additional ethical authorization or a form of informed consent.

Table 1. GWAS data sources of this MR study.

Exposure/Outcome	Dataset		Sample Size or Case/Control	NSNP	Unit	Population	Consortium/Cohort	Year
	GWAS ID	PMID						
Exposure								
$PM_{2.5}$	ukb-b-10817	——	423,796	9,851,867	SD	European	MRC-IEU	2018
$PM_{2.5}$ absorbance	ukb-b-11312	——	423,796	9,851,867	SD	European	MRC-IEU	2018
$PM_{2.5–10}$	ukb-b-12963	——	423,796	9,851,867	SD	European	MRC-IEU	2018
PM_{10}	ukb-b-18469	——	423,796	9,851,867	SD	European	MRC-IEU	2018
NO_2	ukb-b-9942	——	456,380	9,851,867	SD	European	MRC-IEU	2018
NO_x	ukb-b-12417	——	456,380	9,851,867	SD	European	MRC-IEU	2018
Alcohol intake frequency	ukb-b-5779	——	462,346	9,851,867	SD	European	MRC-IEU	2018
Outcome								
NAFLD	ebi-a-GCST90054782	34535985	4,761/373,227	9,097,254	Event	European	UK Biobank	2021
NAFLD	ebi-a-GCST90091033	34841290	8,434/770,180	6,784,388	Event	European	eMERGE, UK Biobank, FinnGen and Estonian Biobank	2021
NAFLD	finn-b-NAFLD	——	894/217,898	16,380,466	Event	European	FinnGen	2021

NSNP, number of Single Nucleotide Polymorphisms; PMID, PubMed ID; SD, standard deviation.

2.3. Selection of Instrumental Variables

To satisfy assumption 1, we implemented a selection procedure for the relevant SNPs for exposure, utilizing a widely recognized threshold of genome-wide significance ($p < 5 \times 10^{-8}$). However, only NO_2 and NO_x exposures yielded an adequate number of

SNPs. Previous research has suggested a limited potential for weak instrumental variable bias in MR analysis when employing linear regression of each genetic variant on risk variables at a screening threshold of $p < 1 \times 10^{-5}$ [21]. Based on the extant literature on MR studies related to $PM_{2.5}$, we discovered that the threshold values for screening IVs were set at $p < 1 \times 10^{-6}$, $p < 5 \times 10^{-6}$, or even $p < 1 \times 10^{-5}$, which exceeded the usual range. As a result, we performed MR operations under two different threshold conditions ($p < 1 \times 10^{-6}$ and $p < 1 \times 10^{-5}$) to acquire a sufficient quantity of SNPs. The independence of SNPs was verified by implementing rigorous inclusion criteria ($r^2 \leq 0.001$; clumping window, 10,000 kb) without a proxy SNP in linkage disequilibrium. A harmonization procedure was undertaken to ascertain positive strand alleles and employ allele frequencies for palindromes as a means of quality control by R software.

To fulfill assumption 2, we used the PhenoScanner (http://www.phenoscanner.medschl.cam.ac.uk/) and GWASCatalog (https://www.ebi.ac.uk/gwas/) tools (accessed on 25 December 2023) to determine if there was a significant correlation between IVs and the risk factors associated with NAFLD, including smoking, alcohol, BMI, T2DM, blood pressure, education, and other factors that had been confirmed to have a causal relationship with NAFLD in MR analyses published so far. For detailed information, please refer to Table S3. When one SNP was mixed with multiple variables, only the variable with the lowest p-value or the strongest level of clinical evidence was listed in the table.

To meet assumption 3, we used the above tools and conducted MR Steiger filtering to monitor the direction of causation [22] and calculated the proportions of variance explained by exposures (R^2) relying on prior investigations. In addition, the F-statistic ($F = \beta^2/SE^2$) for each SNP listed in Table S2 was calculated to present the strength of IVs, and a value greater than 10 was deemed satisfactory, indicating poor chances of weak instrumental bias [23].

2.4. Mendelian Randomization Analysis

The primary approach used for evaluating the causal relationship was the inverse variance weighted (IVW) method, which employed an odds ratio (OR) as the effect value. In MR analysis, IVW employs a single genetic IV to estimate the causal effect using the Wald ratio. After that, several evaluations are meta-analyzed using a fixed-effect model, ensuring a reliable estimation of causality without directed pleiotropy. This approach is commonly employed and referenced in studies [21,24]. To improve accuracy and stability, we enhanced our verification by incorporating the MR-Egger regression, weighted median, weighted mode, simple mode, and MR Robust Adjusted Profile Score (MR-RAPS). By utilizing MR-RAPS, it becomes possible to incorporate numerous weak instruments that fall below the typical GWAS threshold, thereby enhancing the dependability of Cochran's Q-statistic in detecting heterogeneity caused by pleiotropy. This is especially beneficial in reducing the false positive (or type I error) rate. Online calculations were performed to estimate the bias and type I error rate of MR with sample overlap (https://sb452.shinyapps.io/overlap/, accessed on 31 December 2023). Post hoc power calculations [25] for IVW-MR estimates were produced using an online MR power calculation tool (https://sb452.shinyapps.io/power/, accessed on 31 December 2023). Moreover, to mitigate the influence of variables that may distort the results in UVMR, MVMR was utilized to assess the relationship among exposures, confounding factors, and outcomes.

2.5. Sensitivity Analysis

Sensitivity analyses encompassed three components and were executed using several methods. Initially, we assessed the heterogeneity by employing Cochran's Q test for the IVW approach, and a p-value less than 0.05 indicated the presence of heterogeneity among the chosen IVs [21,26]. In addition, we assessed horizontal pleiotropy by employing MR-Egger regression and MR-pleiotropy residual sum and outlier (MR-PRESSO) [27] to ensure compliance with assumptions 2 or 3. The MR-Egger regression model enables the estimation of corrected pleiotropic effects in a causal manner, assessing the null causality assumption based on the InSIDE (instrument strength independent of direct effect) assumption. When the p-value of the MR-Egger intercept was less than 0.05, we deemed the impact of SNPs linked to exposure factors on outcomes to be untrustworthy. The MR-PRESSO algorithm allows for a systematic evaluation of the impact of pleiotropy and identifies exceptional SNPs, while also offering a causal estimation by eliminating associated outliers. Thirdly, we employed the leave-one-out permutation test [28] to test if our findings were impacted by a specific SNP in order to eliminate chance errors from the selection of IVs. If the results of the MR study were significantly altered by excluding a single SNP, it suggests that this particular SNP might have a direct association with the results, thereby violating assumption 3.

If heterogeneity was detected without pleiotropy, the weight median method or the multiplicative random-effects inverse variance weighting (mre-IVW) method was chosen for analysis. If there was identification of horizontal pleiotropy but no heterogeneity, the MR-Egger method was chosen. While the MR-Egger method is recognized for its resilience against pleiotropy, it is also influenced by diminished statistical accuracy and increased likelihood of Type I error in practical applications [29]. Therefore, if the IVW approach yielded a significant outcome without any detected pleiotropy or heterogeneity, while the outcomes of alternative methods were not significant but exhibited beta values in the same direction, it could be considered a favorable outcome. Additionally, to provide further clarification, scatter plots, forest plots, and funnel plots were generated.

2.6. Statistical Analysis

R software (version 4.3.0) was utilized for all analyses, employing the packages "TwoSampleMR" (version 0.5.7), "MRPRESSO," and "MR.RAPS". The level of statistical significance for evidence was established at $p < 0.05$. It is important to acknowledge that no correction methods for multiple testing were employed. After taking into account the possible constraints of implementing corrections, such as the Bonferroni correction, this choice was made, as it may severely limit the detection of causal relationships. Multiple test corrections are not always applicable, particularly in exploratory studies [30]. Due to the investigative character of our study, which sought to reveal fresh associations and impacts, the application of various test adjustment techniques was considered unsuitable for accomplishing our goals.

3. Results

3.1. UVMR Results in the Derivation Dataset

In the UVMR analysis of the derivation set, the screening threshold was set at $p < 1{\times}10^{-6}$ (as indicated in Table 2), and SNPs associated with confounding factors or NAFLD were excluded. The genetic prediction indicated that $PM_{2.5}$ was linked to a higher risk of NAFLD (OR = 4.83, 95% CI = [1.03–22.65], Pweighted median = 0.046), with heterogeneity observed and no evidence of pleiotropy. Based on the leave-one-out plot illustrated in Figure 2, it was observed that rs1318845 stood out as an anomalous SNP. After removing it, the UVMR calculation was performed again. Currently, the IVW approach yielded a positive outcome (OR = 4.26, 95% CI = [1.24–14.64], P_{IVW} = 0.021), with the absence of heterogeneity or pleiotropy. Figure 2 displays the scatter plots, funnel plots, and leave-one-out plots.

In the analysis of the derivation set using the UVMR set at $p < 1 \times 10^{-5}$ (shown in Table 3 and Figure 3), it was observed that $PM_{2.5}$ and NO_2 had a connection with NAFLD (OR = 1.99, 95% CI = [1.22–3.22], P_{IVW} = 0.005; OR = 2.08, 95% CI = [1.27–3.40], $P_{IVW\text{-}mre}$ = 0.004, respectively).

Moreover, there was no observed association between NAFLD and $PM_{2.5}$ absorbance, which served as a substitute for carbonaceous elements in $PM_{2.5}$. Table S4 showed that, when using the IVW, weighted median, MR-Egger, simple mode, weighted mode, and MR-RAPS methods, there was no indication of a causal connection between NAFLD and other air pollutants (IVW method, $PM_{2.5}$ absorbance: $p = 0.503$; $PM_{2.5\text{–}10}$: $p = 0.813$;

PM_{10}: $p = 0.124$; IVW-mre method, NO_x: $p = 0.159$). Table S4 displays the outcomes of the prejudice and type I error rates in MR with sample overlap, along with post hoc power calculations. Steiger-MR found that the SNPs accounted for a greater amount of variability in exposure compared to the outcome.

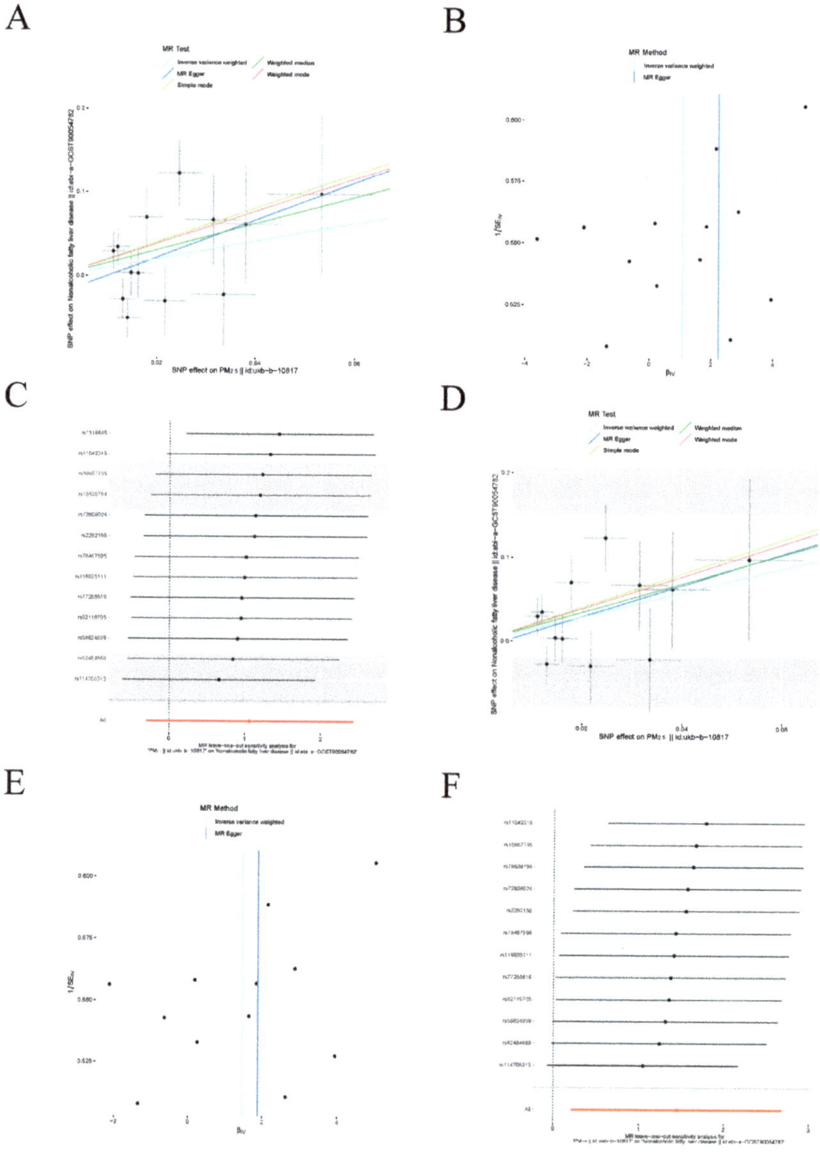

Figure 2. Scatter plots, funnel plots, and leaveone-out plots for causal SNP effects of $PM_{2.5}$ on non-alcoholic fatty liver disease in the derivation dataset at level $p < 1 \times 10^{-6}$. (**A**) Scatter plot (**B**) Funnel plot (**C**) Leave-one-out plot for the exposure of $PM_{2.5}$ before removing outlier-SNP. (**D**) Scatter plot (**E**) Funnel plot (**F**) Leave-one-out plot for the exposure of $PM_{2.5}$ after removing outlier-SNP. The error bars indicate the 95% confidence interval (CI).

Table 2. MR analytical results of air pollution on NAFLD in the derivation dataset at level $p < 1 \times 10^{-6}$.

Exposure	Method	OR (95% CI)	p	NSNP	F Statistic Median (Min, Max)	p (Cochran's Q Heterogeneity Test)	p (MR-Egger Intercept Test)	p (MR-PRESSO Global Test)
$PM_{2.5}$	IVW	2.88 (0.73–11.33)	0.129	13	26.0 (24.1, 30.1)	0.027	0.504	0.030
	MR Egger	9.33 (0.25–347.19)	0.251					
	Weighted median	4.83 (1.03–22.65)	0.046					
	IVW-mre	2.88 (0.73–11.33)	0.129					
	MR-RAPS	3.11 (1.12–8.60)	0.029					
$PM_{2.5}$ (Outlier-corrected)	IVW	4.26 (1.24–14.64)	0.021	12	25.9 (24.1, 30.1)	0.147	0.783	0.173
	MR Egger	6.53 (0.26–163.21)	0.280					
	Weighted median	5.59 (1.27–24.63)	0.023					
	IVW-mre	4.26 (1.24–14.64)	0.021					
	MR-RAPS	4.59 (1.56–13.44)	0.006					

Note: NSNP, number of Single Nucleotide Polymorphisms.

Table 3. MR analytical results of air pollution on NAFLD in the derivation dataset at level $p < 1 \times 10^{-5}$.

Exposure	Method	OR (95% CI)	p	NSNP	F Statistic Median (Min, Max)	p (Cochran's Q Heterogeneity Test)	p (MR-Egger Intercept Test)	p (MR-PRESSO Global Test)
$PM_{2.5}$	IVW	1.99 (1.22–3.22)	0.005	72	21.1 (19.6, 30.1)	0.321	0.317	0.313
	MR Egger	1.08 (0.30–3.88)	0.908					
	Weighted median	1.94 (0.98–3.80)	0.055					
	IVW-mre	1.99 (1.22–3.22)	0.005					
	MR-RAPS	2.06 (1.26–3.35)	0.004					
NO_2	IVW	2.08 (1.27–3.40)	0.004	89	22.1 (19.5, 37.8)	0.028	0.099	0.031
	MR Egger	5.63 (1.58–20.07)	0.009					
	Weighted median	1.76 (0.92–3.36)	0.085					
	IVW-mre	2.08 (1.27–3.40)	0.004					
	MR-RAPS	2.17 (1.39–3.40)	0.001					

Note: NSNP, number of Single Nucleotide Polymorphisms.

3.2. MVMR Results in the Derivation Dataset

To account for the influence caused by the interaction of $PM_{2.5}$ and NO_2, we conducted an MVMR analysis simultaneously considering $PM_{2.5}$ and NO_2 as exposures. As a result, the causal effects of $PM_{2.5}$ and NO_2 on NAFLD were absent after conducting MVMR analysis (OR = 1.42, 95% CI: 0.24–8.57, $p = 0.701$; OR = 1.49, 95% CI: 0.24–9.33, $p = 0.668$; respectively). At the same time, we accounted for the frequency of alcohol intake as a modifying factor for the relationship between air pollution and NAFLD risk. Subsequently, the MVMR analysis depicted in Figure 4 revealed that the connections between $PM_{2.5}$ and NO_2 with NAFLD (OR = 1.76, 95% CI = [0.98–3.14], $p = 0.057$; OR = 1.54, 95% CI = [0.84–2.80], $p = 0.159$, respectively) contradicted the estimates obtained from the UVMR analysis.

3.3. UVMR Results in the Validation Datasets

For further validation, we used two outcome datasets with different sample overlap ratios to perform UVMR. In the UVMR analysis of validation sets at $p < 1 \times 10^{-5}$, we found no causal relationship between $PM_{2.5}$, NO_2, and NAFLD using all MR methods (shown in Table S4). Steiger-MR found that the SNPs accounted for a greater amount of variability in exposure compared to the outcome.

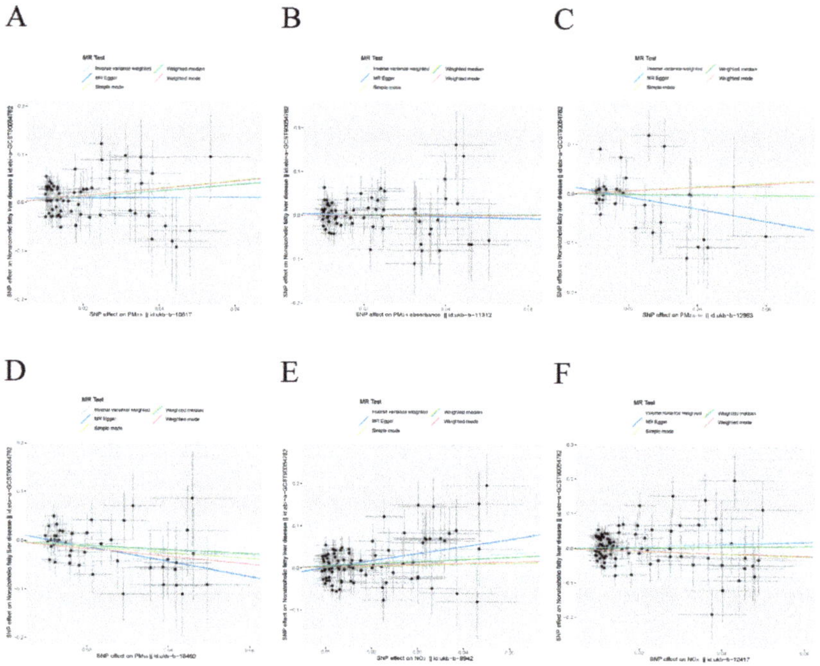

Figure 3. Scatter plots for visualizing the causal effects of air pollution on NAFLD in the derivation dataset at level $p < 1 \times 10^{-5}$. (**A–F**) Scatter plots for the exposure of $PM_{2.5}$, $PM_{2.5}$ absorbance, $PM_{2.5-10}$, PM_{10}, nitrogen dioxide, and nitrogen oxides, respectively. Each black point representing each SNP effect on the exposure (horizontal-axis) and outcome (vertical-axis) is plotted with error bars corresponding to standard error. The slope of each line corresponds to the combined estimate using different methods: inverse variance weighted (light blue line), MR-Egger (blue line), simple mode (light green line), weighted median (green line), and weighted mode (pink line).

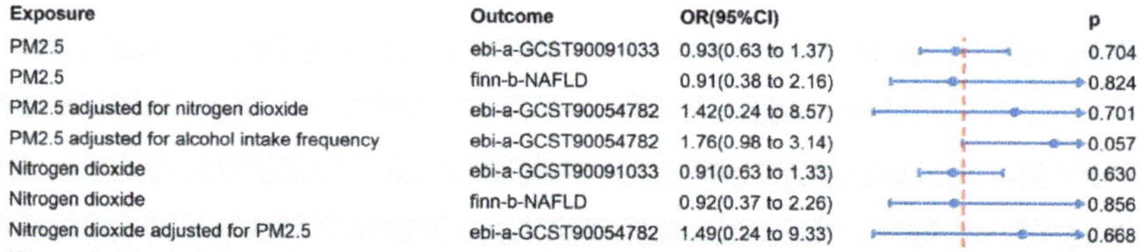

Figure 4. UVMR results of $PM_{2.5}$ and Nitrogen dioxide on NAFLD in the validation datasets and MVMR results in the derivation dataset at level $p < 1 \times 10^{-5}$. UVMR, univariable Mendelian randomization; MVMR, multivariable Mendelian randomization.

4. Discussion

Epidemiological studies on air pollution and NAFLD have been conducted around the world. Research from Asia presented consistent results. In two separate studies, which included 23,170 and 90,086 Chinese individuals, it was discovered that different air pollutants were linked to advanced liver fibrosis (ALF) in patients with metabolic-associated fatty liver disease (MAFLD) and increased odds of MAFLD itself. Notably, $PM_{2.5}$ emerged as the primary factor in these associations [31,32]. A study conducted in Taiwan involving around 35,000 Chinese Taiwanese individuals revealed that being exposed to $PM_{2.5}$ was linked to a higher chance of developing NAFLD [33]. Additionally, a separate study with 351,852 participants discovered that prolonged exposure to $PM_{2.5}$ might lead to higher levels of liver enzymes, particularly alanine aminotransferase (ALT) and γ-glutamyl transferase (γ-GT) [34]. Liver enzyme increases were also found to be linked to exposure to PM_{10} and CO in Korea [35]. Research from western countries presented contradictory results. According to research involving 2513 individuals from the Framingham (Massachusetts) Offspring Study and Third Generation Cohort, residing in proximity to main highways, instead of $PM_{2.5}$, was found to have a probable connection with liver fat [36]. Conversely, a study conducted in Germany involving 4814 inhabitants indicated a positive correlation between prolonged exposure to air pollution and NAFLD. The study found that the most reliable connections were observed between $PM_{2.5}$ and NAFLD. However, it did not establish a consistent link between air pollution exposure and an increased likelihood of advanced fibrosis [37]. Similarly, research involving 456,687 individuals residing in the United Kingdom discovered that the presence of $PM_{2.5}$, $PM_{2.5–10}$, PM_{10}, NO_2, and NO_x in the environment contributed to the additional hazard of NAFLD linked to air pollution scores. Furthermore, the impact of alcohol consumption acted as a modifying factor in the connection between these factors, as revealed by subgroup analysis. After adjusting for alcohol consumption and other covariates in the past 10 years, the majority of associations remained [15]. The derivation set of our study used the same sample source as the observational study and obtained similar results during the UVMR process. However, after adjusting for alcohol intake frequency as a confounding factor through MVMR, the previously discovered association disappeared. One possible reason was that the exposure sets and derivation outcome set used in this study were both from the UKB, so the results were affected by confounding factors during the UVMR process, which often occurred in single-sample Mendelian studies. Although we used parameter estimates to evaluate possible biases caused by sample overlap, and the results showed no unacceptable biases or inflated Type I error rates (Table S4), combining the MVMR results of the derivation set and the UVMR results of the validation sets, we still considered that the results in the derivation queue were false positive. In other words, the available data failed to substantiate the hypothesis of a causal association between air pollutants and NAFLD within the European population. Perhaps this was also the reason why $PM_{2.5}$ absorbance, representing the composition of carbon elements, was not found to have a causal relationship with NAFLD in this study.

However, even so, we cannot completely deny the potential impact of air pollutants on NAFLD. One possible inference is that there exists a threshold effect, which has sparked discussion in the field of cardiovascular disease [38]. The $PM_{2.5}$ level in the UKB datasets was 9.99 ± 1.06 μg/m^3 (Table S1), with 50% falling below 10 μg/m^3 and 90% below 12 μg/m^3, which are limits established by the European Union and the United States Environmental Protection Agency, respectively. The baseline level of air pollutant concentrations might influence the analysis results, so regional differences may lead to different results.

The significant results in animal models may also be due to this reason. Researchers found obvious changes in liver morphology and function in mice after short-term exposure to large amounts of inhalable pollutants, with doses far exceeding those that humans could come into contact with in their daily lives. For a period of 30 days, Leah J. Schneider et al. subjected three-month-old male C57Bl/6 mice to either a low-fat or high-fat (HF) diet and exposed them to either filtered air (FA) or MVE (30 μg/m^3 gasoline engine emissions + 70 μg/m^3 diesel engine emissions) for 6 h per day. Histology findings showed that MVE exposure alone resulted in mild microvesicular steatosis and hepatocyte hypertrophy, compared to FA controls. Additionally, the mixed effect of HF diet and MVE exposure led to increased lipid accumulation, inflammatory infiltrates, and hepatocyte hypertrophy [39]. Hui-Hui Tan et al. exposed mice to $PM_{2.5}$ at an average level of 85 μg/m^3 for 6 weeks; it was discovered that exposure to PM significantly enhanced the secretion of IL-6 by isolated wild-type Kupffer cells. The increase in IL-6 secretion was up to seven times higher and showed a dependence on the dosage, whereas $TLR4^{-/-}$ Kupffer cells did not exhibit the same response. The progression of NAFLD is significantly influenced by the activation of

TLR in Kupffer cells, which are macrophages residing in the liver, leading to the production of pro-inflammatory cytokines. Dongxiao Ding et al. verified that a 3-day exposure to liposoluble extracts of $PM_{2.5}$ at a concentration of 25 $\mu g/cm^2$ caused the accumulation of lipids in HepG2 cells. This accumulation was linked to a reduction in the expression of miR-26a and a subsequent increase in the levels of fatty acid translocase (FAT, or CD36), whose increase resulted in enhanced uptake of free fatty acids (FFAs) [40].

At present, the disease progression of NAFLD from simple steatosis is elucidated by the "two-hit" theory. The "first hit" involves reversible and simple fat accumulation (fatty liver or steatosis). Excessive buildup of triglycerides (TG) in liver cells occurs due to heightened absorption of lipids and the synthesis of new lipids, inadequate breakdown of fatty acids oxidation (FAO), and diminished release of lipids [41]. The "second hit" encompasses various damages and conditions, such as inflammatory cytokines, oxidative stress, and toxins, promoting the advancement of NAFLD to non-alcoholic steatohepatitis (NASH), fibrosis, and hepatocellular carcinoma [42]. For example, augmented lipid content and impaired FAO facilitate the generation of reactive oxygen species and lipophilic lipid intermediates in hepatic cells, promoting oxidative stress and endoplasmic reticulum stress. Chronic oxidative stress initiates an inflammatory reaction, primarily through the activation of the JNK and NF-κB signaling pathways. This results in an increased production of pro-inflammatory proteins (i.e., IL-6 and TNF-α) transmitted by liver cells and non-parenchymal cells [43]. The continuous stimulation of pro-inflammatory reactions sustains a persistent state of inflammation, leading to the enlistment of additional immune cells and the initiation of cellular apoptosis and other mechanisms of cell demise. Cell damage and apoptosis can be promoted by non-triglyceride lipid substances, including long-chain fatty acids, and their products, such as ceramides and diacylglycerols, leading to the harmful effects of lipid accumulation in liver cells known as lipotoxicity [44]. Extended exposure to PM2.5 resulted in elevated insulin resistance, impaired glucose tolerance, peripheral inflammation, and dysarteriotony in mice induced by $PM_{2.5}$. Moreover, the hepatic function and lipid accumulation in the liver were significantly influenced by the inflammation response and oxidative stress, as indicated by previous research [45]. This phenomenon can be described as a "second hit" for NAFLD. Other air pollutants have also been tested in animal models. Female mice exposed to NO_2 experienced elevated levels of hepatic enzymes in their serum, resulting in liver dysfunction. However, this effect was not observed in male mice. Furthermore, NO_2 disrupted the process of glucose metabolism by decreasing the synthesis of hepatic glycogen and increasing the production of glucose, while also promoting lipid deposition through increased lipogenesis and uptake. As a result, it led to elevated levels of lipid oxidation and secretion [46].

Over the last three years, there has been widespread utilization of Mendelian randomization to establish a causal relationship between the two diseases. Recently, there has been a growing application of this method to investigate the link between pollutants and diseases. Liu C.X. et al. discovered casual links between $PM_{2.5}$ and high blood pressure, T2D, and obesity [47]. Similarly, Li W.J. et al. identified positive associations between NO_x exposure and squamous cell lung cancer as well as esophageal cancer; between NO_2 exposure and endometrial cancer as well as ovarian cancer; between $PM_{2.5}$ exposure and ER+ breast cancer as well as ER- breast cancer; between PM_{course} exposure and glioma; and between PM_{10} exposure and mesothelioma as well as esophageal cancer [48]. Ning P.P. et al. found that PM_{10} was associated with an increased risk of Alzheimer's disease [49]. Qiu S.Z. et al. found that, while the link between $PM_{2.5}$ levels and lifespan was not statistically significant, $PM_{2.5}$ exposure indirectly impacts lifespan through factors such as diastolic blood pressure (DBP), high blood pressure, angina pectoris, high cholesterol, and Alzheimer's disease [50].

Our MR study has several advantages. Although there have been clinical cohort studies focused on air pollutants and NAFLD in various regions, as well as animal studies using different modeling methods, this is the first study to explore the influence of air pollutants on NAFLD using human GWAS data. Based on previously published authoritative epidemiological studies, the derivation set and validation sets were selected within the same race with different sample overlap rates, making the results comparable. Moreover, we used different MR methods and threshold conditions in the derivation set for discovery. At the same time, MVMR was used in the derivation set and UVMR was used in the validation sets for checking, which deepened the credibility of the results.

This study is subject to certain limitations. Recently, some researchers have questioned the use of MR to explore the relationship between air pollution and other diseases. The estimation of air pollutants was typically conducted by utilizing an individual's residential address. Au Yeung believes that the use of MR is inappropriate because any genetic associations with air pollutants could easily be a reflection of hidden confounding, rendering the positive findings uninterpretable in relation to the research questions originally posed [51]. The application of MR in this article may also face such doubts, but it is still meaningful due to different study designs and assumption directions. Different from traditional MR, which attaches importance to evaluating the biological plausibility of genetics, MR in this article is only used as a mathematical statistical inference method, compared with traditional regression analysis methods used in epidemiology using the same exposure dataset. Presently, the prevailing techniques for sampling environmental air pollution rely on fixed-location and time-sampling methods, with the UKB serving as the most extensively utilized and expansive database in traditional epidemiological research. There may be varying degrees of confusion bias due to exposure and outcome datasets coming from the same source, so this article used two different outcome datasets as validation sets to reduce the interference of confounding factors. Meanwhile, when traditional epidemiology corrects confounding factors, the results may also be disrupted due to incomplete correction, so this article applied MVMR with confounding factor data from the same source as an exposure dataset for adjustment and obtained different results from the traditional epidemiology. Different statistical inference methods were used for the same dataset, resulting in different results and opposite conclusions, which made the finding valuable despite the use of MR potentially violating the assumption of biocompatibility to some extent. In addition, the MR analysis was conducted solely on individuals with European heritage, and this association might vary in individuals of different ancestries such as a South-East Asian population exposed to different levels of outdoor and indoor air pollution and with different distributions of confounders. Additionally, the data sets employed in our research had constraints regarding the air pollutant constituents. For instance, the absence of explicit $PM_{2.5}$ component data in the summarized data hindered our ability to carry out additional subgroup analyses. Therefore, more research is still needed to determine whether different air pollutants can increase the risk of NAFLD and how.

5. Conclusions

In conclusion, this MR study provides genetic evidence for a null causal relationship between air pollution and NAFLD in the European population. Perhaps confounding elements have played an undeniable role in epidemiological studies that have found atmospheric pollutants were positively bound up with NAFLD. More human data and animal experiments are warranted to enhance our understanding in this area.

Supplementary Materials: The following supporting information can be downloaded at: https://www.mdpi.com/article/10.3390/toxics12030228/s1, Table S1: Detailed information about exposure and outcome in the MR study; Table S2: Characteristics of the genetic instrument variables for the air pollution on NAFLD in the derivation dataset in the MR study at the genome-wide significance level ($p < 1 \times 10^{-5}$); Table S3: Characteristics of the SNPs correlated with the confounding factors for NAFLD or NAFLD directly at genome-wide significance level ($p < 1 \times 10^{-5}$); Table S4: MR analytical results of air pollution on NAFLD at different significance levels; STROBE-MR checklist.

Author Contributions: J.Y. and Y.Z. designed and conducted the analysis of the data. J.Y. and Y.Y. drafted the manuscript. Z.X. and L.L. revised the manuscript. All authors have read and agreed to the published version of the manuscript.

Funding: Grant from Zhejiang Province Basic Public Welfare Research Program (LQ23H030006).

Institutional Review Board Statement: This study was based on published databases and did not require ethical approval.

Informed Consent Statement: Not applicable.

Data Availability Statement: Only publicly available data were used in this study. Data sources and handling of these data are described in the Materials and Methods, Table 1, and Supplementary Tables S1–S4. The corresponding author can provide all the necessary data and materials supporting the findings of this work upon a reasonable request.

Acknowledgments: We thank the IEU Open GWAS project, UK Biobank, and Finngen consortium, as well as the research groups led by Benoit J. Arsenault and Ewen M. Harrison, for generously supplying the summary results data utilized in the analyses.

Conflicts of Interest: The authors affirm that they do not have any conflicting interests to disclose.

Abbreviations

PM	particulate matter
NO_2	nitrogen dioxide
NO_x	nitrogen oxides
NAFLD	non-alcoholic fatty liver disease
MAFLD	metabolic-associated fatty liver disease
MR	Mendelian randomization
UVMR	univariable Mendelian randomization
MVMR	multivariable Mendelian randomization
GWAS	Genome-Wide Association Study
SNPs	single nucleotide polymorphisms
IVs	instrumental variables
OR	odds ratio
CI	confidence interval
UKB	UK Biobank
MRC-IEU	UK Medical Research Council Integrative Epidemiology Unit
EGCUT	Estonian Genome Center of the University of Tartu
STROBE-MR	Strengthening observational studies using Mendelian randomization
MR-RAPS	MR-Robust Adjusted Profile Score
MR-PRESSO	MR-Pleiotropy RESidual Sum and Outlier
mre-IVW/IVW-mre	multiplicative random-effects inverse variance weighting

References

1. Younossi, Z.; Anstee, Q.M.; Marietti, M.; Hardy, T.; Henry, L.; Eslam, M.; George, J.; Bugianesi, E. Global Burden of NAFLD and NASH: Trends, Predictions, Risk Factors and Prevention. *Nat. Rev. Gastroenterol. Hepatol.* **2018**, *15*, 11–20. [CrossRef] [PubMed]
2. Mantovani, A.; Scorletti, E.; Mosca, A.; Alisi, A.; Byrne, C.D.; Targher, G. Complications, Morbidity and Mortality of Nonalcoholic Fatty Liver Disease. *Metab. Clin. Exp.* **2020**, *111*, 154170. [CrossRef]
3. Targher, G.; Corey, K.E.; Byrne, C.D.; Roden, M. The Complex Link between NAFLD and Type 2 Diabetes Mellitus—Mechanisms and Treatments. *Nat. Rev. Gastroenterol. Hepatol.* **2021**, *18*, 599–612. [CrossRef] [PubMed]
4. Cazac, G.; Lăcătușu, C.-M.; Mihai, C.; Grigorescu, E.-D.; Onofriescu, A.; Mihai, B. New Insights into Non-Alcoholic Fatty Liver Disease and Coronary Artery Disease: The Liver-Heart Axis. *Life* **2022**, *12*, 1189. [CrossRef] [PubMed]
5. Jo, S.; Kim, Y.-J.; Park, K.W.; Hwang, Y.S.; Lee, S.H.; Kim, B.J.; Chung, S.J. Association of NO2 and Other Air Pollution Exposures With the Risk of Parkinson Disease. *JAMA Neurol.* **2021**, *78*, 800–808. [CrossRef]
6. Jones, R.R.; Fisher, J.A.; Hasheminassab, S.; Kaufman, J.D.; Freedman, N.D.; Ward, M.H.; Sioutas, C.; Vermeulen, R.; Hoek, G.; Silverman, D.T. Outdoor Ultrafine Particulate Matter and Risk of Lung Cancer in Southern California. *Am. J. Respir. Crit. Care Med.* **2024**, *209*, 307–315. [CrossRef] [PubMed]
7. Chen, J.; Dan, L.; Sun, Y.; Yuan, S.; Liu, W.; Chen, X.; Jiang, F.; Fu, T.; Zhang, H.; Deng, M.; et al. Ambient Air Pollution and Risk of Enterotomy, Gastrointestinal Cancer, and All-Cause Mortality among 4,708 Individuals with Inflammatory Bowel Disease: A Prospective Cohort Study. *Environ. Health Perspect.* **2023**, *131*, 77010. [CrossRef]
8. Kentros, P.A.; Huang, Y.; Wylie, B.J.; Khoury-Collado, F.; Hou, J.Y.; de Meritens, A.B.; St Clair, C.M.; Hershman, D.L.; Wright, J.D. Ambient Particulate Matter Air Pollution Exposure and Ovarian Cancer Incidence in the USA: An Ecological Study. *BJOG* **2023**, *131*, 690–698. [CrossRef]

9. Li, Y.; Fan, Z.; Lu, W.; Xu, R.; Liu, T.; Liu, L.; Chen, G.; Lv, Z.; Huang, S.; Zhou, Y.; et al. Long-Term Exposure to Ambient Fine Particulate Matter-Bound Polycyclic Aromatic Hydrocarbons and Cancer Mortality: A Difference-in-Differences Approach. *Chemosphere* **2023**, *340*, 139800. [CrossRef]
10. Cohen, A.J.; Brauer, M.; Burnett, R.; Anderson, H.R.; Frostad, J.; Estep, K.; Balakrishnan, K.; Brunekreef, B.; Dandona, L.; Dandona, R.; et al. Estimates and 25-Year Trends of the Global Burden of Disease Attributable to Ambient Air Pollution: An Analysis of Data from the Global Burden of Diseases Study 2015. *Lancet* **2017**, *389*, 1907–1918. [CrossRef]
11. Zhao, N.; Wu, W.; Feng, Y.; Yang, F.; Han, T.; Guo, M.; Ren, Q.; Li, W.; Li, J.; Wang, S.; et al. Polymorphisms in Oxidative Stress, Metabolic Detoxification, and Immune Function Genes, Maternal Exposure to Ambient Air Pollution, and Risk of Preterm Birth in Taiyuan, China. *Environ. Res.* **2021**, *194*, 110659. [CrossRef]
12. Kim, J.H.; Lee, S.; Hong, Y.-C. Modification Effect of PARP4 and ERCC1 Gene Polymorphisms on the Relationship between Particulate Matter Exposure and Fasting Glucose Level. *Int. J. Environ. Res. Public. Health* **2022**, *19*, 6241. [CrossRef]
13. Yang, S.-I.; Kim, B.-J.; Lee, S.-Y.; Kim, H.-B.; Lee, C.M.; Yu, J.; Kang, M.-J.; Yu, H.-S.; Lee, E.; Jung, Y.-H.; et al. Prenatal Particulate Matter/Tobacco Smoke Increases Infants' Respiratory Infections: COCOA Study. *Allergy Asthma Immunol. Res.* **2015**, *7*, 573–582. [CrossRef]
14. Emdin, C.A.; Khera, A.V.; Kathiresan, S. Mendelian Randomization. *JAMA* **2017**, *318*, 1925–1926. [CrossRef]
15. Li, F.-R.; Liao, J.; Zhu, B.; Li, X.; Cheng, Z.; Jin, C.; Mo, C.; Wu, X.; Li, Q.; Liang, F. Long-Term Exposure to Air Pollution and Incident Non-Alcoholic Fatty Liver Disease and Cirrhosis: A Cohort Study. *Liver Int.* **2023**, *43*, 299–307. [CrossRef] [PubMed]
16. Skrivankova, V.W.; Richmond, R.C.; Woolf, B.A.R.; Davies, N.M.; Swanson, S.A.; VanderWeele, T.J.; Timpson, N.J.; Higgins, J.P.T.; Dimou, N.; Langenberg, C.; et al. Strengthening the Reporting of Observational Studies in Epidemiology Using Mendelian Randomisation (STROBE-MR): Explanation and Elaboration. *BMJ* **2021**, *375*, n2233. [CrossRef] [PubMed]
17. Eeftens, M.; Beelen, R.; de Hoogh, K.; Bellander, T.; Cesaroni, G.; Cirach, M.; Declercq, C.; Dėdelė, A.; Dons, E.; de Nazelle, A.; et al. Development of Land Use Regression Models for PM(2.5), PM(2.5) Absorbance, PM(10) and PM(Coarse) in 20 European Study Areas; Results of the ESCAPE Project. *Environ. Sci. Technol.* **2012**, *46*, 11195–11205. [CrossRef]
18. Fairfield, C.J.; Drake, T.M.; Pius, R.; Bretherick, A.D.; Campbell, A.; Clark, D.W.; Fallowfield, J.A.; Hayward, C.; Henderson, N.C.; Joshi, P.K.; et al. Genome-Wide Association Study of NAFLD Using Electronic Health Records. *Hepatol. Commun.* **2022**, *6*, 297–308. [CrossRef]
19. Ghodsian, N.; Abner, E.; Emdin, C.A.; Gobeil, É.; Taba, N.; Haas, M.E.; Perrot, N.; Manikpurage, H.D.; Gagnon, É.; Bourgault, J.; et al. Electronic Health Record-Based Genome-Wide Meta-Analysis Provides Insights on the Genetic Architecture of Non-Alcoholic Fatty Liver Disease. *Cell Rep. Med.* **2021**, *2*, 100437. [CrossRef] [PubMed]
20. Kurki, M.I.; Karjalainen, J.; Palta, P.; Sipilä, T.P.; Kristiansson, K.; Donner, K.M.; Reeve, M.P.; Laivuori, H.; Aavikko, M.; Kaunisto, M.A.; et al. FinnGen Provides Genetic Insights from a Well-Phenotyped Isolated Population. *Nature* **2023**, *613*, 508–518. [CrossRef]
21. Burgess, S.; Butterworth, A.; Thompson, S.G. Mendelian Randomization Analysis with Multiple Genetic Variants Using Summarized Data. *Genet. Epidemiol.* **2013**, *37*, 658–665. [CrossRef]
22. Hemani, G.; Tilling, K.; Davey Smith, G. Orienting the Causal Relationship between Imprecisely Measured Traits Using GWAS Summary Data. *PLoS Genet.* **2017**, *13*, e1007081. [CrossRef]
23. Thompson, S.B.; Simon, G. *Mendelian Randomization: Methods for Causal Inference Using Genetic Variants*, 2nd ed.; Chapman and Hall/CRC: New York, NY, USA, 2021; ISBN 978-0-429-32435-2.
24. Slob, E.A.W.; Burgess, S. A Comparison of Robust Mendelian Randomization Methods Using Summary Data. *Genet. Epidemiol.* **2020**, *44*, 313–329. [CrossRef] [PubMed]
25. Brion, M.-J.A.; Shakhbazov, K.; Visscher, P.M. Calculating Statistical Power in Mendelian Randomization Studies. *Int. J. Epidemiol.* **2013**, *42*, 1497–1501. [CrossRef]
26. Greco, M.F.D.; Minelli, C.; Sheehan, N.A.; Thompson, J.R. Detecting Pleiotropy in Mendelian Randomisation Studies with Summary Data and a Continuous Outcome. *Stat. Med.* **2015**, *34*, 2926–2940. [CrossRef] [PubMed]
27. Verbanck, M.; Chen, C.-Y.; Neale, B.; Do, R. Detection of Widespread Horizontal Pleiotropy in Causal Relationships Inferred from Mendelian Randomization between Complex Traits and Diseases. *Nat. Genet.* **2018**, *50*, 693–698. [CrossRef] [PubMed]
28. Burgess, S.; Bowden, J.; Fall, T.; Ingelsson, E.; Thompson, S.G. Sensitivity Analyses for Robust Causal Inference from Mendelian Randomization Analyses with Multiple Genetic Variants. *Epidemiology* **2017**, *28*, 30–42. [CrossRef] [PubMed]
29. Burgess, S.; Thompson, S.G. Interpreting Findings from Mendelian Randomization Using the MR-Egger Method. *Eur. J. Epidemiol.* **2017**, *32*, 377–389. [CrossRef]
30. Gelbard, R.B.; Cripps, M.W. Pitfalls in Study Interpretation. *Surg. Infect. (Larchmt)* **2021**, *22*, 646–650. [CrossRef]
31. Xing, Y.; Gao, X.; Li, Q.; Li, X.; Wang, Y.; Yang, Y.; Yang, S.; Lau, P.W.C.; Zeng, Q.; Wang, H. Associations between Exposure to Ambient Particulate Matter and Advanced Liver Fibrosis in Chinese MAFLD Patients. *J. Hazard. Mater.* **2023**, *460*, 132501. [CrossRef]
32. Guo, B.; Guo, Y.; Nima, Q.; Feng, Y.; Wang, Z.; Lu, R.; Baimayangji; Ma, Y.; Zhou, J.; Xu, H.; et al. Exposure to Air Pollution Is Associated with an Increased Risk of Metabolic Dysfunction-Associated Fatty Liver Disease. *J. Hepatol.* **2022**, *76*, 518–525. [CrossRef]
33. Sun, S.; Yang, Q.; Zhou, Q.; Cao, W.; Yu, S.; Zhan, S.; Sun, F. Long-Term Exposure to Air Pollution, Habitual Physical Activity and Risk of Non-Alcoholic Fatty Liver Disease: A Prospective Cohort Study. *Ecotoxicol. Environ. Saf.* **2022**, *235*, 113440. [CrossRef] [PubMed]

34. Zhang, Z.; Guo, C.; Chang, L.-Y.; Bo, Y.; Lin, C.; Tam, T.; Hoek, G.; Wong, M.C.; Chan, T.-C.; Lau, A.K.; et al. Long-Term Exposure to Ambient Fine Particulate Matter and Liver Enzymes in Adults: A Cross-Sectional Study in Taiwan. *Occup. Environ. Med.* **2019**, *76*, 488–494. [CrossRef] [PubMed]
35. Kim, H.-J.; Min, J.-Y.; Seo, Y.-S.; Min, K.-B. Association of Ambient Air Pollution with Increased Liver Enzymes in Korean Adults. *Int. J. Environ. Res. Public. Health* **2019**, *16*, 1213. [CrossRef]
36. Li, W.; Dorans, K.S.; Wilker, E.H.; Rice, M.B.; Long, M.T.; Schwartz, J.; Coull, B.A.; Koutrakis, P.; Gold, D.R.; Fox, C.S.; et al. Residential Proximity to Major Roadways, Fine Particulate Matter, and Hepatic Steatosis. *Am. J. Epidemiol.* **2017**, *186*, 857–865. [CrossRef]
37. Matthiessen, C.; Glaubitz, L.; Lucht, S.; Kälsch, J.; Luedde, T.; Erbel, R.; Stang, A.; Schmidt, B.; Friedman, S.L.; Canbay, A.; et al. Long-Term Exposure to Air Pollution and Prevalent Nonalcoholic Fatty Liver Disease. *Environ. Epidemiol.* **2023**, *7*, e268. [CrossRef]
38. Liang, X.; Liang, L.; Fan, Y. Two-Sample Mendelian Randomization Analysis Investigates Ambient Fine Particulate Matter's Impact on Cardiovascular Disease Development. *Sci. Rep.* **2023**, *13*, 20129. [CrossRef]
39. Schneider, L.J.; Santiago, I.; Johnson, B.; Stanley, A.H.; Penaredondo, B.; Lund, A.K. Histological Features of Non-Alcoholic Fatty Liver Disease Revealed in Response to Mixed Vehicle Emission Exposure and Consumption of a High-Fat Diet in Wildtype C57Bl/6 Male Mice. *Ecotoxicol. Environ. Saf.* **2023**, *261*, 115094. [CrossRef]
40. Ding, D.; Ye, G.; Lin, Y.; Lu, Y.; Zhang, H.; Zhang, X.; Hong, Z.; Huang, Q.; Chi, Y.; Chen, J.; et al. MicroRNA-26a-CD36 Signaling Pathway: Pivotal Role in Lipid Accumulation in Hepatocytes Induced by PM2.5 Liposoluble Extracts. *Environ. Pollut.* **2019**, *248*, 269–278. [CrossRef] [PubMed]
41. Powell, E.E.; Wong, V.W.-S.; Rinella, M. Non-Alcoholic Fatty Liver Disease. *Lancet* **2021**, *397*, 2212–2224. [CrossRef]
42. Luci, C.; Bourinet, M.; Leclère, P.S.; Anty, R.; Gual, P. Chronic Inflammation in Non-Alcoholic Steatohepatitis: Molecular Mechanisms and Therapeutic Strategies. *Front. Endocrinol.* **2020**, *11*, 597648. [CrossRef]
43. Monserrat-Mesquida, M.; Quetglas-Llabrés, M.; Abbate, M.; Montemayor, S.; Mascaró, C.M.; Casares, M.; Tejada, S.; Abete, I.; Zulet, M.A.; Tur, J.A.; et al. Oxidative Stress and Pro-Inflammatory Status in Patients with Non-Alcoholic Fatty Liver Disease. *Antioxidants* **2020**, *9*, 759. [CrossRef] [PubMed]
44. Mendez-Sanchez, N.; Cruz-Ramon, V.C.; Ramirez-Perez, O.L.; Hwang, J.P.; Barranco-Fragoso, B.; Cordova-Gallardo, J. New Aspects of Lipotoxicity in Nonalcoholic Steatohepatitis. *Int. J. Mol. Sci.* **2018**, *19*, 2034. [CrossRef] [PubMed]
45. Xu, M.-X.; Ge, C.-X.; Qin, Y.-T.; Gu, T.-T.; Lou, D.-S.; Li, Q.; Hu, L.-F.; Feng, J.; Huang, P.; Tan, J. Prolonged PM2.5 Exposure Elevates Risk of Oxidative Stress-Driven Nonalcoholic Fatty Liver Disease by Triggering Increase of Dyslipidemia. *Free Radic. Biol. Med.* **2019**, *130*, 542–556. [CrossRef]
46. Li, D.; Ji, S.; Guo, Y.; Sang, N. Ambient NO2 Exposure Sex-Specifically Impairs Myelin and Contributes to Anxiety and Depression-like Behaviors of C57BL/6J Mice. *J. Hazard. Mater.* **2021**, *416*, 125836. [CrossRef]
47. Liu, C.-X.; Liu, Y.-B.; Peng, Y.; Peng, J.; Ma, Q.-L. Causal Effect of Air Pollution on the Risk of Cardiovascular and Metabolic Diseases and Potential Mediation by Gut Microbiota. *Sci. Total Environ.* **2023**, *912*, 169418. [CrossRef] [PubMed]
48. Li, W.; Wang, W. Causal Effects of Exposure to Ambient Air Pollution on Cancer Risk: Insights from Genetic Evidence. *Sci. Total Environ.* **2023**, *912*, 168843. [CrossRef]
49. Ning, P.; Guo, X.; Qu, Q.; Li, R. Exploring the Association between Air Pollution and Parkinson's Disease or Alzheimer's Disease: A Mendelian Randomization Study. *Environ. Sci. Pollut. Res. Int.* **2023**, *30*, 123939–123947. [CrossRef]
50. Qiu, S.; Hu, Y.; Liu, G. Mendelian Randomization Study Supports the Causal Effects of Air Pollution on Longevity via Multiple Age-Related Diseases. *npj Aging* **2023**, *9*, 29. [CrossRef]
51. Au Yeung, S.L.; Gill, D. Concerns over Using the Mendelian Randomization Design to Investigate the Effect of Air Pollution. *Sci. Total Environ.* **2024**, *917*, 170474. [CrossRef]

toxics

MDPI

Article

Lipid Dysregulation Induced by Gasoline and Diesel Exhaust Exposure and the Interaction with Age

Yutong Gao [1], Xinzhuo Zhang [2], Xinting Li [1], Jinsheng Zhang [1], Zongyan Lv [1], Dongping Guo [1], Hongjun Mao [1] and Ting Wang [1,*]

1 Tianjin Key Laboratory of Urban Transport Emission Research, State Environmental Protection Key Laboratory of Urban Ambient Air Particulate Matter Pollution Prevention and Control, College of Environmental Science and Engineering, Nankai University, Tianjin 300071, China
2 Department of Visual Optics Medicine, Tianjin Medical University, Tianjin 300070, China
* Correspondence: wangting@nankai.edu.cn

Abstract: Limited knowledge exists regarding gasoline and diesel exhaust effects on lipid metabolism. This study collected gasoline and diesel exhaust under actual driving conditions and conducted inhalation exposure on male young and middle-aged C57BL/6J mice for 4 h/day for 5 days to simulate commuting exposure intensity. Additionally, $PM_{2.5}$ from actual roadways, representing gasoline and diesel vehicles, was generated for exposure to human umbilical vein endothelial cells (HUVECs) and normal liver cells (LO2) for 24, 48, and 72 h to further investigate exhaust particle toxicity. Results showed that diesel exhaust reduced total cholesterol and low-density lipoprotein cholesterol levels in young mice, indicating disrupted lipid metabolism. Aspartate aminotransferase and alanine aminotransferase levels increased by 53.7% and 21.7%, respectively, suggesting potential liver injury. Diesel exhaust exposure decreased superoxide dismutase and increased glutathione peroxidase levels. Cell viability decreased, and reactive oxygen species levels increased in HUVECs and LO2 following exposure to exhaust particles, with dose- and time-dependent effects. Diesel exhaust particles exhibited more severe inhibition of cell proliferation and oxidative damage compared to gasoline exhaust particles. These findings provide novel evidence of the risk of disrupted lipid metabolism due to gasoline and diesel exhaust, emphasizing the toxicity of diesel exhaust.

Keywords: gasoline exhaust; diesel exhaust; lipid metabolism; liver function; oxidative stress

1. Introduction

Road traffic represents a major source of air pollutants in cities, exposing pedestrians and vehicle passengers to high concentrations of locally generated pollutants [1]. Various air pollutants are emitted from road vehicles, including but not limited to black carbon (BC), elemental carbon (EC), carbon monoxide (CO), hydrocarbons (HC), nitrogen oxides (NOx), nitrogen dioxide (NO_2), fine particulate matter ($PM_{2.5}$, aerodynamic diameter of $\leq$2.5 μm), etc., which contribute to the complexity of pollution compositions and concentrations of vehicle exhausts. Fuel type is one of the main influence factors of air pollutants derived from vehicle emission [2,3]. The most common fuel in private road passenger transport is gasoline, whereas diesel is the most common fuel in public road passenger and freight transit [4]. Most of the existing heavy-duty vehicles and some types of medium- and light-duty vehicles, including public buses, trucks, machinery, etc., are run with diesel [5]. Diesel vehicles emit a higher proportion of BC and NOx compared to gasoline vehicles [6]. The study in an exemplary emission hotspot of Germany's North Rhine-Westphalia has shown that diesel vehicles contribute 71% of PM_{10} (of an aerodynamic diameter of $\leq$10 μm) emissions and 91% of NOx emissions, while gasoline vehicles contribute 29% of PM_{10} emissions and 9% of NOx emissions [7]. In China, it is reported that gasoline vehicles are responsible for 80.9% of CO, 77.6% of HC and 4.8% of NOx from total vehicle emissions, while 18.0% of CO, 11.4% of HC, 88.8% of NOx and >99% of PM are produced by diesel vehicles, according to the China Mobile Source Environmental Management Annual Report in 2021 (https://www.mee.gov.cn/hjzl/sthjzk/ydyhjgl/202109/t20210910_920787.shtml accessed on 1 August 2023).

Epidemiological studies have suggested the adverse health effects of diesel and gasoline exhaust exposure [8–12]. Recent experimental studies have mainly focused on the health impacts induced by diesel exhaust particles. In a study by Vesterdal et al. [13], in vivo and in vitro experiments using liver cells demonstrated oxidative stress and lipid accumulation following exposure to diesel exhaust particles. Through an in vitro cell study, Tseng et al. [14] found that inhalation of diesel exhaust particles induced oxidative stress in endothelial cells, leading to endothelial cell apoptosis. Lung exposure to diesel engine exhaust particles (DEP) has been associated with oxidative stress and lipid accumulation in the livers of obese diabetic mice [15]. In vivo studies by Miller et al. [16] demonstrated increased atherosclerotic plaque size and plasma lipid peroxidation in mice exposed to DEP. An in vitro cell study on gasoline exhaust particles showed that ultrafine particles present in gasoline exhaust also induced significant oxidative stress, lipid peroxidation, and cell inflammation [17]. In summary, the primary mechanism may involve the induction of inflammation and oxidative stress [18,19], with reactive oxygen species (ROS) generated by oxidative stress leading to the release of vascular permeability factor/vascular endothelial growth factor A, which affects the permeability of intercellular adhesion junctions [20]. Subsequently, particles may pass through the vascular endothelial-calcium-VE-cadherin network and enter the circulatory system [21], potentially affecting lipid metabolism in the human body. In actual situations, the penetration of gasoline and diesel fuels is diverse among on-road vehicle fleets in different regions. The different fuel-type compositions of vehicle fleets cause spatial variability in exhaust emissions, which may result in varying degrees of health effects [22]. In the downtown area, the vehicle fleet is mainly composed of gasoline vehicles, while there is a considerable proportion of diesel vehicles in the suburban area [23]. Therefore, in the real world, there are significant differences in the health effects of traffic-related air pollution on people living in downtown and suburban areas. However, there is still a lack of direct and comprehensive comparison of the health effects of gasoline and diesel emissions exposure under actual traffic exposure levels.

Lipid metabolism plays a critical role in the synthesis, breakdown, and utilization of fats in the human body, which is crucial for maintaining energy balance and storing body fat. Abnormal lipid metabolism is closely associated with metabolic diseases such as diabetes [24] and cardiovascular diseases, including coronary heart disease, myocardial infarction, and stroke [25], potentially leading to lipid deposition in arterial walls and the development of atherosclerosis. Lipid metabolism abnormalities may interact with inflammatory and oxidative stress conditions [25], forming a vicious cycle that accelerates disease progression. In addition, the lipid metabolism undergoes alteration with advancing age [26,27]. With the aging process, the cell's protective ability degrades. The aging process induces the progressive degeneration of cell protective ability, leading to well-defined phenotypic changes in blood vessels and a heightened susceptibility to cardiovascular system diseases [28]. Moreover, young individuals are in a developmental stage characterized by hormonal fluctuations and rapid maturation of organ systems; their lipid metabolism systems are typically more sensitive, which implies that metabolic processes are vulnerable to environmental perturbations during puberty [29]. Existing evidence has proven that age is one of the most important factors in the health effects of environmental pollutants [30,31]. However, the comparative study of the impacts of exposure to diesel and gasoline exhaust on lipid metabolism remains unclear. Furthermore, study of the interaction effect between vehicle exhaust and age is still lacking. Therefore, young and middle-aged C57BL/6J mice were exposed to diesel and gasoline exhaust from vehicles on a chassis dynamometer under actual traffic exposure levels. The effects on blood lipids, liver function, and oxidative stress levels were investigated to evaluate the impacts of diesel and gasoline exhaust on lipid metabolism. Furthermore, based on the results of the in vivo experiment, in vitro experiments using human umbilical vein endothelial cells (HUVECs) and human normal liver cells (LO2) were conducted to investigate the potential mechanisms of diesel and gasoline exhaust exposure. This research will provide scientific evidence for understanding the link between diesel and gasoline exhaust exposure and metabolic diseases.

2. Materials and Methods

2.1. Mouse Exposure

2.1.1. Experimental Animals

Young (8-week-old) and middle-aged (24-week-old) male C57BL/6J mice were purchased from the Laboratory Animal Center of the Academy of Military Medical Sciences (Beijing, China). After 1-week acclimation, all mice were exposed to gasoline/diesel vehicle exhaust by inhalation exposure. The young mice were divided into three groups: the gasoline exhaust (GE) group, the diesel exhaust (DE) group, and the control group (exposed to ambient air) ($n = 6$ in each group). Middle-aged mice were grouped in the same manner as young mice. To simulate the average intensity of personal exposure to traffic-related air pollution in daily commutes, inhalation exposure experiments were conducted for 4 h/day for 5 days in an exposure chamber. The mice were provided with water and food *ad libitum*. All procedures were approved by the Animal Experiments Ethical Committee of Nankai University and carried out in conformity with the Guide for Care and Use of Laboratory Animals.

2.1.2. Exposure Process in Mice

Gasoline and diesel vehicle exhaust was emitted from the experimental vehicles on the chassis dynamometer (Figure S1A). During the 4 h exposure period, the experimental vehicle was operated under a 1 h New European Driving Cycle (NEDC), including acceleration, deceleration, constant speed, and idle speed modes; 1 h idle speed; 1 h 40 km/h constant speed; and 1 h 80 km/h speed modes to simulate the actual average commuting driving conditions. The collected exhaust was diluted eight times with ambient air and introduced into the exposure chamber at a rate of 15–20 L/min. The concentrations of pollutants in the exposure chamber were measured using scanning mobility particle sizers and aerodynamic particle sizers.

The exposure chamber was made of medical-grade stainless steel (316L MS) and had a volume of 40 L [500 (L) × 400 (W) × 200 (H) mm]. There were four multi-functional openings in the chamber, which were used for air intake, air outlet, and detection of concentrations of $PM_{2.5}$ or gaseous pollutants. The exposure chamber could accommodate two standard independent ventilation cages for mice. The temperature was controlled at 20–25 °C during the exposure period (Figure S1). Twelve hours after the final exposure, mice were sacrificed.

The concentrations of $PM_{2.5}$ in the exposure chamber were continuously measured by a scanning mobility particle sizer (SMPS, 3898) spectrometer (TSI Inc., Shoreview, MN, USA) and an aerodynamic particle sizer (APS, 3321) spectrometer (TSI Inc., Shoreview, MN, USA). The concentrations of gaseous pollutant emissions were measured by a SEMTECH-DS Portable Emission Measurement System (PEMS) (Sensors Inc., Saline, MI, USA). The concentrations of gaseous pollutants and the mass concentrations of $PM_{2.5}$ in the chamber are shown in Table 1.

Table 1. Concentrations of gaseous pollutants and the mass concentrations of $PM_{2.5}$ in the chamber during the exposure period.

	$PM_{2.5}$ (μg/m³)	CO (μg/m³)	NO (μg/m³)	NO_2 (μg/m³)
GE group	50	25	2	-
DE group	370	50	20	4
Control group	6	-	-	-

2.1.3. Biochemical Analysis of Serum

Blood samples were collected from the retro-orbital veins of mice while they were under isoflurane anesthesia. To extract supernatant serum, blood samples were placed into 1.5 mL microcentrifuge tubes and centrifuged at 3000 rpm for 10 min. Serum samples (100 μL/sample) were transferred to a new tube and tested using an automated biochemical analyzer (Model 7020, Hitachi, Tokyo, Japan). Total cholesterol (TC), triglyceride (TG), high-density lipoprotein cholesterol (HDLc), low-density lipoprotein cholesterol (LDLc), alkaline phosphatase (ALP), alanine aminotransferase (ALT), and aspartate aminotransferase (AST) levels were analyzed.

2.1.4. Determination of Oxidative Stress Indicators

The aortic and liver tissues of mice were pretreated to obtain supernatant, and the supernatant and serum were taken to measure the oxidative parameters. The tissue samples were stored in liquid nitrogen until assayed for superoxide dismutase (SOD), glutathione peroxidase (GSH-Px), and malondialdehyde (MDA). All parameters were measured using enzyme-linked immunosorbent assay (ELISA) kits as directed by the manufacturer (Beyotime Biotechnology Co. Ltd., Beijing, China).

2.2. In Vitro Experiment

2.2.1. $PM_{2.5}$ Collection

To investigate the in vivo toxicity of gasoline and diesel exhaust particles, $PM_{2.5}$ samples were collected in two traffic micro-environments, including the Wujinglu Tunnel located in the urban area of Tianjin City and the typical collection and distribution port highway Teda Street located in Tianjin Port. According to our previous research [32], the Wujinglu Tunnel traffic is mainly composed of gasoline vehicles (with diesel vehicles accounting for only about 2%). As an important gathering and distribution channel for Tianjin Port, which has the eighth largest cargo volume in the world, Teda Street traffic is mainly composed of diesel vehicles transporting goods [33]. Therefore, the Wujinglu Tunnel and Teda Street can represent the actual traffic pollution exposure levels of gasoline and diesel vehicles as the main vehicle types, respectively. $PM_{2.5}$ was sampled from 06:30 to 21:30 and 22:00 to 06:00 from 28 August to 7 September in 2021 in Wujinglu Tunnel and from 7:30 to 17:00 and 17:20 to 7:20 from 12 to 22 June 2021 on Teda Street, respectively. The sampling height was approximately 1.5 m above ground level, within the average human respiratory zone, and approximately 1.5 m away from road traffic. The quartz fiber filters (90 mm diameter, PALL) for $PM_{2.5}$ collection were baked at 600 °C in a muffle furnace for 2 h and then equilibrated for up to 72 h at a constant temperature (22 ± 1 °C) and relative humidity (35 ± 1%). Air samples were collected at a speed of approximately 100 L/min using a medium-volume sampler (TH-150AII, Tianhong, Wuhan, China) with a $PM_{2.5}$ size-selective inlet. The sampled filters were wrapped with annealed aluminum foil and stored in a refrigerator at −18 °C until analysis. Particle size distribution was measured using a Dekati® Electrical Low-Pressure Impactor (Dekati® ELPI+, Kangasala, Finland). The ELPI+ continuously monitored the number and concentration of particles. The typical quantity size distribution of $PM_{2.5}$ from Wujinglu Tunnel and Teda Street is shown in Table S1.

The sampled filters were cut to sizes of 2 cm × 1 cm, which were then put in the sample bottle, and 100 mL of deionized distilled water was added to soak them. Extraction by ultrasonic sonication was performed for 2 h after soaking for 30 min. The liquid containing $PM_{2.5}$ was filtered through six layers of sterile gauze and centrifuged at 12,000 rpm at 4 °C for 30 min. Detached $PM_{2.5}$ was then vacuum-freeze dried, and the mass was weighed [34]. $PM_{2.5}$ was resuspended in a certain amount of sterile saline to achieve $PM_{2.5}$ suspensions and stored at −20 °C until further experimentation. During the sonication process, the container was covered to minimize the risk of contamination and loss of volatile components; further, the freeze-drying process was conducted under low temperature and reduced pressure conditions to directly sublime the water content from the solid state without passing through the liquid phase. This method helped to maximize the retention of volatile and water-soluble components in the sample, thereby reducing their loss and ensuring long-term stability. The preparation method for this $PM_{2.5}$ particle suspension has been widely used in existing relevant studies and has been proven effective [35–37].

2.2.2. Cell Culture

Human umbilical vein endothelial cells (HUVECs) and human normal liver cells (LO2) were obtained from ScienCell (Carlsbad, CA, USA) and cultured in a humidified incubator at 37 °C with 5% CO_2. HUVECs were cultured in endothelial cell medium (EndoCM), while RPMI 1640 medium was used for LO2 cell culture. For all of the experiments, HUVECs between passages 7 and 9 were utilized. The cells were divided into three groups: (1) the control group (medium only); (2) gasoline exhaust particles (GE particles in medium); and (3) diesel exhaust particles (DE particles in medium). The human daily inhalation dose of $PM_{2.5}$ was calculated based on actual $PM_{2.5}$ measurements (~30 μg/m^3), as described in our previous study [34]. According to the formula shown in Text S1, the daily inhaled mass of $PM_{2.5}$ for humans was determined to be 345.9 μg. In the preliminary experiments, exposure to estimated human daily intake doses of $PM_{2.5}$ caused severe inhibition of cell viability. Therefore, we conducted in vitro experiments using doses equivalent to 1/100 and 1/50 of the estimated human daily intake of $PM_{2.5}$. Each well was cultured with 200 μL of cell culture medium containing HUVECs and LO2 cells. Thus, the doses administered in vitro were 17.3 μg/mL and 34.6 μg/mL, respectively.

2.2.3. CCK-8 Assay for Cell Viability

Cell viability was assessed using Cell Counting Kit-8 (CCK-8, Beyotime Biotechnology Co., Ltd., Shanghai, China) assays. HUVECs and LO2 cells in the logarithmic growth phase were seeded in 48-well plates at a density of 4×10^3 cells per well. Each well was supplemented with 200 μL of medium containing the corresponding pollutants, and the medium was changed every 24 h during the incubation period. After culturing for 24, 48, and 72 h under the experimental conditions, the cells were incubated with CCK-8 reagent (10 μL/well) for 4 h [38]. Following the kit instructions, CCK-8 optical density (OD) absorbance at 450 nm was measured to judge the effect of exhaust particulate matter on cell viability.

2.2.4. Reactive Oxygen Species (ROS) Levels

HUVECs and LO2 cells in the logarithmic growth phase were seeded in 6-well plates at a density of 5×10^6 cells per well. Each well was supplemented with 1 mL of medium containing the corresponding pollutants, and the medium was changed every 24 h during the incubation period. After culturing for 24, 48, and 72 h, 10 μM DCFH-DA (Sigma-Aldrich, Saint Louis, MO, USA) was added to each well and incubated at 37 °C for 45 min. Subsequently, the average fluorescence intensity was measured using a FACS Calibur flow cytometer (BD, San Jose, CA, USA) after collection to assess the impact of exhaust particles on cellular ROS levels.

2.3. *Statistical Analysis*

GraphPad Prism Software Version 8.3.4 (San Diego, CA, USA) was used for the statistical analysis. A student's *t*-test and one-way analysis of variance (ANOVA) with a subsequent Bonferroni's multiple comparisons test were performed for the statistical significance test. A P-value of less than 0.05 was considered statistically significant. Experimental data were presented as the mean and standard error of the mean.

3. Results

3.1. Effect on Biochemical Parameters in Mice

As shown in Figure 1a, exposure to diesel exhaust significantly reduced the body weight of young mice ($p < 0.05$), while the body weight of middle-aged mice was significantly reduced in all of the groups.

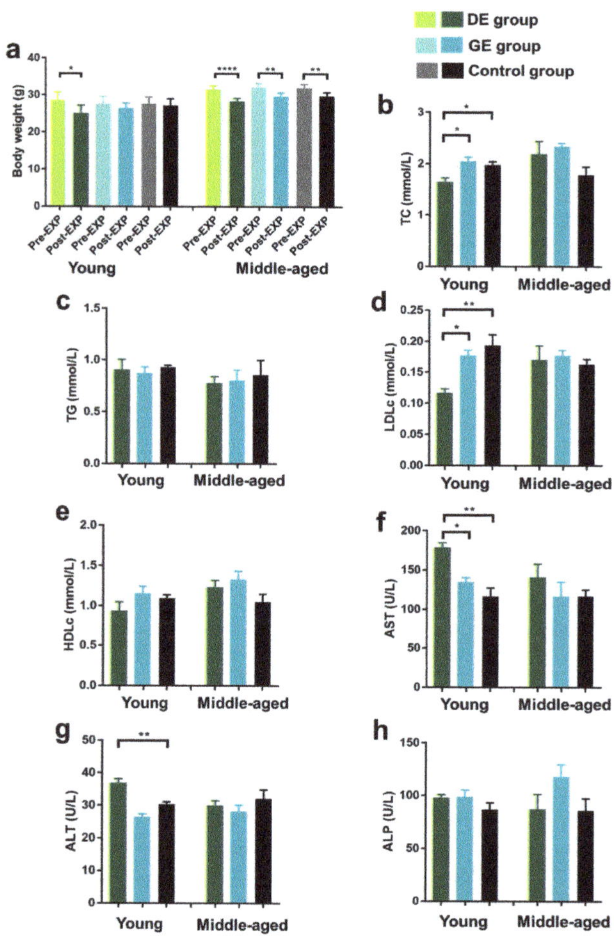

Figure 1. Effect of gasoline and diesel exhaust exposure on lipid profiles and liver function in C57BL/6 mice. (**a**) Body weight; (**b**) Serum total cholesterol level (TC); (**c**) Serum triglyceride level (TG); (**d**) Serum LDL-cholesterol level (LDLc); (**e**) Serum HDL-cholesterol level (HDLc); (**f**) Aspartate aminotransferase (AST); (**g**) Alanine aminotransferase (ALT); (**h**) Alkaline phosphatase (ALP) (Control group: exposure to ambient air; GE group: exposure to gasoline exhaust; DE group: exposure to diesel exhaust) (n = 6 in each group) (* $p < 0.05$; ** $p < 0.01$; **** $p < 0.0001$).

Serum samples were obtained to evaluate the effects of exhaust particles on lipid metabolism and liver function in mice, and TC, TG, LDLc, HDLc, AST, ALT, and ALP were determined. Blood lipid levels in the mice are shown in Figure 1b–e. For young mice, the TC and LDLc levels decreased significantly in the DE group ($p < 0.01$) compared with the control group, while there were no significant differences in all the lipid indicators between the GE and control groups. For middle-aged mice, there were no significant differences in TC, TG, LDLc, and HDLc level variations between the DE/GE and control groups.

The AST, ALT, and ALP levels are shown in Figure 1f–h. For young mice, diesel exhaust exposure elevated the AST and ALT levels by 53.7% and 21.7% ($p < 0.01$), respectively, compared to control group. Furthermore, compared to the GE group, the AST levels increased significantly in the DE group ($p < 0.05$). However, there were no significant differences in AST, ALT, and ALP level variations between the GE and control groups. For middle-aged mice, there were no significant differences in all of the liver function indicators between the DE/GE and control groups.

3.2. *Effect on Oxidative Stress in Mice*

Considering the negative effects of gasoline and diesel vehicle exhaust on the lipid mechanisms and liver function of mice, the oxidative stress of vehicle exhaust exposure on serum, aorta, and liver tissues was investigated. The SOD, GSH-Px, and MDA levels were measured.

3.2.1. Serum

As shown in Figure 2a,b, for young mice, the SOD activity in serum decreased significantly after exposure to both gasoline (GE group) and diesel exhaust (DE group) in comparison with the control group, while the GSH-Px activity increased significantly in the DE group. Moreover, there was a significant increase in GSH-Px levels in the DE group compared to the GE group. For middle-aged mice, the SOD levels decreased, and the GSH-Px activity in serum increased significantly in the DE group compared to the control and GE groups. Moreover, all of the effects of diesel exhaust exposure on SOD and GSH-Px activities were more pronounced than those caused by gasoline exhaust exposure. There were no significant differences in MDA levels among all of the groups of young and middle-aged mice (Figure 2c).

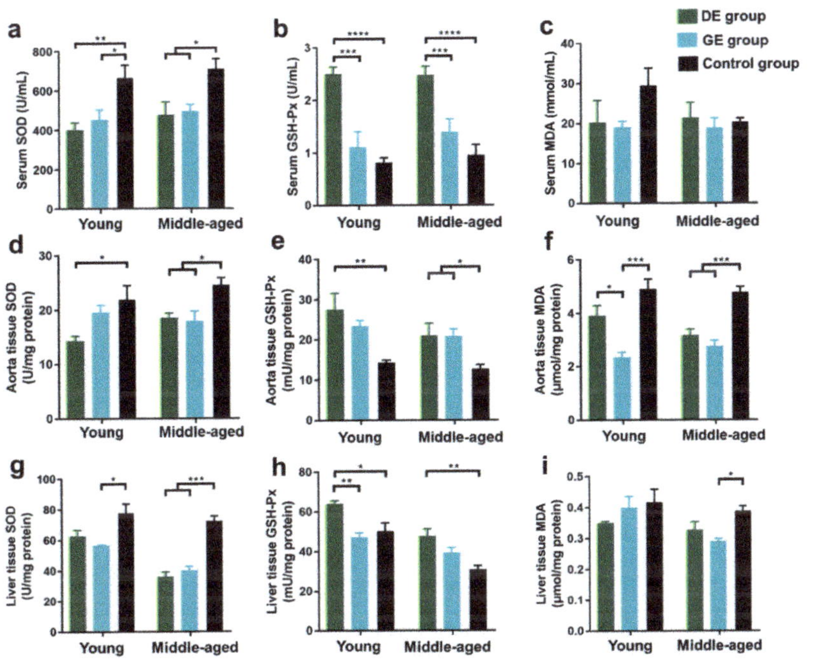

Figure 2. Effect of gasoline and diesel exhaust exposure on oxidative stress in C57BL/6 mice. (**a**) Serum superoxide dismutase (SOD); (**b**) Serum glutathione peroxidase (GSH-Px); (**c**) Serum malondialdehyde

(MDA); (**d**) Aorta SOD; (**e**) Aorta GSH-Px; (**f**) Aorta MDA; (**g**) Liver SOD; (**h**) Liver GSH-Px; (**i**) Liver MDA. (Control group: exposure to ambient air; GE group: exposure to gasoline exhaust; DE group: exposure to diesel exhaust) (n = 6 in each group) (* $p < 0.05$; ** $p < 0.01$; *** $p < 0.001$; **** $p < 0.0001$).

3.2.2. Aorta

The SOD, GSH-Px, and MDA levels in aorta tissues after exposure to gasoline and diesel exhaust are shown in Figure 2d–f. For young mice, compared to the control group, the SOD level decreased, and the GSH-Px level increased significantly in the DE group, while the MDA level significantly decreased in the GE group. In addition, there was a more significant decrease in MDA levels in the GE group than in the DE group. For middle-aged mice, the SOD and MDA levels decreased, and the GSH-Px level increased significantly in both the GE and DE groups compared to the control group.

3.2.3. Liver

The SOD, GSH-Px, and MDA levels in liver tissues after exposure to gasoline and diesel exhaust are shown in Figure 2g–i. For young mice, compared to the control group, the SOD activity decreased significantly in the GE group, and the GSH-Px activity increased significantly in the DE group. Furthermore, the increase in GSH-Px level in the DE group was more significant than that in the GE group. For the middle-aged group, the SOD levels decreased significantly in both the GE and DE groups compared to the control group, while the GSH-Px level increased significantly in the DE group, and the MDA level decreased significantly in the GE group.

3.3. *Effect on Cell Viability of HUVECs and LO2*

Based on the results of in vivo experiments concerning the effect on vascular and hepatic function, HUVECs and LO2 cells were incubated to explore the impacts and potential mechanisms of gasoline and diesel exhaust exposure. In addition, as shown in Table 1, the gaseous pollutants (CO, NO, and NO_2) were below the Chinese National Air Quality Standard Grade II. However, the $PM_{2.5}$ concentrations in the chamber during gasoline and diesel vehicle exhaust exposure periods were 50 and 370 $\mu g/m^3$, respectively, which exceeded 0.43 and 9.57 times the standard. Therefore, $PM_{2.5}$ samples emitted from gasoline and diesel vehicles were collected to conduct the in vitro exposure experiment.

Figure 3a,b illustrates the effects of gasoline and diesel exhaust $PM_{2.5}$ on the viability of HUVECs and LO2 cells. As shown in Figure 3a, both gasoline and diesel exhaust particles significantly reduced HUVEC viability at 72 h ($p < 0.001$), with dose–effect dependence. In addition, diesel exhaust particles exhibited a more pronounced inhibitory effect on cell proliferation of HUVECs ($p < 0.01$) than gasoline exhaust particles. As depicted in Figure 3b, the cell viability of LO2 decreased significantly in both the GE and DE groups at 72 h ($p < 0.001$), but no significant difference was observed in the inhibitory effect on liver cell proliferation between the groups of different particle types and concentrations.

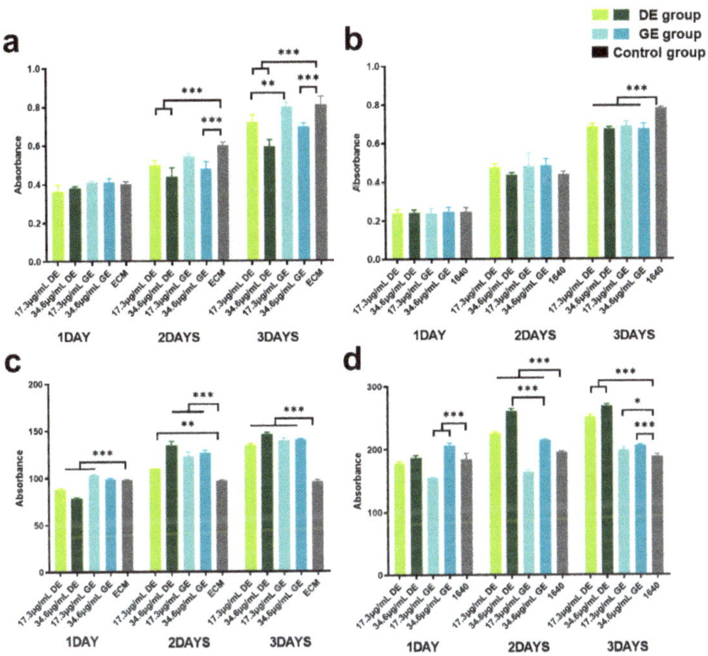

Figure 3. Effect of gasoline and diesel exhaust particle exposure on cell viability and ROS levels. (**a**) human umbilical vein endothelial cells (HUVECs) Cell Viability; (**b**) normal liver cells (LO2) Cell Viability; (**c**) HUVEC ROS Levels; (**d**) LO2 ROS Levels. (Control group: cells cultured in the respective medium only; Gasoline group: cells co-cultured with GE particles in the respective medium; Diesel group: cells co-cultured with DE particles in the respective medium.) (* $p < 0.05$; ** $p < 0.01$; *** $p < 0.001$).

3.4. Effect on ROS Level

Figure 3c,d illustrates the impacts of gasoline and diesel exhaust particles on the oxidative stress levels in HUVECs and LO2. Significant increments in ROS levels in HUVECs and LO2 cells ($p < 0.01$) were observed. Moreover, the diesel exhaust particles exhibited more severe oxidation stress on liver cells than gasoline exhaust particles ($p <.0.001$) (Figure 3d).

4. Discussion

Vehicular emissions have been recognized as one of the most important sources of air pollutants [39,40]. The fuel type is the most important influence factor for air pollutants derived from vehicle emissions [2]. Gasoline- and diesel-fueled engines are the major constituent parts of on-road vehicles. Vehicular exhaust can rapidly enter the systemic circulation upon inhalation, induce systemic pathologies, affect lipid metabolism, and lead to various diseases [41–45]. Moreover, gasoline and diesel vehicle exhaust have great health impacts on people living in downtown and suburban areas, respectively. Therefore, to investigate the health impact of exposure to gasoline and diesel vehicle exhaust, in vivo experiments in C57BL/6J mice and in vitro experiments using human umbilical vein endothelial cells (HUVECs) and human normal liver cells (LO2) were conducted. In addition, the interaction effects between age and vehicle exhaust were evaluated in this study.

Regarding the analysis of blood lipids in mice, exposure to diesel exhaust led to a significant reduction in TC and LDLc levels in young mice. However, for middle-aged mice, there were no significant differences in all of the lipid indicators between the DE/GE and control groups. Previous studies have indicated a slight decrease in serum cholesterol after sub-chronic exposure to diesel exhaust in 10–12-week-old rats [46], with no significant impact observed in short-term exposures [47]. Furthermore, regarding the effects of $PM_{2.5}$ on blood lipids, a group study conducted in Wuhan, China, targeting healthy young adults aged 18–30, revealed that for every 10 μg/m³ increase in $PM_{2.5}$ concentration, the changes in TC and LDLc were −0.33% (95% *CI*: −0.64%, −0.01%) and −0.94% (95% *CI*: −1.53%, −0.35%), respectively [48]. Cholesterol is the sole precursor to all steroid hormones, like glucocorticoids responsible for blood sugar regulation and mineral corticoids required to regulate mineral balance and blood pressure [49,50]. In addition, cholesterol serves as a precursor for the biosynthesis of bile acids and vitamin D [49]. TC level is related to the regulation of stress responses, immune responses, electrolyte homeostasis, and the maintenance of secondary sexual characteristics, skeletal development, and bone homeostasis [51–53]. Furthermore, cholesterol can be obtained from circulating LDLc [54], and a decrease in LDLc levels is related to a low TC level. Lower TC and LDLc levels may impact cellular functions and hinder nutrient absorption and utilization. Therefore, exposure to diesel exhaust may have adverse effects on the growth and development of adolescents.

Regarding the analysis of liver function in mice, exposure to diesel exhaust significantly increased AST and ALT levels in young mice, while the effects of gasoline exhaust were not significant. Meanwhile, there was no significant influence of both gasoline and diesel vehicle exhaust exposure on all of the liver function indicators in middle-aged mice. The AST and ALT reflect the extent of hepatocellular injury [55]. Increments in serum AST and ALT were found in people with hepatosis compared to fit people [56]. The decrease in TC and LDL-C in serum is related to the liver, where liver cells are the site of cholesterol synthesis, and LDL-C transports cholesterol from the liver to other tissues. The decrement in TC and LDLc, as well as the increment in AST and ALT, are clinical diagnostic indicators of liver cell damage, suggesting possible acute injury to the liver [57,58]. Liver cells play a significant role in cholesterol synthesis, and LDLc transports cholesterol from the liver to other tissues. The liver is a central hub for balancing cholesterol from all sources and plays a pivotal role in modulating plasma LDLc [59]. It is possible that exposure to diesel exhaust may have an impact on the liver. Low LDLc levels could be caused by abnormalities in liver function or thyroid function [60,61]. Moreover, a study conducted by J. A. Bond et al. [62] suggested that the liver might serve as the primary site for the metabolism of carcinogens, such as 1-nitropyrene (1-NP), carried by diesel exhaust. Consistent with our findings, a cohort study conducted by Lin Xu et al. [63] on young adult males around the age of 35 found that exposure to diesel engine exhaust particles led to a significant increase in ALT and AST levels in participants, thereby increasing the risk of liver damage. Another study investigating the impact of nanoparticle rich-diesel exhaust (NR-DE) on the livers of 8-week-old male F344 rats revealed that NR-DE exposure led to increased AST and ALT activity in rats, and high concentrations of NR-DE further activated hepatic inflammatory signaling [64].

Therefore, exposure to vehicle exhaust, especially diesel vehicle exhaust, had a greater impact on young mice than on middle-aged mice in terms of blood lipid levels and liver function. Previous studies have classified the age of mice to correspond to different stages in the human lifecycle, where mice aged 6–8 weeks correspond to human adolescence and mice aged 24–26 weeks have fully matured in all aspects and have transitioned from adulthood to middle age [65]. Consistent with our findings, Ali K. Hamade et al. [66] observed that combined exposure to ozone and carbon black led to a decrease in heart rate and an increase in heart rate variability in mice, with these effects being more pronounced in young mice and relatively weaker in older mice. This difference in response may be attributed to the fact that the immune system of young mice has not fully developed, making them more sensitive to environmental pollutants and having a higher permeability of the respiratory epithelium to these pollutants [67,68]. Furthermore, both young and middle-aged mice were exposed to the same concentration of exhaust during the experiment, but due to the lighter body weight of young mice, their relative exposure to pollutants was greater, possibly resulting in more significant biological effects. Research by P.U. Simioni et al. [69] demonstrated that the aging process affects humoral and cellular-mediated immune responses, rendering older mice less sensitive to environmental challenges.

In order to further investigate the impact of gasoline and diesel exhaust on oxidative stress in mice, we measured oxidative stress markers, including SOD, GSH-Px, and MDA, in serum, aorta tissues, and liver tissues. Oxidative stress can be defined as an increase over physiological values in the steady-state concentrations of ROS. Antioxidant enzymes, such as SOD and GSH-Px, are identified as the first line of defense against the production and/or accumulation of ROS [70]. The SOD is a scavenger of endogenous ROS. Reduced SOD activity not only leads to inadequate removal of oxygen radicals but also induces MDA synthesis, resulting in protein and cellular damage and apoptosis [71,72]. GSH-Px is an essential enzyme for peroxide degradation, protecting the structural and functional integrity of cell membranes against peroxide damage [73]. MDA is a product of cellular membrane lipid peroxidation [74], which is commonly known as a marker of oxidative stress. Our results demonstrated that after exposure to gasoline and diesel emissions, SOD levels in the serum of young mice decreased significantly, and SOD levels in the aortic tissues and liver of adult mice also decreased significantly, with a greater impact observed from diesel exhaust. Both young and middle-aged mice showed significant increments in GSH-Px levels after diesel exhaust exposure and significant reductions in MDA levels in the aorta tissues after gasoline exhaust exposure. In existing studies, after instilling diesel exhaust particles into the trachea of mice, the ROS levels in the lungs first rose to a peak and began to decrease after 24 h [75]. Xu et al. [76] administered 50 μL of $PM_{2.5}$ suspension (7.8 μg/g) via nasal drip to 8-week-old C57BL/6 mice. After three consecutive weeks of exposure, the total SOD level in the lung tissue of the mice decreased, and the GSH-Px level decreased after nine consecutive weeks of exposure. It can be inferred that short-term exhaust exposure leads to transient oxidative stress in the body, and the decrease in SOD levels and the increase in GSH-Px levels indicate that the body is recovering from tissue and organ damage. The rapid increase in GSH-Px activity in mice under stress led to a decrease in MDA levels. Overall, these results suggest that the degree of lipid oxidative damage caused by short-term acute exposure is relatively mild. This may be attributed to the timely activation of the endogenous antioxidant defense system, which effectively clears harmful oxidative substances and prevents their accumulation within the body, thereby mitigating severe oxidative damage. Young mice exhibited greater sensitivity to acute stimulation with a more pronounced oxidative stress response compared to middle-aged mice, which is consistent with the results observed for blood lipids and liver function.

These findings suggest that exposure to gasoline and diesel exhaust induces oxidative stress in the body, with diesel exhaust having a greater impact on oxidative stress compared to gasoline exhaust. A study by Fen Yin et al. [77] similarly reported increased levels of 9- and 13-hydroxyoctadecadienoic levels in the livers of mice exposed to diesel exhaust, indicating increased oxidative stress. Previous research has demonstrated that diesel exhaust emissions are more toxic than gasoline exhaust emissions when considering engines with equal horsepower [78]. Diesel vehicle emissions contain 2 to 40 times more particulate matter and 20 to 30 times more nitro-polycyclic aromatic hydrocarbons compared to gasoline vehicle emissions [79]. As shown in Table 1, in this study, the gaseous pollutants (CO, NO, and NO_2) in the chamber during gasoline and diesel vehicle exhaust exposure periods were below the Chinese National Air Quality Standard Grade II. However, the measured concentrations of $PM_{2.5}$ were 50 and 370 $\mu g/m^3$, respectively, which exceeded 0.43 and 9.57 times the standard. Therefore, $PM_{2.5}$ was assumed to be the major constituent in diesel and gasoline exhaust. In addition, based on the negative effects of gasoline and diesel exhaust exposure on vascular and liver function in in vivo experiments, HUVECs and LO2 cells were cultured in in vitro experiments to further explore the effects and potential mechanisms of $PM_{2.5}$ in gasoline and diesel exhaust.

The results of the in vitro experiments demonstrated that exposure to diesel and gasoline vehicle exhaust particles resulted in decreased cell viability and increased ROS levels in both cell types with dose and time dependence, leading to inhibited cell proliferation, cellular oxidative damage, and impaired cellular functions. These findings are consistent with the current research results, suggesting that internalization of diesel engine exhaust particles into the cytoplasm of cells can induce oxidative stress [80], promoting cell apoptosis. Wang et al. [81] demonstrated that diesel engine exhaust particles induce oxidative stress and autophagy in endothelial cells, with cells attempting to eliminate the particles and generate free radicals after 2 h, followed by cell senescence and apoptosis after 12 h.

Furthermore, compared to gasoline vehicle exhaust particles, diesel vehicle exhaust particles exhibited more severe inhibition of HUVEC viability but higher oxidative stress in LO2 cells. HUVECs play a crucial role in forming the vascular barrier of blood vessels, preventing the entry of cells and large molecules from the blood into surrounding tissues, and regulating the exchange of fluids, gases, and solutes. The reduced cell viability of HUVECs caused by diesel exhaust particles may alter the permeability of blood vessel walls, leading to the leakage of blood components and extracellular fluid into surrounding tissues. This condition could increase intracellular oxidative stress, potentially initiating lipid oxidation reactions and lipid peroxidation damage, resulting in edema and inflammatory responses. Liver cells are one of the main sites for lipid breakdown and are central to cholesterol synthesis and metabolism. The reduced cell viability of liver cells induced by diesel exhaust particle exposure may slow down lipid breakdown, disturb cholesterol metabolism, and lead to the accumulation of fat in the liver, causing fatty liver and impacting lipid metabolism [77]. Grace V. Aquino et al. [82] found that ultrafine particles (UFPs) from diesel vehicle engine exposure caused concentration-dependent increases in ROS production in rat blood–brain barrier endothelial cells and perivascular microglia. Li et al. [83] demonstrated that UFPs affect signaling pathways in vascular endothelial cells and induce vascular endothelial oxidative stress via JNK activation.

However, this present study has limitations. The primary focus was to investigate the effects of gasoline and diesel exhaust emissions on lipid metabolism through biochemical and cellular experiments, without evaluating histopathological changes. Moreover, in our study, vehicle exhaust exposure induced oxidative damage in vivo and in vitro. Therefore, it is likely that inflammatory events could be caused. In future research, we will further incorporate pathological analysis and inflammatory indicator analysis.

In summary, combined with the in vitro and in vivo results, compared to gasoline vehicle exhaust, exposure to diesel vehicle exhaust had more substantial negative impacts on lipid metabolism and liver function via oxidative stress in live cells and cell injury in vascular cells. Moreover, the diesel exhaust exposure induced lipid metabolism dysfunction and acute liver injury in young mice, which revealed that puberty exhibited more instability and irregular regulation ability and more sensitivity to traffic emissions.

5. Conclusions

This study conducted in vivo and in vitro toxicological experiments on exposure to gasoline and diesel vehicle exhaust. The aim was to explore the impact of actual traffic exposure levels of gasoline and diesel vehicle exhaust on lipid metabolism. The results revealed that diesel exhaust exposure significantly decreased serum levels of TC and LDLc in young mice, suggesting potential disruptions in lipid homeostasis. Furthermore, it significantly elevated the levels of AST and ALT in young mice, indicative of potential acute liver injury. These effects were more pronounced in young mice, emphasizing the heightened susceptibility of adolescents to adverse impacts from vehicle emissions. Additionally, both gasoline and diesel exhaust exposure were found to decrease the viability of endothelial cells and liver cells, accompanied by elevated levels of ROS, implying cellular oxidative damage. Strikingly, the effects of exposure to diesel exhaust were more pronounced, indicating that diesel exhaust possesses greater toxicity, potentially exerting a more substantial influence on lipid metabolism and oxidative stress in the body compared to gasoline exhaust. Overall, our research provides evidence of the complex relationship between vehicle emissions from gasoline and diesel engines in actual traffic environments and lipid metabolism, oxidative stress, and age-related vulnerabilities. These findings are of paramount importance for mitigating health risks associated with vehicle emissions.

Supplementary Materials: The following supporting information can be downloaded at: https://www.mdpi.com/article/10.3390/toxics12040303/s1, Figure S1: (A) The exposure chamber; (B) The exposure process; Table S1: Typical quantity-size distribution of PM2.5.

Author Contributions: Conceptualization, X.L. and T.W.; methodology, T.W.; software, J.Z.; validation, Y.G. and X.L.; resources, Z.L., D.G. and H.M.; data curation, X.Z.; writing—original draft preparation, Y.G.; writing—review and editing, Y.G. and T.W.; visualization, X.L.; supervision, T.W. All authors have read and agreed to the published version of the manuscript.

Funding: This study was supported by the National Natural Science Foundation of China (No. 42377424); and the Fundamental Research Funds for the Central Universities of China (No. ZB23003425, 63211075).

Institutional Review Board Statement: All procedures were approved by the Animal Experiments Ethical Committee of Nankai University and carried out in conformity with the Guide for Care and Use of Laboratory Animals.

Informed Consent Statement: Not applicable.

Data Availability Statement: Data are contained within the article.

Conflicts of Interest: The authors declare that they have no competing interests.

Abbreviations

BC	black carbon;
EC	elemental carbon;
CO	carbon monoxide;
HC	hydrocarbons;
NOx	nitrogen oxides;
NO_2	nitrogen dioxide;
PM	Particulate Matter;
OR	Odds Ratio;
DEP	diesel engine exhaust particles;
ROS	reactive oxygen species;
HUVECs	human umbilical vein endothelial cells;
LO2	human normal liver cells;
GE	gasoline exhaust;
DE	diesel exhaust;
NEDC	New European Driving Cycle;
SMPS	Scanning Mobility Particle Sizer;
APS	Aerodynamic Panicle Sizer;
TC	Total Cholesterol;
TG	Total Triglycerides;
HDLc	High-Density Lipoprotein Cholesterol;
LDLc	Low-Density Lipoprotein Cholesterol;
ALP	alkaline phosphatase;
ALT	alanine aminotransferase;
AST	aspartate aminotransferase;
SOD	Superoxide Dismutase;
MDA	Malondialdehyde;
GSH-Px	Glutathione Peroxidase;
ELISA	enzyme-linked immunosorbent assay;
CCK-8	Cell Counting Kit-8;
OD	optical density.

References

1. Wei, P.; Brimblecombe, P.; Yang, F.H.; Anand, A.; Xing, Y.; Sun, L.; Sun, Y.X.; Chu, M.Y.; Ning, Z. Determination of local traffic emission and non-local background source contribution to on-road air pollution using fixed-route mobile air sensor network. *Environ. Pollut.* **2021**, *290*, 118055. [CrossRef]
2. Tolis, E.I.; Karanotas, T.; Svolakis, G.; Panaras, G.; Bartzis, J.G. Air quality in cabin environment of different passenger cars: Effect of car usage, fuel type and ventilation/infiltration conditions. *Environ. Sci. Pollut. Res.* **2021**, *28*, 51232–51241. [CrossRef]
3. Wang, Y.; Xing, Z.; Xu, H.; Du, K. Emission factors of air pollutants from CNG-gasoline bi-fuel vehicles: Part I. Black carbon. *Sci. Total Environ.* **2016**, *572*, 1161–1165. [CrossRef]
4. Malla, S. Assessment of mobility and its impact on energy use and air pollution in Nepal. *Energy* **2014**, *69*, 485–496. [CrossRef]
5. Li, T.; Yang, H.-L.; Xu, L.-T.; Zhou, Y.-T.; Min, Y.-J.; Yan, S.-C.; Zhang, Y.-H.; Wang, X.-M. Comprehensive treatment strategy for diesel truck exhaust. *Environ. Sci. Pollut. Res.* **2023**, *30*, 54324–54332. [CrossRef]
6. Lund, M.T.; Berntsen, T.K.; Heyes, C.; Klimont, Z.; Samset, B.H. Global and regional climate impacts of black carbon and co-emitted species from the on-road diesel sector. *Atmos. Environ.* **2014**, *98*, 50–58. [CrossRef]
7. Breuer, J.L.; Samsun, R.C.; Peters, R.; Stolten, D. The impact of diesel vehicles on NOx and PM10 emissions from road transport in urban morphological zones: A case study in North Rhine-Westphalia, Germany. *Sci. Total Environ.* **2020**, *727*, 138583. [CrossRef]
8. Niu, Y.; Zhang, X.; Meng, T.; Wang, H.; Bin, P.; Shen, M.; Chen, W.; Yu, S.; Leng, S.; Zheng, Y. Exposure characterization and estimation of benchmark dose for cancer biomarkers in an occupational cohort of diesel engine testers. *J. Expo. Sci. Env. Epidemiol.* **2018**, *28*, 579–588. [CrossRef]
9. Pan, W.C.; Yeh, S.Y.; Wu, C.D.; Huang, Y.T.; Chen, Y.C.; Chen, C.J.; Yang, H.I. Association Between Traffic Count and Cardiovascular Mortality: A Prospective Cohort Study in Taiwan. *J. Epidemiol.* **2021**, *31*, 343–349. [CrossRef]
10. Habert, C.; Garnier, R. Health effects of diesel exhaust: A state of the art. *Rev. Des Mal. Respir.* **2015**, *32*, 138–154. [CrossRef]
11. Parent, M.E.; Rousseau, M.C.; Boffetta, P.; Cohen, A.; Siemiatycki, J. Exposure to diesel and gasoline engine emissions and the risk of lung cancer. *Am. J. Epidemiol.* **2007**, *165*, 53–62. [CrossRef]
12. Andersen, M.H.G.; Frederiksen, M.; Saber, A.T.; Wils, R.S.; Fonseca, A.S.; Koponen, I.K.; Johannesson, S.; Roursgaard, M.; Loft, S.; Møller, P.; et al. Health effects of exposure to diesel exhaust in diesel-powered trains. *Part Fibre Toxicol* **2019**, *16*, 21. [CrossRef]
13. Vesterdal, L.K.; Danielsen, P.H.; Folkmann, J.K.; Jespersen, L.F.; Aguilar-Pelaez, K.; Roursgaard, M.; Loft, S.; Moller, P. Accumulation of lipids and oxidatively damaged DNA in hepatocytes exposed to particles. *Toxicol. Appl. Pharmacol.* **2014**, *274*, 350–360. [CrossRef]
14. Tseng, C.Y.; Wang, J.S.; Chang, Y.J.; Chang, J.F.; Chao, M.W. Exposure to High-Dose Diesel Exhaust Particles Induces Intracellular Oxidative Stress and Causes Endothelial Apoptosis in Cultured In Vitro Capillary Tube Cells. *Cardiovasc. Toxicol.* **2015**, *15*, 345–354. [CrossRef]
15. Tomaru, M.; Takano, H.; Inoue, K.I.; Yanagisawa, R.; Osakabe, N.; Yasuda, A.; Shimada, A.; Kato, Y.; Uematsu, H. Pulmonary exposure to diesel exhaust particles enhances fatty change of the liver in obese diabetic mice. *Int. J. Mol. Med.* **2007**, *19*, 17–22. [CrossRef]
16. Miller, M.R.; Shaw, C.A.; Langrish, J.P. From particles to patients: Oxidative stress and the cardiovascular effects of air pollution. *Future Cardiol.* **2012**, *8*, 577–602. [CrossRef]
17. Durga, M.; Nathiya, S.; Rajasekar, A.; Devasena, T. Effects of ultrafine petrol exhaust particles on cytotoxicity, oxidative stress generation, DNA damage and inflammation in human A549 lung cells and murine RAW 264.7 macrophages. *Environ. Toxicol. Pharmacol.* **2014**, *38*, 518–530. [CrossRef]
18. Brook, R.D.; Rajagopalan, S.; Pope, C.A.; Brook, J.R.; Bhatnagar, A.; Diez-Roux, A.V.; Holguin, F.; Hong, Y.L.; Luepker, R.V.; Mittleman, M.A.; et al. Particulate Matter Air Pollution and Cardiovascular Disease An Update to the Scientific Statement From the American Heart Association. *Circulation* **2010**, *121*, 2331–2378. [CrossRef]
19. Delfino, R.J.; Staimer, N.; Vaziri, N.D. Air pollution and circulating biomarkers of oxidative stress. *Air Qual. Atmos. Health* **2011**, *4*, 37–52. [CrossRef]
20. Tseng, C.-Y.; Chang, J.-F.; Wang, J.-S.; Chang, Y.-J.; Gordon, M.K.; Chao, M.-W. Protective Effects of N-Acetyl Cysteine against Diesel Exhaust Particles-Induced Intracellular ROS Generates Pro-Inflammatory Cytokines to Mediate the Vascular Permeability of Capillary-Like Endothelial Tubes. *PLoS ONE* **2015**, *10*, e0131911. [CrossRef]
21. Chao, M.W.; Kozlosky, J.; Po, I.P.; Strickland, P.O.; Svoboda, K.K.H.; Cooper, K.; Laumbach, R.J.; Gordon, M.K. Diesel exhaust particle exposure causes redistribution of endothelial tube VE-cadherin. *Toxicology* **2011**, *279*, 73–84. [CrossRef]
22. Huang, Y.X.; Unger, N.; Harper, K.; Heyes, C. Global Climate and Human Health Effects of the Gasoline and Diesel Vehicle Fleets. *GeoHealth* **2020**, *4*, e2019GH000240. [CrossRef]
23. Wu, Y.-C.; Batterman, S.A. Proximity of schools in Detroit, Michigan to automobile and truck traffic. *J. Expo. Sci. Environ. Epidemiol.* **2006**, *16*, 457–470. [CrossRef]
24. Athyros, V.G.; Doumas, M.; Imprialos, K.P.; Stavropoulos, K.; Georgianou, E.; Katsimardou, A.; Karagiannis, A. Diabetes and lipid metabolism. *Hormones* **2018**, *17*, 61–67. [CrossRef]
25. Noels, H.; Lehrke, M.; Vanholder, R.; Jankowski, J. Lipoproteins and fatty acids in chronic kidney disease: Molecular and metabolic alterations. *Nat. Rev. Nephrol.* **2021**, *17*, 528–542. [CrossRef]
26. Averyanova, I.V. Age-related blood biochemical changes (lipid metabolism) in healthy young and mature men living under the North conditions. *Klin. Lab. Diagn.* **2021**, *66*, 728–732. [CrossRef]

27. Wu, J.; Bu, D.D.; Wang, H.Q.; Shen, D.; Chong, D.Y.; Zhang, T.Y.; Tao, W.W.; Zhao, M.F.; Zhao, Y.; Fang, L.; et al. The rhythmic coupling of Egr-1 and Cidea regulates age-related metabolic dysfunction in the liver of male mice. *Nat. Commun.* **2023**, *14*, 1634. [CrossRef]
28. Gradinaru, D.; Borsa, C.; Ionescu, C.; Prada, G.I. Oxidized LDL and NO synthesis-Biomarkers of endothelial dysfunction and ageing. *Mech. Ageing Dev.* **2015**, *151*, 101–113. [CrossRef]
29. Perng, W.; Watkins, D.J.; Cantoral, A.; Mercado-García, A.; Meeker, J.D.; Téllez-Rojo, M.M.; Peterson, K.E. Exposure to phthalates is associated with lipid profile in peripubertal Mexican youth. *Environ. Res.* **2017**, *154*, 311–317. [CrossRef]
30. Lee, S.W.; Yon, D.K.; James, C.C.; Lee, S.; Koh, H.Y.; Sheen, Y.H.; Oh, J.W.; Han, M.Y.; Sugihara, G. Short-term effects of multiple outdoor environmental factors on risk of asthma exacerbations: Age-stratified time-series analysis. *J. Allergy Clin. Immunol.* **2019**, *144*, 1542–1550. [CrossRef]
31. Wang, N.; Mengersen, K.; Tong, S.; Kimlin, M.; Zhou, M.; Wang, L.; Yin, P.; Xu, Z.; Cheng, J.; Zhang, Y.; et al. Short-term association between ambient air pollution and lung cancer mortality. *Environ. Res.* **2019**, *179*, 108748. [CrossRef]
32. Song, A.; Peng, J.; Guo, J.; Zhang, J.; Tong, H.; Lv, Z.; Yang, N.; Tang, M.; Mao, H. Interannual variations of vehicle emissions and evaluation of emission control policies based on tunnel measurements in a typical megacity in China. *Acta Sci. Circumstantiae* **2023**, *43*, 166–178.
33. Zhang, Y.; Andre, M.; Liu, Y.; Ren, P.; Yang, Z.; Yuan, Y.; Mao, H. Research on vehicle activity characteristies of typical roads in Tianjin. *Environ. Pollut. Control* **2018**, *40*, 365–372.
34. Zhao, J.B.; Mi, X.Y.; Zhao, L.L.; Midgley, A.C.; Tang, H.Y.; Tian, M.Y.; Yan, H.Y.; Wang, K.; Wang, R.; Wan, Y.J.; et al. Validation of PM2.5 model particle through physicochemical evaluation and atherosclerotic plaque formation in ApoE(-/-) mice. *Ecotoxicol. Environ. Saf.* **2020**, *192*, 110308. [CrossRef]
35. Meng, Z.; Zhang, Q. Damage effects of dust storm $PM_{2.5}$ on DNA in alveolar macrophages and lung cells of rats. *Food Chem. Toxicol.* **2007**, *45*, 1368–1374. [CrossRef]
36. Wang, H.T.; Wang, G.S.; Meng, Y.F.; Liu, Y.Q.; Yao, X.Q.; Feng, C.L. Modified Guo-Min decoction ameliorates PM2.5-induced lung injury by inhibition of PI3K-AKT and MAPK signaling pathways. *Phytomedicine* **2024**, *123*, 155211. [CrossRef]
37. Wang, X.F.; Jiang, S.F.; Liu, Y.; Du, X.Y.; Zhang, W.B.; Zhang, J.; Shen, H.Q. Comprehensive pulmonary metabolome responses to intratracheal instillation of airborne fine particulate matter in rats. *Sci. Total Environ.* **2017**, *592*, 41–50. [CrossRef]
38. Zhang, Y.; Zhao, J.; Hu, Q.; Mao, H.; Wang, T. Nitro substituent caused negative impact on occurrence and development of atherosclerotic plaque by PM2.5-bound polycyclic aromatic compounds. *Sci. Total Environ.* **2023**, *906*, 167700. [CrossRef]
39. González, C.M.; Gómez, C.D.; Rojas, N.Y.; Acevedo, H.; Aristizábal, B.H. Relative impact of on-road vehicular and point-source industrial emissions of air pollutants in a medium-sized Andean city. *Atmos. Environ.* **2017**, *152*, 279–289. [CrossRef]
40. Tong, Z.; Chen, Y.; Malkawi, A.; Adamkiewicz, G.; Spengler, J.D. Quantifying the impact of traffic-related air pollution on the indoor air quality of a naturally ventilated building. *Environ. Int.* **2016**, *89–90*, 138–146. [CrossRef]
41. Aragon, M.J.; Chrobak, I.; Brower, J.; Roldan, L.; Fredenburgh, L.E.; McDonald, J.D.; Campen, M.J. Inflammatory and Vasoactive Effects of Serum Following Inhalation of Varied Complex Mixtures. *Cardiovasc. Toxicol.* **2016**, *16*, 163–171. [CrossRef]
42. Campen, M.; Robertson, S.; Lund, A.; Lucero, J.; McDonald, J. Engine exhaust particulate and gas phase contributions to vascular toxicity. *Inhal. Toxicol.* **2014**, *26*, 353–360. [CrossRef]
43. Schisler, J.C.; Ronnebaum, S.M.; Madden, M.; Channell, M.; Campen, M.; Willis, M.S. Endothelial inflammatory transcriptional responses to an altered plasma exposome following inhalation of diesel emissions. *Inhal. Toxicol.* **2015**, *27*, 272–280. [CrossRef]
44. Vedal, S.; Campen, M.J.; McDonald, J.D.; Larson, T.V.; Sampson, P.D.; Sheppard, L.; Simpson, C.D.; Szpiro, A.A. National Particle Component Toxicity (NPACT) initiative report on cardiovascular effects. *Res. Rep. (Health Eff. Inst.)* **2013**, *178*, 5–8.
45. Elder, A.; Oberdorster, G. Translocation and effects of ultrafine particles outside of the lung. *Clin. Occup. Environ. Med.* **2006**, *5*, 785–796.
46. Reed, M.D.; Gigliotti, A.P.; McDonald, J.D.; Seagrave, J.C.; Seilkop, S.K.; Mauderly, J.L. Health effects of subchronic exposure to environmental levels of diesel exhaust. *Inhal. Toxicol.* **2004**, *16*, 177–193. [CrossRef]
47. Conklin, D.J.; Kong, M.; Committee, H.E.I.H.R. Part 4. Effects of subchronic diesel engine emissions exposure on plasma markers in rodents: Report on 1- and 3-month exposures in the ACES bioassay. *Res. Rep. (Health Eff. Inst.)* **2012**, *166*, 189–223.
48. Sun, J.H.; Peng, S.X.; Li, Z.Y.; Liu, F.F.; Wu, C.X.; Lu, Y.A.; Xiang, H. Association of Short-Term Exposure to $PM_{2.5}$ with Blood Lipids and the Modification Effects of Insulin Resistance: A Panel Study in Wuhan. *Toxics* **2022**, *10*, 663. [CrossRef]
49. Rastogi, L.; Dash, K.; Sashidhar, R.B. Selective and sensitive detection of cholesterol using intrinsic peroxidase-like activity of biogenic palladium nanoparticles. *Curr. Res. Biotechnol.* **2021**, *3*, 42–48. [CrossRef]
50. Moon, J.-Y.; Moon, M.H.; Kim, K.T.; Jeong, D.H.; Kim, Y.N.; Chung, B.C.; Choi, M.H. Cytochrome P450-mediated metabolic alterations in preeclampsia evaluated by quantitative steroid signatures. *J. Steroid Biochem. Mol. Biol.* **2014**, *139*, 182–191. [CrossRef]
51. Bochem, A.E.; Holleboom, A.G.; Romijn, J.A.; Hoekstra, M.; Dallinga-Thie, G.M.; Motazacker, M.M.; Hovingh, G.K.; Kuivenhoven, J.A.; Stroes, E.S.G. High density lipoprotein as a source of cholesterol for adrenal steroidogenesis: A study in individuals with low plasma HDL-C. *J. Lipid Res.* **2013**, *54*, 1698–1704. [CrossRef]
52. Ding, L.; Yang, L.; Wang, Z.; Huang, W. Bile acid nuclear receptor FXR and digestive system diseases. *Acta Pharm. Sin. B* **2015**, *5*, 135–144. [CrossRef]

53. Luo, W.; Liu, L.; Yang, L.; Dong, Y.; Liu, T.; Wei, X.; Liu, D.; Gu, H.; Kong, J.; Yuan, Z.; et al. The vitamin D receptor regulates miR-140-5p and targets the MAPK pathway in bone development. *Metabolism* **2018**, *85*, 139–150. [CrossRef]
54. Schade, D.S.; Shey, L.; Eaton, R.P. Cholesterol Review: A Metabolically Important Molecule. *Endocr. Pract.* **2020**, *26*, 1514–1523. [CrossRef]
55. Minuk, G.Y. Canadian Association of Gastroenterology Practice Guidelines: Evaluation of abnormal liver enzyme tests. *Can. J. Gastroenterol.* **1998**, *12*, 417–421. [CrossRef]
56. Dai, S.; Wang, Z.; Yang, Y.; Du, P.; Li, X. PM2.5 induced weight loss of mice through altering the intestinal microenvironment: Mucus barrier, gut microbiota, and metabolic profiling. *J. Hazard. Mater.* **2022**, *431*, 128653. [CrossRef]
57. De Silva, N.M.G.; Borges, M.C.; Hingorani, A.D.; Engmann, J.; Shah, T.; Zhang, X.S.; Luan, J.A.; Langenberg, C.; Wong, A.; Kuh, D.; et al. Liver Function and Risk of Type 2 Diabetes: Bidirectional Mendelian Randomization Study. *Diabetes* **2019**, *68*, 1681–1691. [CrossRef]
58. Kavishankar, G.B.; Moree, S.S.; Lakshmidevi, N. Hepatoprotective and antioxidant activity of N-Trisaccharide in different experimental rats. *Phytomedicine* **2014**, *21*, 1026–1031. [CrossRef]
59. Xu, X.; Dong, Y.; Ma, N.; Kong, W.; Yu, C.; Gong, L.; Chen, J.; Ren, J. MiR-337-3p lowers serum LDL-C level through targeting PCSK9 in hyperlipidemic mice. *Metabolism* **2021**, *119*, 154768. [CrossRef]
60. Surakka, I.; Hornsby, W.E.; Farhat, L.; Rubenfire, M.; Fritsche, L.G.; Hveem, K.; Chen, Y.E.; Brook, R.D.; Willer, C.J.; Weinberg, R.L. A Novel Variant in APOB Gene Causes Extremely Low LDL-C Without Known Adverse Effects. *JACC. Case Rep.* **2020**, *2*, 775–779. [CrossRef]
61. Wang, D.F.; Tan, K.S.; Zeng, W.P.; Li, S.X.; Wang, Y.Q.; Xu, F.P.; Tan, W. Hepatocellular BChE as a therapeutic target to ameliorate hypercholesterolemia through PRMT5 selective degradation to restore LDL receptor transcription. *Life Sci.* **2022**, *293*, 120336. [CrossRef]
62. Bond, J.A.; Medinsky, M.A.; Dutcher, J.S. Metabolism of 1- 14C nitropyrene in isolated perfused rat livers. *Toxicol. Appl. Pharmacol.* **1984**, *75*, 531–538. [CrossRef]
63. Xu, L.; Li, Y.; Ma, W.; Sun, X.; Fan, R.; Jin, Y.; Chen, N.; Zhu, X.; Guo, H.; Zhao, K.; et al. Diesel exhaust particles exposure induces liver dysfunction: Exploring predictive potential of human circulating microRNAs signature relevant to liver injury risk. *J. Hazard. Mater.* **2023**, *458*, 132060. [CrossRef] [PubMed]
64. Ito, Y.; Yanagiba, Y.; Ramdhan, D.H.; Hayashi, Y.; Li, Y.F.; Suzuki, A.K.; Kamijima, M.; Nakajima, T. Nanoparticle-Rich Diesel Exhaust-Induced Liver Damage via Inhibited Transactivation of Peroxisome Proliferator-Activated Receptor Alpha. *Environ. Toxicol.* **2016**, *31*, 1985–1995. [CrossRef] [PubMed]
65. Dutta, S.; Sengupta, P. Men and mice: Relating their ages. *Life Sci.* **2016**, *152*, 244–248. [CrossRef]
66. Hamade, A.K.; Misra, V.; Rabold, R.; Tankersley, C.G. Age-related changes in cardiac and respiratory adaptation to acute ozone and carbon black exposures: Interstrain variation in mice. *Inhal. Toxicol.* **2010**, *22*, 84–94. [CrossRef] [PubMed]
67. Oliveira, M.; Slezakova, K.; Delerue-Matos, C.; Pereira, M.C.; Morais, S. Children environmental exposure to particulate matter and polycyclic aromatic hydrocarbons and biomonitoring in school environments: A review on indoor and outdoor exposure levels, major sources and health impacts. *Environ. Int.* **2019**, *124*, 180–204. [CrossRef]
68. Salvi, S. Health effects of ambient air pollution in children. *Paediatr. Respir. Rev.* **2007**, *8*, 275–280. [CrossRef]
69. Simioni, P.U.; Costa, E.H.; Tamashiro, W. Aging reduces the primary humoral response and the in vitro cytokine production in mice. *Braz. J. Med. Biol. Res.* **2007**, *40*, 1111–1120. [CrossRef]
70. Muthumani, M.; Prabu, S.M. Silibinin potentially protects arsenic-induced oxidative hepatic dysfunction in rats. *Toxicol. Mech. Methods* **2012**, *22*, 277–288. [CrossRef]
71. Li, Q.L.; Wu, Y.H.; Niu, M.; Lu, X.J.; Huang, Y.H.; He, D.H. Protective effects of tacalcitol against oxidative damage in human epidermal melanocytes. *Int. J. Dermatol.* **2017**, *56*, 232–238. [CrossRef] [PubMed]
72. Shi, M.H.; Wu, Y.; Li, L.; Cai, Y.F.; Liu, M.; Gao, X.H.; Chen, H.D. Meta-analysis of the association between vitiligo and the level of superoxide dismutase or malondialdehyde. *Clin. Exp. Dermatol.* **2017**, *42*, 21–29. [CrossRef]
73. Karsli, N.; Akcali, C.; Ozgoztasi, O.; Kirtak, N.; Inaloz, S. Role of oxidative stress in the pathogenesis of vitiligo with special emphasis on the antioxidant action of narrowband ultraviolet B phototherapy. *J. Int. Med. Res.* **2014**, *42*, 799–805. [CrossRef] [PubMed]
74. Liu, H.H.; Shih, T.S.; Chen, I.J.; Chen, H.L. Lipid Peroxidation and Oxidative Status Compared in Workers at a Bottom Ash Recovery Plant and Fly Ash Treatment Plants. *J. Occup. Health* **2008**, *50*, 492–497. [CrossRef] [PubMed]
75. Zheng, X.M.; Wang, G.L.; Bin, P.; Meng, T.; Niu, Y.; Yang, M.; Zhang, L.P.; Duan, H.W.; Yu, T.; Dai, Y.F.; et al. Time-course effects of antioxidants and phase II enzymes on diesel exhaust particles-induced oxidative damage in the mouse lung. *Toxicol. Appl. Pharmacol.* **2019**, *366*, 25–34. [CrossRef]
76. Xu, M.M.; Wang, X.H.; Xu, L.; Zhang, H.; Li, C.F.; Liu, Q.; Chen, Y.Q.; Chung, K.F.; Adcock, I.M.; Li, F. Chronic lung inflammation and pulmonary fibrosis after multiple intranasal instillation of $PM_{2.5}$ in mice. *Environ. Toxicol.* **2021**, *36*, 1434–1446. [CrossRef]
77. Yin, F.; Driscoll, W.; Sulaiman, D.; Vergnes, L.; Ricks, J.; Ramanathan, G.; Stewart, J.; Mehrabian, M.; Beaven, S.W.; Reue, K.; et al. Diesel Exhaust Induces Mitochondrial Dysfunction, Hyperlipidemia and Liver Steatosis. *Circulation* **2018**, *138*, A17401. [CrossRef]
78. Krivoshto, I.N.; Richards, J.R.; Albertson, T.E.; Derlet, R.W. The toxicity of diesel exhaust: Implications for primary care. *J. Am. Board Fam. Med.* **2008**, *21*, 55–62. [CrossRef] [PubMed]

79. IARC Working Group on the Evaluation of Carcinogenic Risks to Humans, International Agency for Research on Cancer. Diesel and gasoline engine exhausts and some nitroarenes. iarc monographs on the evaluation of carcinogenic risks to humans. *IARC Monogr. Eval. Carcinog. Risks Hum.* **2014**, *105*, 9–699.
80. Tseng, C.Y.; Wang, J.S.; Chao, M.W. Causation by Diesel Exhaust Particles of Endothelial Dysfunctions in Cytotoxicity, Pro-inflammation, Permeability, and Apoptosis Induced by ROS Generation. *Cardiovasc. Toxicol.* **2017**, *17*, 384–392. [CrossRef]
81. Wang, J.S.; Tseng, C.Y.; Chao, M.W. Diesel Exhaust Particles Contribute to Endothelia Apoptosis via Autophagy Pathway. *Toxicol. Sci.* **2017**, *156*, 72–83. [CrossRef] [PubMed]
82. Aquino, G.V.; Dabi, A.; Odom, G.J.; Zhang, F.; Bruce, E.D. Evaluating the endothelial-microglial interaction and comprehensive inflammatory marker profiles under acute exposure to ultrafine diesel exhaust particles in vitro. *Toxicology* **2021**, *454*, 152748. [CrossRef] [PubMed]
83. Li, R.S.; Ning, Z.; Ai, L.S.; Sioutas, C.; Hsiai, T. Atmospheric Nanoparticles Induce Vascular Oxidative Stress via JNK Activation. *Circulation* **2008**, *118*, S318.

toxics

MDPI

Article

Independent and Joint Effects of Prenatal Incense-Burning Smoke Exposure and Children's Early Outdoor Activity on Preschoolers' Obesity

Meimei Chen [1], Esben Strodl [2], Weikang Yang [3,*], Xiaona Yin [3], Guomin Wen [3], Dengli Sun [3], Danxia Xian [3], Yafen Zhao [3] and Weiqing Chen [1,4,*]

1 Department of Epidemiology, School of Public Health, Sun Yat-sen University, Guangzhou 510080, China; chenmm29@mail2.sysu.edu.cn
2 School of Psychology and Counselling, Queensland University of Technology, Brisbane, QLD 4059, Australia; e.strodl@qut.edu.au
3 Women's and Children's Hospital of Longhua District of Shenzhen, Shenzhen 518110, China
4 School of Health Management, Xinhua College of Guangzhou, Guangzhou 510080, China
* Correspondence: yangweikang@lhfywork.com (W.Y.); chenwq@mail.sysu.edu.cn (W.C.)

Abstract: Incense burning is a significant source of indoor air pollution in many Asian regions. There is emerging evidence that maternal prenatal exposure to incense-burning smoke may be a risk factor for childhood obesity. We aimed to extend this new line of research by investigating the independent and joint effect of incense-burning smoke exposure, and children's outdoor activity in early life, on preschoolers' obesity. A total of 69,637 mother–child dyads were recruited from all kindergartens in the Longhua District of Shenzhen, China. Information on sociodemographic characteristics, maternal exposure to incense-burning smoke (IBS) during pregnancy, and frequency and duration of outdoor activity at the age of 1–3 years was collected by a self-administered questionnaire. In addition, the heights and weights of the children were measured by the research team. Logistic regression models and cross-over analyses were conducted to investigate the independent and combined effects of maternal exposure to incense-burning smoke during pregnancy and children's early outdoor activity on obesity in preschoolers. We found that prenatal exposure to incense-burning smoke increased the risk of the presence of obesity in preschoolers' (AOR = 1.13, 95% CI = 1.03–1.23). Additionally, lower frequencies (<3 times/week) or shorter durations (<60 min/time) of outdoor activity from the age of 1–3 years were significantly associated with the presence of obesity, with AORs of 1.24 (95% CI =1.18–1.32) and 1.11 (95% CI = 1.05–1.17), respectively. Furthermore, the cross-over analysis showed that prenatal exposure to IBS combined with a lower frequency of early outdoor activity (AOR = 1.47, 95% CI = 1.31–1.66) or a shorter duration of outdoor activity during ages of 1–3 years (AOR = 1.22, 95% CI = 1.07–1.39) increased the risk of obesity in preschoolers. Finally, additive interactions between prenatal exposure to IBS and postnatal outdoor activity on obesity were identified. Our study indicates that maternal exposure to incense-burning smoke during pregnancy and early lower postanal outdoor activity may independently and jointly increase the risk of obesity among preschoolers.

Keywords: incense-burning smoke; early outdoor activity; joint effect; obesity; preschool child

1. Introduction

The prevalence of childhood overweight and obesity has reached alarmingly high levels in the past decades worldwide. Globally, 124 million children and adolescents aged 5–19 years are affected by obesity, with the prevalence climbing from 0.7% to 5.6% in girls and from 0.9% to 7.8% in boys from 1975 to 2016, respectively [1]. In addition, according to the World Health Organization, approximately 38.2 million children under the age of five years were overweight or obese in 2019 [2]. According to the Global Burden of Disease study in 2015, China has the highest number of obese children in the world [3]. These statistics raise significant public health concerns given that there is mounting evidence that childhood obesity is a risk factor for numerous physical and mental health conditions in children [4,5] and that the persistence of obesity into adulthood is a significant risk factor for chronic diseases, such as diabetes, hypertension, hyperlipidemia [6], cardio cerebral vascular disease [7], and certain tumors in adults [8]. As such, early childhood is a critical period for preventing persistent obesity [9,10] and the subsequent health conditions associated with it. To guide the development of targeted public health interventions, it is therefore essential to identify significant risk and protective factors for childhood obesity.

While the etiology of childhood obesity is not yet fully understood, it is well known that childhood obesity is the result of a complex interplay of genetic, prenatal, and postnatal environmental factors. Moreover, there is increasing evidence showing that the programming of obesity begins prenatally and early postnatally [11]. For instance, previous research has identified the following prenatal risk factors for offspring obesity: high maternal prepregnancy BMI, maternal excessive weight gain during pregnancy, gestational diabetes, maternal physical activity during pregnancy, maternal smoking in pregnancy [12–16], and prenatal exposure to air pollution [17,18], as well as adverse birth outcomes of preterm birth, low birth weight, and macrosomia [19,20]. Additionally, prior studies have shown that early infants' and toddlers' health behaviors, such as nonbreastfeeding, consumption of high-sugar foods, fast eating pace, excessive screen time, and lack of physical activity, are risk factors for childhood obesity [19–23]. Conversely, playing outdoors, particularly in natural play spaces, boosts children's physical activity, decreasing childhood obesity [24].

Based on the theory of developmental origins of health and disease (DOHaD), fetuses exposed to malnutrition and environmental hazards can experience heightened susceptibility to fetal origin of adult disease (FOAD), with this susceptibility further enhanced by postnatal exposure to hazardous environmental factors [25,26]. It is now widely accepted that exposure to hazardous in utero environments plays significant roles in fetal development and initiation of FOAD that may involve epigenetic alterations in the development of FOAD [25,26]. For example, Rueda-Clausen et al. found that prenatal hypoxia and postnatal high-fat diets in offspring were associated with an increased myocardial susceptibility to ischemia [27]. In addition, our recent study found that prenatal mosquito coil smoke exposure and early postnatal nutrition status can independently and jointly increase the risk of preschoolers' obesity [28].

Incense burning, a practice widely observed in Asia and the Middle East, has been identified as a potential source of indoor air pollution, with the burning of incense releasing enormous levels of fine particles, polycyclic aromatic hydrocarbon (PAH), high concentrations of detrimental gases, and other toxic chemical compounds [29–32]. Previous studies have reported the potentially harmful health effects associated with incense burning, such as respiratory problems [33], neurobehavioral development [34], cardiovascular mortality [35], cancer [36,37], and adverse birth outcomes [38]. However, few studies have investigated the effect of exposure to incense burning on obesity. A cross-sectional study in Guangzhou reported that children exposed to three or more types of indoor air pollutants (cooking oil fumes, home decoration, secondhand smoke, and incense burning) had higher obesity anthropometric indices and increased odds of being overweight/obese [39]. However, the study found no statistical significance between incense burning and overweight/obesity. As such, there is a need for further research to clarify the key prenatal and postnatal factors linking exposure to indoor air pollutants with different childhood obesity measures.

Given the emerging evidence that exposure to indoor air pollution may be a risk factor for early childhood obesity, this study aimed to test the theory of DOHaD by examining whether maternal prenatal exposure to incense-burning smoke and early childhood physical activity levels independently and jointly predict the presence of childhood obesity in preschoolers. The aims of this study are important not only in terms of identifying significant risk factors for childhood obesity but also in terms of providing evidence to support the hypothesis that childhood health conditions are affected by an interaction of both prenatal and postnatal factors. Identifying these complex interactions is critical to enhancing the sophistication of our understanding of the biopsychosocial factors contributing to childhood ill health, thereby improving the effectiveness of public health interventions.

2. Materials and Methods

2.1. Study Population

The Longhua Child Cohort Study (LCCS) is an ongoing prospective study that has involved the administration of a population-based survey once a year in the Longhua District of Shenzhen since September 2014. The aim of this study is to examine the influence of environmental factors during a preschooler's early life on childhood psychobehavioral development. The LCCS recruits children when they enter preschool and invites their mothers to complete a self-administered structured questionnaire every year. A total of 69,637 child–mother dyads were recruited during the LCCS 2021 survey. After excluding children (1) with missing information on important sociodemographic characteristics (i.e., birth weight, gestational age, and present height and weight); (2) whose mothers did not report information of exposure to IBS during pregnancy; and (3) who were nonsingleton births and whose gestational age was low (under 24 weeks) or high (42 weeks or greater) (data from 64,889 (93.2%) child–mother dyads were included in this study (Figure 1)). We employed multiple imputation (MI) to fill in the missing data or outliers for covariates among 8868 (13.7%) participants whose questionnaires did not contain information on at least one chosen covariate.

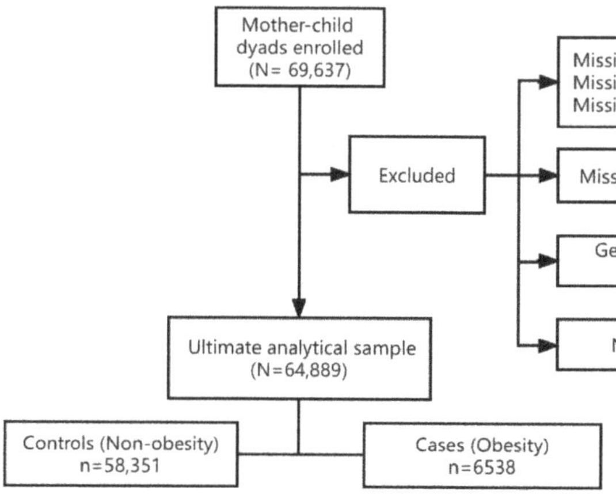

Figure 1. Flow diagram of the participant selection.

This study was approved by the Ethics Committee of the School of Public Health at Sun Yat-Sen University and was conducted in accordance with the Declaration of Helsinki. Written informed consent was obtained from mothers.

2.2. Data Collection

The mothers were asked to complete a self-administered structured questionnaire regarding the sociodemographic characteristics of the parents (family monthly income, age at childbirth, marital status, parental education level, mother's height and weight before prepregnancy, weight gain during pregnancy), as well as the child's age, sex, gestational age, birth weight, and present height and weight.

2.3. Prenatal IBS Exposure Measurement

In addition, the questionnaire included three questions for the mother regarding incense-burning smoke exposure during pregnancy: "Did your household have the habit of burning incense at home during your pregnancy in 1–13 weeks (the first trimester)"? (2) "Did your household have the habit of burning incense at home during your pregnancy in 14–27 weeks (the second trimester)"? (3) "Did your household have the habit of burning incense at home during your pregnancy after 28 weeks (the third trimester)"? [(the response format was "no", "sometimes (1 time per week)", "often" (at least 2 times per week)",)]. If the answer was "sometimes" or "often", then prenatal exposure to IBS was considered present. Moreover, to identify the potentially sensitive period, we divided the participants into 8 subgroups according to the different combinations of IBS exposure status (No or Yes) in each trimester.

2.4. Early Frequency and Duration of Outdoor Activity Measurement

The frequency and duration of outdoor activity of children were evaluated by the following questions: (1) How often did your baby go outdoors for physical activity during the year of 1–3 years old? [(the response options were "0 = ≥3 times/week", or "1 = <3 times/week",)]; (2) How much time did your baby spend outdoors for physical activity on average during the year of 1–3 years old? [(the possible responses were 0 = ≥60 min/time", or "1 = <60 min/time",)]. The answers were transformed into the following variables that illustrated the children's outdoor activity from birth to three years old: (1) the frequency of outdoor activity and (2) the duration of outdoor activity.

2.5. Measurement and Definition of Obesity

Children's height and weight were measured by skilled nurses at the Longhua Maternity and Child Healthcare Hospital. A portable electronic weight scale (fractional value = 0.01 kg), placed on the ground level, was used to measure the weight of each preschooler, who was required to stand in the center of the scale bareheaded, barefooted, and dressed in close-fitting light clothes. The value was read and accurately recorded to 0.1 kg by nurses after stabilizing. A column human altimeter (fractional value = 0.1 cm), that was placed vertically against the wall on horizontal ground, was used to measure the weight of the preschoolers with each asked to stand on the pedal, with their heels close together, feet spaced at an angle of 60 degrees, chest raised, abdomen pulled in, and eyes looking straight ahead. With their line of sighting the same height as the slide board, the measurements were read by slider to the apex of the measured child's skull.

The body mass index (BMI) was determined by dividing the weight in kilograms by the square of height in meters (kg/m^2). Childhood obesity was defined as having a BMI higher than the specified thresholds based on age and gender, as per the BMI growth curves designed for Chinese children [40].

2.6. Potential Confounding Variables

In light of previously published studies [16,39,41], the potential covariates selected were children's gender and age, birth weight, single child or not, premature birth, feeding pattern, early nutritional status, parental age at conception, maternal marital status and prepregnancy BMI, family income, maternal folic acid intake during pregnancy, prenatal exposure to environmental tobacco smoke, mosquito coil smoke, and cooking oil fumes.

2.7. Statistical Analyses

Frequencies and proportions were used to describe the categorical variables, and the chi-square test was applied to test and describe associations of subjects' characteristics with childhood obesity.

A series of binary logistic regression analyses were utilized to evaluate the independent and joint associations of prenatal exposure to incense-burning smoke, postnatal early frequency, and duration of outdoor activity with obesity in preschoolers after adjusting for the aforementioned covariates. The multiplicative interaction was examined by the interaction of odds ratio (IOR) in the logistic regression models. If the 95% CI of the IOR spanned 1, the multiplicative interaction was considered nonsignificant. Furthermore, relative excess risk due to interaction (RERI) and attributable proportion due to interaction (AP) were calculated. If the 95% CIs of RERI and AP did not span 0, the additive interaction was considered significant [42]. A cross-over analysis was performed to elucidate the possible sensitivity period. Additionally, sensitivity analyses were conducted after excluding children who were preterm birth (gestational age < 37 weeks) or low birth weight (birth weight < 2500 g).

All statistical analyses were performed using R Studio version 4.3.1, with two-sided $p < 0.05$ deemed significant.

3. Results

3.1. Population Characteristics

Table 1 describes the comparison of demographic characteristics between obese and nonobese children. Of the 64,889 preschoolers included in this study, 6538 (10.0%) of them were obese, with the prevalence of obesity in boys being 11.7% and 8.2% in girls. Of the total sample, 6117 (9.4%) mothers reported that they had experienced prenatal exposure to IBS. Obese and nonobese preschoolers differed significantly on sex, age, single child or not, family income, marital status, maternal prepregnancy BMI, maternal gained weight during pregnancy, maternal folic acid intake during pregnancy, prenatal exposure to mosquito coil smoke and cooking oil fumes, education level of parents, feeding pattern, early nutritional status, birth weight, gestational age, and preterm birth or not.

Table 1. Characteristics of the study participants.

Characteristics	Total (N = 64,889)	Obesity (n = 6538)	Prevalence (%)	p
Gender				<0.001
Boys	34,647	4070	11.7	
Girls	30,242	2468	8.2	
Age (years)				<0.001
<3	185	18	9.7	
3–4	12,527	1076	8.6	
4–5	22,313	2279	10.2	
≥5	29,864	3165	10.6	
Single child				<0.001
No	21,162	1759	8.3	
Yes	43,727	4779	10.9	
Family income (USD/month)				<0.001
<3077	32,246	3396	10.5	
3077~6154	21,781	2089	9.6	
≥6154	10,862	1053	9.7	
Marital status				<0.001
Married	63,225	6308	10.0	
Others	1664	230	13.8	
Maternal prepregnancy BMI				<0.001
Underweight (<18.5)	13,356	1059	7.9	
Normal (18.5~23.9)	45,976	4675	10.2	
Overweight (>24)	5557	804	14.5	
Maternal occupation				0.006
Full-time housewife	10,545	948	9.0	
others	54,344	5411	9.9	
Maternal gestational weight gain				<0.001
<5kg	3141	431	13.7	
5–10 kg	21,857	2223	10.2	
11–15 kg	25,598	2296	9.0	
16–20 kg	10,921	1168	10.7	
>20 kg	3372	420	12.5	

Table 1. *Cont.*

Characteristics	Total (N = 64,889)	Obesity (n = 6538)	Prevalence (%)	p
Folic acid intake during pregnancy				<0.001
No	38,198	4097	10.7	
Yes	26,691	2441	9.1	
Environmental tobacco smoke (ETS)				0.121
No	53,922	5388	10.0	
Yes	10,967	1150	10.5	
Mosquito coil smoke (MCS)				<0.001
No	45,092	4352	9.7	
Yes	19,797	2186	11.0	
Home renovated				0.026
No	61,363	6194	10.1	
Yes	2131	185	8.7	
Unclear	1395	159	11.4	
Cooking oil fumes				<0.001
No	13,597	1498	11.0	
Yes	51,292	5040	9.8	
Heavy metal exposure				0.831
No	64,392	6486	10.1	
Yes	497	52	10.5	
Benzene exposure				0.155
No	64,438	6483	10.1	
Yes	451	55	12.2	
Maternal education level				<0.001
Junior high school or lower	9498	1063	11.2	
High school	13,117	1391	10.6	
College or higher	42,274	4084	9.7	
Paternal education level				<0.001
Junior high school or lower	8532	980	11.5	
High school	13,256	1402	10.6	
College or higher	43,101	4156	9.6	
Maternal age at childbirth (years)				0.559
<35	58,481	5879	10.1	
≥35	6408	659	10.3	
Paternal age at childbirth (years)				0.03
<35	39,847	3926	9.9	
≥35	25,042	2612	10.4	
Feeding pattern				0.007
Breastfeeding	38,094	3864	10.1	
Artificial feeding	6424	706	11.0	
Mixed feeding	20,371	1968	9.7	
Nutritional status at 0–1 years old				<0.001
Poorly nourished	856	77	9.0	
Medium-nourished	15,949	13,689	8.6	
Well-nourished	48,084	5093	10.6	
Nutritional status at 1–3 years old				<0.001
Poorly nourished	996	81	8.1	
Medium-nourished	20,520	1592	7.8	
Well-nourished	43,373	4865	11.2	
Birth weight (g)				<0.001
<2500	3022	335	11.1	
2500–4000	55,763	5351	9.6	
≥4000	6104	852	14.0	
Preterm birth				<0.001
No	60,309	5982	9.9	
Yes	4580	556	12.1	

3.2. Association between Maternal Exposure to IBS during Pregnancy and Obesity among Preschoolers

As shown in Table 2, compared with the nonexposed group, maternal exposure to IBS during the whole pregnancy significantly increased the risk of offspring obesity after controlling for a range of confounding factors (AOR = 1.13, 95% CI = 1.03~1.23). However, when the pregnancy was divided into three trimesters, there was a nonsignificant trend for maternal exposure to IBS in specific trimesters (the 1st trimester: AOR = 1.14, 95% CI = 0.96~1.34; the 2nd trimester: AOR = 1.19, 95% CI = 0.94~1.51; the 3rd trimester: AOR = 0.84, 95% CI = 0.68~1.04)

Table 2. Associations of maternal IBS exposure during pregnancy with children's obesity.

Prenatal IBS Exposure	Total (N = 64,889)	Obesity (n, %)	AOR (95% CI) [a]	AOR (95% CI) [b]
The whole pregnancy				
No	58,772	5837 (9.9)	1.00	1.00
Yes	6117	701 (11.5)	1.13 (1.03, 1.23) **	1.13 (1.03, 1.23) **
1st trimester				
No	59,732	5933 (9.9)	1.00	1.00
Yes	5157	605 (11.7)	1.15 (1.05, 1.26) **	1.14 (0.96, 1.34)
2nd trimester				
No	60,243	5999 (10.0)	1.00	1.00
Yes	4646	539 (11.6)	1.14 (1.03, 1.26) **	1.19 (0.94, 1.51)
3rd trimester				
No	60,222	6019 (10.0)	1.00	1.00
Yes	4667	519 (11.1)	1.09 (0.99, 1.20)	0.84 (0.68, 1.04)

Model a: adjusted for child's gender and age, birth weight, single child or not, premature birth, parental age at conception, maternal marital status and prepregnancy BMI, family income, prenatal exposure to ETS, MCS, cooking oil fumes, child's feeding pattern, early nutritional status, folic acid intake during pregnancy. Model b: 1st trimester: adjusted for Model a + prenatal exposure to 2nd trimester and 3rd trimester; 2nd trimester: adjusted for Model a + prenatal exposure to 1st trimester and 3rd trimester; 3rd trimester: adjusted for Model a + prenatal exposure to 1st trimester and 2nd trimester. ** $p < 0.01$.

With regard to the frequency of IBS exposure during the different trimesters, after controlling for confounding factors, only maternal prenatal exposure to IBS ≥ 2 times/week in the 1st trimester (AOR = 1.31, 95% CI = 1.01~1.70) was significantly associated with an increased the risk of childhood obesity. Nonsignificant trends were found for the associations between those prenatally exposed to IBS with 1 time/week in the 1st trimester (AOR = 1.11, 95% CI = 0.94~1.31) and with both 1 time/week (AOR = 1.19, 95% CI = 0.94~1.51) and 2 times/week (AOR = 1.20, 95% CI = 0.84~1.69) in the 2nd trimester increased the risk of childhood obesity (Table 3).

Table 3. Associations of frequency of trimester-specific IBS exposure during pregnancy with children obesity.

Frequency of IBS Exposure	Total (N = 64,889)	Obesity (n, %)	AOR (95% CI) [a]	AOR (95% CI) [b]
1st trimester				
Never	59,732	5933 (9.9)	1.00	1.00
1 time/week	4481	516 (11.5)	1.12 (1.01, 1.24) *	1.11 (0.94, 1.31)
≥2 times/week	676	89 (13.2)	1.33 (1.06, 1.67) *	1.31 (1.01, 1.70) *
2nd trimester				
Never	60,243	5999 (10.0)	1.00	1.00
1 time/week	4094	474 (11.6)	1.14 (1.03, 1.26) *	1.19 (0.94, 1.51)
≥2 times/week	552	65 (11.8)	1.15 (0.87, 1.48)	1.20 (0.84, 1.69)
3rd trimester				
Never	60,222	6019 (10.0)	1.00	1.00
1 time/week	4086	458 (11.2)	1.10 (0.99, 1.22)	0.85 (0.68, 1.06)
≥2 times/week	581	61 (10.5)	1.01 (0.76, 1.31)	0.77(0.54, 1.06)

Model a: adjusted for child's gender and age, birth weight, single child or not, premature birth, parental age at conception, maternal marital status and prepregnancy BMI, family income, prenatal exposure to ETS, MCS, cooking oil fumes, child's feeding pattern, early nutritional status, folic acid intake during pregnancy. Model b: 1st trimester: adjusted for Model a + prenatal exposure to 2nd trimester and 3rd trimester; 2nd trimester: adjusted for Model a + prenatal exposure to 1st trimester and 3rd trimester; 3rd trimester: adjusted for Model a + prenatal exposure to 1st trimester and 2nd trimester. * $p < 0.05$.

After controlling for confounding factors, the crossover analysis revealed that prenatal exposure to IBS concurrently in the 1st and 2nd trimesters (AOR = 1.50, 95% CI = 1.07~2.07) and in the whole three trimesters (AOR = 1.12, 95% CI = 1.01~1.25) significantly increased the risk of offspring obesity (Table 4).

Table 4. Associations of trimester-specific IBS exposure during pregnancy with children obesity.

Trimester-Specific IBS Exposure			Total (N = 64,889)	Obesity (n, %)	OR (95% CI)	AOR (95% CI) [a]
1st Trimester	2nd Trimester	3rd Trimester				
No	No	No	58,772	5837 (9.9)	1.00	1.00
Yes	No	No	980	118 (12.0)	1.24 (1.02, 1.50) *	1.16 (0.94, 1.40)
No	Yes	No	185	21 (11.4)	1.16 (0.72, 1.79)	1.10 (0.68, 1.71)
No	No	Yes	407	35 (8.6)	0.85 (0.59, 1.19)	0.87 (0.60, 1.21)
Yes	Yes	No	285	43 (15.1)	1.61 (1.15, 2.21) **	1.50 (1.07, 2.07) *
Yes	No	Yes	84	9 (10.7)	1.09 (0.51, 2.06)	1.08 (0.50, 2.06)
No	Yes	Yes	368	40 (10.9)	1.11 (0.78, 1.52)	1.13 (0.80, 1.56)
Yes	Yes	Yes	3808	435 (11.4)	1.17 (1.05, 1.30) **	1.12 (1.01, 1.25) *

[a]: adjusted for child's gender and age, birth weight, single child or not, premature birth, parental age at conception, maternal marital status and prepregnancy BMI, family income, prenatal exposure to ETS, MCS, cooking oil fumes, child's feeding pattern, early nutritional status, folic acid intake during pregnancy. * $p < 0.05$, ** $p < 0.01$.

3.3. Association of Frequency and Duration of Outdoor Activity from 1 to 3 Years of Age with Children Obesity

Table 5 presents the associations of the frequency and duration of outdoor activity from 1 to 3 years of age with children obesity. After adjusting for confounding factors, compared with children whose mothers reported that their child frequently went outdoors (≥3 times/week) at the age of 1~3 years, those who had a paucity of frequent outdoor activity had significantly greater odds of experiencing obesity during preschool (AOR = 1.24, 95% CI = 1.18~1.32). Additionally, a shorter duration of outdoor activity (<60 min/time) (AOR = 1.11, 95% CI = 1.05~1.17) was significantly associated with a higher risk of offspring obesity compared with children who had a longer duration of outdoor activity. Furthermore, compared with children with both the higher frequency (≥3 times/week) and the longer duration of outdoor activity at the age of 1~3 years, those with lower frequencies and longer durations, as well as those with lower frequencies (AOR = 1.13, 95% CI = 1.04~1.21) or with shorter durations of outdoor activity (AOR = 1.36, 95% CI =1.05~1.17), were significantly associated with preschool obesity.

Table 5. Associations of frequency and duration of outdoor activity from 1 to 3 years of age with children's obesity.

Outdoor Activity during 1–3 Years Old	Total (N = 64,889)	Obesity (n, %)	OR (95% CI)	AOR (95% CI) [a]
Frequency				
≥3 times/week	45,060	4261 (9.5)	1.00	1.00
<3 times/week	19,829	2277 (11.5)	1.24 (1.18, 1.31) ***	1.24 (1.18, 1.32) ***
Duration				
≥60 min/time	42,596	4175 (9.8)	1.00	1.00
<60 min/time	22,293	2363 (10.6)	1.09(1.03, 1.15) **	1.11 (1.05, 1.17) ***
Combination of Frequency and duration				
≥3 times/week + ≥60 min/time	32,402	3099 (9.6)	1.00	1.00
≥3 times/week + <60 min/time	12,658	1162 (9.2)	0.96 (0.89, 1.03)	0.98 (0.92, 1.06)
<3 times/week + ≥60 min/time	10,194	1076 (10.6)	1.12 (1.04, 1.20) **	1.13 (1.04, 1.21) **
<3 times/week + <60 min/time	9635	1201 (12.5)	1.35 (1.25, 1.44) ***	1.36 (1.26, 1.46) ***

[a]: adjusted for child's gender and age, birth weight, single child or not, premature birth, parental age at conception, maternal marital status and prepregnancy BMI, family income, prenatal exposure to ETS, MCS, cooking oil fumes, child's feeding pattern, early nutritional status, folic acid intake during pregnancy. ** $p < 0.01$, *** $p < 0.001$.

3.4. Combination Effect between Maternal IBS Exposure during Pregnancy and Outdoor Activity from 1 to 3 Years of Age on Preschool Obesity

Table 6 presents the combined effect of maternal IBS exposure during pregnancy and outdoor activity during 1 to 3 years old on children's obesity.

Table 6. Combination effect between maternal IBS exposure during pregnancy and outdoor activity from 1 to 3 years of age on children's obesity.

IBS Exposure	Outdoor Activity	AOR (95% CI) *	IOR (95% CI)	RERI (95% CI) *	AP (95% CI) [a]
Pregnancy	Frequency				
No	≥3 times/week	1.00			
No	<3 times/week	1.21 (1.14, 1.29) ***			
Yes	≥3 times/week	1.01 (0.90, 1.14)			
Yes	<3 times/week	1.47 (1.31, 1.66) ***	1.21 (1.01, 1.42) *	0.08 (0.03, 0.13)	0.06 (0.03, 0.09)
Pregnancy	Duration				
No	≥60 min/time	1.00			
No	<60 min/time	1.11 (1.05, 1.17) ***			
Yes	≥60 min/time	1.14 (1.02, 1.27) *			
Yes	<60 min/time	1.22 (1.07, 1.39) **	0.96 (0.81, 1.14)	0.07 (0.03, 0.11)	0.05 (0.03, 0.08)

[a]: adjusted for child's gender and age, birth weight, single child or not, premature birth, parental age at conception, maternal marital status and prepregnancy BMI, family income, prenatal exposure to ETS, MCS, cooking oil fumes, child's feeding pattern, early nutritional status, folic acid intake during pregnancy. * $p < 0.05$, ** $p < 0.01$, *** $p < 0.001$.

Compared with children with no prenatal maternal IBS exposure and a higher frequency of outdoor activity, children with a combination of no prenatal exposure to IBS and lower frequencies of outdoor activity (AOR = 1.22, 95% CI = 1.07~1.39) and a combination between prenatal exposure to IBS and lower frequencies of outdoor activity (<60 min/time) (AOR = 1.47, 95% CI = 1.31~1.66) were both significantly more likely to experience obesity during preschool. Furthermore, there was a significant multiplicative interaction between prenatal maternal exposure to IBS and less frequent outdoor activity (<3 times/week) on obesity, with an IOR of 1.21 (95% CI = 1.01, 1.42). We also found a significant additive interaction between the frequency of outdoor activity and IBS exposure, with an RERI of 0.08 (95% CI = 0.03~0.13) and AP of 0.06 (95% CI = 0.03~0.09).

Compared with children with no prenatal IBS exposure and a longer duration of outdoor activity (≥60 min/time), children's obesity was significantly associated with a combination of no prenatal exposure to IBS and shorter durations of outdoor activity (<60 min/time) (AOR = 1.11, 95% CI = 1.05~1.17), a combination of prenatal exposure to IBS and longer durations of outdoor activity (≥60 min/time) (AOR = 1.14, 95% CI = 1.02~1.27), and a combination of prenatal exposure to IBS and shorter durations of outdoor activity (<60 min/time) (AOR = 1.22, 95% CI = 1.07~1.39). Similarly, we found a significant additive interaction between prenatal maternal exposure to IBS and shorter durations of outdoor activity on obesity with an RERI of 0.07 (95% CI = 0.03~0.11) and an AP of 0.05 (95% CI = 0.03~0.08).

3.5. Sensitivity Analysis

Sensitivity analyses were performed after excluding participants who were preterm birth or low birth weight (n = 13,079), and the main results are still similar to the aforementioned findings. More details are shown in Tables S1–S6.

4. Discussion

To the best of our knowledge, this is the first large-scale study on the association between maternal exposure to incense-burning smoke during pregnancy and obesity in Chinese preschoolers. Our results identify a significant association between maternal exposure to IBS during pregnancy and offspring obesity with a dose-response relationship between frequency of trimester-specific IBS exposure and children's obesity. That is, mothers exposed to prenatal IBS in both the first and second trimesters concurrently and in all three trimesters were more likely to have offspring who experienced obesity in preschool. In addition, we observed that a low level of early outdoor activity was associated with a higher risk of obesity in preschoolers. Importantly, we also found both a multiplicative and an additive interaction between maternal prenatal IBS exposure and lower frequency of outdoor activity of children from 1 to 3 years old. Similarly, we found an additive interaction between maternal prenatal IBS exposure and a shorter duration of outdoor activity from 1 to 3 years old on the risk of childhood obesity.

In the past few decades, a series of studies have found associations between prenatal exposure to outdoor air pollution and childhood obesity. For instance, a prospective study in Boston found a positive relationship between exposure to ambient $PM_{2.5}$ in utero, and from conception to 2nd years, and the risk of children between two and nine years being overweight and obese [43]. The Colorado-based Healthy Start study showed that second-trimester $PM_{2.5}$ exposure was associated with a higher percent fat mass, and residential proximity to a highway during pregnancy was associated with higher odds of offspring being overweight at age 4~6 years [44]. Additionally, a study of 239 children born at $\geq$37 weeks gestation, from the Asthma Coalition on Community, Environment and Social Stress (ACCESS) project, indicated that increased $PM_{2.5}$ exposure in early-to-mid pregnancy was more strongly associated with increased fat mass and higher BMI z-score in boys and with increased waist-to-hip ratio (WHR) in girls [45]. Recently, a review by Shi et al. concluded that exposure to air pollution during pregnancy might increase the risk of childhood obesity [17], while another review by Sun et al. indicated that perinatal exposure to $PM_{2.5}$ could cause obesity in progeny [18]. Similarly, a systematic review by Qureshi et al. reported an association between prenatal exposure to environmental tobacco smoke and childhood obesity (OR = 1.91, 95% CI = 1.23~2.94) [46]. In line with these previous findings, our study found that maternal prenatal exposure to indoor air pollution of IBS was significantly linked with the presence of obesity in preschoolers, with a dose–response relationship between the frequency of trimester-specific IBS exposure in the 1st trimester and children obesity. Similarly, another recent study of ours found that prenatal exposure to indoor air pollution of mosquito coil smoke (MCS) was significantly positively associated with preschoolers' obesity [28]. In this current study, the cross-over analysis highlighted the positive association of prenatal IBS exposure in the first and second trimesters concurrently and in the whole pregnancy with obesity in preschoolers, and it indicated a dose–response relationship between maternal exposure to IBS during pregnancy and offspring obesity. Based on the definition of the sensitivity period/critical window [47], given that no significant association was found for the first trimester after adjusting for covariates, we speculated that there may not exist a critical period for prenatal IBS exposure causing offspring obesity in childhood.

Obesity is typically considered as an abnormal or excessive fat accumulation caused by excessive energy intake or insufficient energy consumption. In the case of the same nutritional status, children with insufficient energy consumption are more likely to be obese. While limited studies reported the relationships between outdoor activity and childhood obesity, research has indicated that time spent outdoors is associated with increased physical activity, which has been reported to have a negative association with childhood obesity [48–50]. One study among children aged 10 to 12 found that for every additional hour spent outdoors, physical activity increased by 27 min a week, and the prevalence of overweight dropped from 41% to 27% [51]. The parents of preschool children reported that physical activity usually occurs during outdoor playtime as opposed to during indoor activities [52]. One systematic review revealed overall positive effects of outdoor time on physical activity compared with sedentary behavior [53]. Additionally, several researchers have proposed that increasing outdoor time could be an effective measure for limiting sedentary behavior and increasing physical activity and fitness in children [54,55]. The ecological model, as described by Davison et al., suggests that physical activity is one of the risk factors for children's obesity [56]. The World Health Organization

(WHO) recommends moderate-to-vigorous physical activity for children and adolescents for at least 60 min per day [57]. Consistent with these studies, we found that preschool children with less frequency or shorter durations of outdoor physical activity during 1–3 years old had a higher risk of obesity.

Consistent with the theory of DOHaD, the combination of maternal lifestyle during pregnancy and the early nutritional environment of the offspring is considered important for the development of obesity [16]. For example, an epidemiological study indicated that elevated exposure to mercury in utero was associated with a higher risk of the offspring being overweight or obese in childhood, with this risk being reduced by adequate maternal folate supplementation [58]. Additionally, an animal study suggested that prenatal dexamethasone and postnatal high-fat diet treatment caused dysregulation of nutrient-sensing molecules and circadian clock genes in visceral adipose tissue in rats [59]. Similarly, another animal study found that prenatal low-protein diets followed by postnatal high-fat diets resulted in a rapid increase in subcutaneous adipose tissue mass in the offspring, contributing to the development of obesity and insulin resistance [60]. In line with these findings, our study observed that children with mothers exposed to IBS during pregnancy had a much higher risk of obesity, especially when they experienced lower frequency or shorter durations of outdoor physical activity at ages of 1 to 3 years, with significant multiple and additive interactions between prenatal and postnatal variables. Taken together, all these findings proved the First-hit/Second-hit Framework of DOHaD [25,26].

Based upon the findings of prior studies, three possible pathways are proposed as explanations for the combination effect of prenatal IBS exposure and postnatal early childhood outdoor physical activity causing childhood obesity [25,61–63]. First, air pollution exposure may result in changes in metabolic hormones, such as leptin and adiponectin. A prospective study reported that maternal exposure to $PM_{2.5}$ and NO_2 during pregnancy increased umbilical cord blood adiponectin levels [64]. Second, oxidative stress and inflammation may be potential mediators. A Dutch study reported that maternal higher PM_{10} and NO_2 exposure during pregnancy were associated with higher levels of C-reactive protein in cord blood at delivery [65]. Likewise, the Healthy Start study found that exposure to $PM_{2.5}$ during midpregnancy had positive associations with maternal IL-6 [66]. Moreover, an animal study found that maternal supplementation with antioxidants reduced oxidative stress and prevented the offspring of Western-diet-fed rats from developing obesity [67]. Third, epigenetic modifications, involving histone modification, miRNA expression, and DNA methylation, are considered to be the most important mediators of developmental programming [25]. The ENVIRONAGE birth cohort found that $PM_{2.5}$ exposure during the second trimester was negatively associated with DNA methylation of the lep promote status in the placenta, and with placental 3-NTp, a marker of oxidative/nitrosative stress [68]. Cai et al. reported that early pregnancy PM_{10} exposure was associated with placental DNA methylation involved in glucocorticoid metabolism in fetal growth [69]. These three pathways could contribute to changes in placental function and fetal intrauterine reprogramming, leading to a reduction in individual metabolic levels and increased susceptibility to obesity [25,55]. Based on this, insufficient fat consumption, such as a lack of outdoor exercise in early life, further exacerbates the development of obesity.

Some limitations should be considered when interpreting these results. First, the assessment of prenatal IBS exposure relied on retrospective self-reporting by mothers. This introduces the potential for recall bias, particularly concerning the accurate timing of exposure during specific trimesters. Second, the actual components and concentration of smoke emitted from burning incense, as well as the average duration of exposure to IBS during each period, were not objectively measured. Third, the recall time frame for mothers ranged from 2 to 7 years, so the validity of a mother's recall regarding the frequency and duration of their child's outdoor activities may have been biased. Fourth, all participants in this study were recruited from the Longhua District of Shenzhen, which may restrict the generalizability of our findings, as there could be variations in the habit of household incense burning across different cultures. Fifth, though a range of covariates were considered in our analysis, there were still unmeasured confounders, such as household ventilation conditions and outdoor air pollution conditions near the residential area, which may potentially influence the findings. Sixth, the assessment of outdoor activity relying on outdoor time and frequency, and the actual physical activity is not so clear, which may impact the findings. Seventh, retrospective studies provide relatively weaker evidence for establishing a causal relationship between the combined impact of prenatal and postnatal factors on childhood obesity. Therefore, it is necessary to conduct a prospective cohort to replicate these findings.

5. Conclusions

In summary, our findings suggest that maternal exposure to incense-burning smoke during pregnancy and low levels of postnatal outdoor physical activity in children, from the age of 1–3 years old, may independently and jointly increase the risk of obesity among preschoolers. In addition, there are dose–response relations between prenatal exposure to incense-burning smoke and childhood obesity. These findings highlight the necessity of implementing public health interventions to avoid maternal exposure to incense-burning smoke during pregnancy and to provide young children with more outdoor physical activity so that childhood obesity may be decreased.

Supplementary Materials: The following supporting information can be downloaded at https://www.mdpi.com/article/10.3390/toxics12050329/s1, Table S1: Associations between maternal incense-burning smoke exposure during pregnancy and children's obesity excluding PTB and LBW; Table S2: Associations between trimester-specific IBS exposure during pregnancy and children's obesity excluding PTB and LBW; Table S3: Associations between frequency of trimester-specific IBS exposure during pregnancy and children's obesity excluding PTB and LBW; Table S4: Associations between frequency of trimester-specific IBS exposure during pregnancy and children's obesity excluding PTB and LBW; Table S5: Associations between frequency and duration of outdoor activity from 1 to 3 years of age on preschool obesity excluding PTB and LBW; Table S6: Combination Effect between maternal IBS exposure during pregnancy and outdoor activity from 1 to 3 years of age on preschool obesity.

Author Contributions: Author Contributions: Conceptualization, W.C. and M.C.; resources, W.C.; methodology, W.C. and M.C.; formal analysis, M.C.; investigation, X.Y., G.W., D.S. and D.X.; data curation, M.C.; writing—original draft preparation, M.C.; writing—review and editing, W.C. and E.S.; visualization, M.C.; supervision, W.C., E.S. and W.Y.; project administration, W.C., W.Y., X.Y., G.W., D.S., D.X. and Y.Z. All authors have read and agreed to the published version of the manuscript.

Funding: The Science and Technology Planning Project of Guangdong Province provided funding for this study under grant number 2019A1515011915. The nonprofit scientific research management and academic institutions that provided the funding did not participate in the study's design, execution, analyses, data interpretation, or decision to submit results.

Institutional Review Board Statement: The Institutional Review Board of the School of Public Health at Sun Yat-sen University in Guang-zhou, China, approved this study in accordance with the Declaration of Helsinki (protocol code: No.2015–016).

Informed Consent Statement: All participants in this study gave their informed consent. Written consent for children was received from their parents or guardians.

Data Availability Statement: Due to participant privacy concerns, the datasets created and/or analyzed in this study cannot be accessed by the general public. However, they can be obtained from the corresponding author upon reasonable request.

Acknowledgments: The Longhua Maternity and Child Healthcare Hospital clinicians who assisted in recruiting participants and collecting data are sincerely appreciated by the authors.

Conflicts of Interest: The authors declare no conflicts of interest.

References

1. NCD Risk Factor Collaboration (NCD-RisC). Worldwide trends in body-mass index, underweight, overweight, and obesity from 1975 to 2016: A pooled analysis of 2416 population-based measurement studies in 128.9 million children, adolescents, and adults. *Lancet* **2017**, *390*, 2627–2642. [CrossRef]
2. World Health Organization. Obesity and Overweight. Available online: https://www.who.int/news-room/fact-sheets/detail/obesity-and-overweight (accessed on 6 July 2023).
3. GBD 2015 Obesity Collaborators; Afshin, A.; Forouzanfar, M.H.; Reitsma, M.B.; Sur, P.; Estep, K.; Lee, A.; Marczak, L.; Mokdad, A.H.; Moradi-Lakeh, M.; et al. Health Effects of Overweight and Obesity in 195 Countries over 25 Years. *N. Engl. J. Med.* **2017**, *377*, 13–27. [CrossRef]
4. Mühlig, Y.; Antel, J.; Föcker, M.; Hebebrand, J. Are bidirectional associations of obesity and depression already apparent in childhood and adolescence as based on high-quality studies? A systematic review. *Obes. Rev.* **2016**, *17*, 235–249. [CrossRef] [PubMed]
5. Milaneschi, Y.; Simmons, W.K.; van Rossum, E.F.C.; Penninx, B.W. Depression and obesity: Evidence of shared biological mechanisms. *Mol. Psychiatry* **2019**, *24*, 18–33. [CrossRef] [PubMed]
6. Weiss, R.; Dziura, J.; Burgert, T.S.; Tamborlane, W.V.; Taksali, S.E.; Yeckel, C.W.; Allen, K.; Lopes, M.; Savoye, M.; Morrison, J.; et al. Obesity and the metabolic syndrome in children and adolescents. *N. Engl. J. Med.* **2004**, *350*, 2362–2374. [CrossRef]
7. Friedemann, C.; Heneghan, C.; Mahtani, K.; Thompson, M.; Perera, R.; Ward, A.M. Cardiovascular disease risk in healthy children and its association with body mass index: Systematic review and meta-analysis. *BMJ* **2012**, *345*, e4759. [CrossRef]
8. Renehan, A.G.; Tyson, M.; Egger, M.; Heller, R.F.; Zwahlen, M. Body-mass index and incidence of cancer: A systematic review and meta-analysis of prospective observational studies. *Lancet* **2008**, *371*, 569–578. [CrossRef]
9. Blake-Lamb, T.L.; Locks, L.M.; Perkins, M.E.; Baidal, J.A.W.; Cheng, E.R.; Taveras, E.M. Interventions for Childhood Obesity in the First 1000 Days A Systematic Review. *Am. J. Prev. Med.* **2016**, *50*, 780–789. [CrossRef]
10. Geserick, M.; Vogel, M.; Gausche, R.; Lipek, T.; Spielau, U.; Keller, E.; Pfäffle, R.; Kiess, W.; Körner, A. Acceleration of BMI in Early Childhood and Risk of Sustained Obesity. *N. Engl. J. Med.* **2018**, *379*, 1303–1312. [CrossRef]
11. Locke, A.E.; Kahali, B.; Berndt, S.I.; Justice, A.E.; Pers, T.H.; Day, F.R.; Powell, C.; Vedantam, S.; Buchkovich, M.L.; Yang, J.; et al. Genetic studies of body mass index yield new insights for obesity biology. *Nature* **2015**, *518*, 197–206. [CrossRef]
12. Aris, I.M.; Bernard, J.Y.; Chen, L.-W.; Tint, M.T.; Pang, W.W.; E Soh, S.; Saw, S.-M.; Shek, L.P.-C.; Godfrey, K.M.; Gluckman, P.D.; et al. Modifiable risk factors in the first 1000 days for subsequent risk of childhood overweight in an Asian cohort: Significance of parental overweight status. *Int. J. Obes.* **2018**, *42*, 44–51. [CrossRef]
13. Whitaker, R.C.; Wright, J.A.; Pepe, M.S.; Seidel, K.D.; Dietz, W.H. Predicting obesity in young adulthood from childhood and parental obesity. *N. Engl. J. Med.* **1997**, *337*, 869–873. [CrossRef]
14. Joubert, B.R.; Felix, J.F.; Yousefi, P.; Bakulski, K.M.; Just, A.C.; Breton, C.; Reese, S.E.; Markunas, C.A.; Richmond, R.C.; Xu, C.-J.; et al. DNA Methylation in Newborns and Maternal Smoking in Pregnancy: Genome-wide Consortium Meta-analysis. *Am. J. Hum. Genet.* **2016**, *98*, 680–696. [CrossRef]
15. Kominiarek, M.A.; Peaceman, A.M. Gestational weight gain. *Am. J. Obstet. Gynecol.* **2017**, *217*, 642–651. [CrossRef]
16. Larqué, E.; Labayen, I.; Flodmark, C.-E.; Lissau, I.; Czernin, S.; Moreno, L.A.; Pietrobelli, A.; Widhalm, K. From conception to infancy—Early risk factors for childhood obesity. *Nat. Rev. Endocrinol.* **2019**, *15*, 456–478. [CrossRef]
17. Shi, X.; Zheng, Y.; Cui, H.; Zhang, Y.; Jiang, M. Exposure to outdoor and indoor air pollution and risk of overweight and obesity across different life periods: A review. *Ecotoxicol. Environ. Saf.* **2022**, *242*, 113893. [CrossRef]
18. Sun, J.; Liu, H.; Zhang, C.; Liu, X.; Sun, X.; Chen, X.; Yang, G.; Wang, N. Predisposed obesity and long-term metabolic diseases from maternal exposure to fine particulate matter ($PM_{2.5}$)—A review of its effect and potential mechanisms. *Life Sci.* **2022**, *310*, 121054. [CrossRef]
19. Pan, X.-F.; Tang, L.; Lee, A.H.; Binns, C.; Yang, C.-X.; Xu, Z.-P.; Zhang, J.-L.; Yang, Y.; Wang, H.; Sun, X. Association between fetal macrosomia and risk of obesity in children under 3 years in Western China: A cohort study. *World J. Pediatr.* **2019**, *15*, 153–160. [CrossRef]
20. Martín-Calvo, N.; Goni, L.; Tur, J.A.; Martínez, J.A. Low birth weight and small for gestational age are associated with complications of childhood and adolescence obesity: Systematic review and meta-analysis. *Obes. Rev.* **2022**, *23* (Suppl. S1), e13380. [CrossRef]
21. Robinson, T.N.; Banda, J.A.; Hale, L.; Lu, A.S.; Fleming-Milici, F.; Calvert, S.L.; Wartella, E. Screen Media Exposure and Obesity in Children and Adolescents. *Pediatrics* **2017**, *140* (Suppl. S2), S97–S101. [CrossRef]
22. Dattilo, A.M. Modifiable Risk Factors and Interventions for Childhood Obesity Prevention within the First 1000 Days. In *Complementary Feeding: Building the Foundations for a Healthy Life*; Karger Publishers: Basel, Switzerland, 2017; Volume 87.
23. Bleich, S.N.; Vercammen, K.A.; Zatz, L.Y.; Frelier, J.M.; Ebbeling, C.B.; Peeters, A. Interventions to prevent global childhood overweight and obesity: A systematic review. *Lancet Diabetes Endocrinol.* **2018**, *6*, 332–346. [CrossRef]
24. Herrington, S.; Brussoni, M. Beyond Physical Activity: The Importance of Play and Nature-Based Play Spaces for Children's Health and Development. *Curr. Obes. Rep.* **2015**, *4*, 477–483. [CrossRef]
25. Padmanabhan, V.; Cardoso, R.C.; Puttabyatappa, M. Developmental Programming, a Pathway to Disease. *Endocrinology* **2016**, *157*, 1328–1340. [CrossRef]

26. Li, X.; Zhang, M.; Pan, X.; Xu, Z.; Sun, M. "Three Hits" Hypothesis for Developmental Origins of Health and Diseases in View of Cardiovascular Abnormalities: "Three Hits" Hypothesis for FOAD. *Birth Defects Res.* **2017**, *109*, 744–757. [CrossRef]
27. Rueda-Clausen, C.F.; Morton, J.S.; Dolinsky, V.W.; Dyck, J.R.B.; Davidge, S.T. Synergistic effects of prenatal hypoxia and postnatal high-fat diet in the development of cardiovascular pathology in young rats. *Am. J. Physiol. Regul. Integr. Comp. Physiol.* **2012**, *303*, R418–R426. [CrossRef]
28. Liang, Y.; Strodl, E.; Lu, Q.; Liu, X.-C.; Hu, B.-J.; Chen, W.-Q. Combined Effect of Prenatal Mosquito Coil Smoke Exposure and Early Postnatal Nutritional Status on Obesity among Preschoolers. *Atmosphere* **2023**, *14*, 1004. [CrossRef]
29. Wang, B.; Lee, S.C.; Ho, K.F.; Kang, Y.M. Characteristics of emissions of air pollutants from burning of incense in temples, Hong Kong. *Sci. Total Environ.* **2007**, *377*, 52–60. [CrossRef]
30. Jetter, J.J.; Guo, Z.; A McBrian, J.; Flynn, M.R. Characterization of emissions from burning incense. *Sci. Total Environ.* **2002**, *295*, 51–67. [CrossRef]
31. Yeatts, K.B.; El-Sadig, M.; Leith, D.; Kalsbeek, W.; Al-Maskari, F.; Couper, D.; Funk, W.E.; Zoubeidi, T.; Chan, R.L.; Trent, C.B.; et al. Indoor air pollutants and health in the United Arab Emirates. *Environ. Health Perspect.* **2012**, *120*, 687–694. [CrossRef]
32. He, J.-R.; Wei, D.-M.; Chan, F.-F.; Luan, Y.-Z.; Tu, S.; Lu, J.-H.; Li, W.-D.; Yuan, M.-Y.; Chen, N.-N.; Chen, Q.-Z.; et al. Associations between maternal exposure to incense burning and blood pressure during pregnancy. *Sci. Total Environ.* **2018**, *610–611*, 1421–1427. [CrossRef]
33. Chen, Y.C.; Ho, W.C.; Yu, Y.H. Adolescent lung function associated with incense burning and other environmental exposures at home. *Indoor Air* **2017**, *27*, 746–752. [CrossRef]
34. Fang, X.-Y.; Strodl, E.; Liu, B.-Q.; Liu, L.; Yin, X.-N.; Wen, G.-M.; Sun, D.-L.; Xian, D.-X.; Jiang, H.; Jing, J.; et al. Association between prenatal exposure to household inhalants exposure and ADHD-like behaviors at around 3 years of age: Findings from Shenzhen Longhua Child Cohort Study. *Environ. Res.* **2019**, *177*, 108612. [CrossRef]
35. Pan, A.; Clark, M.L.; Ang, L.-W.; Yu, M.C.; Yuan, J.-M.; Koh, W.-P. Incense use and cardiovascular mortality among Chinese in Singapore: The Singapore Chinese Health Study. *Environ. Health Perspect.* **2014**, *122*, 1279–1284. [CrossRef]
36. Tang, L.; Lim, W.-Y.; Eng, P.; Leong, S.S.; Lim, T.K.; Ng, A.W.; Tee, A.; Seow, A. Lung cancer in Chinese women: Evidence for an interaction between tobacco smoking and exposure to inhalants in the indoor environment. *Environ. Health Perspect.* **2010**, *118*, 1257–1260. [CrossRef]
37. He, Y.-Q.; Xue, W.-Q.; Shen, G.-P.; Tang, L.-L.; Zeng, Y.-X.; Jia, W.-H. Household inhalants exposure and nasopharyngeal carcinoma risk: A large-scale case-control study in Guangdong, China. *BMC Cancer* **2015**, *15*, 1022. [CrossRef]
38. Chen, L.-Y.; Ho, C. Incense Burning during Pregnancy and Birth Weight and Head Circumference among Term Births: The Taiwan Birth Cohort Study. *Environ. Health Perspect.* **2016**, *124*, 1487–1492. [CrossRef]
39. Jiang, N.; Bao, W.-W.; Gui, Z.-H.; Chen, Y.-C.; Zhao, Y.; Huang, S.; Zhang, Y.-S.; Liang, J.-H.; Pu, X.-Y.; Huang, S.-Y.; et al. Findings of indoor air pollution and childhood obesity in a cross-sectional study of Chinese schoolchildren. *Environ. Res.* **2023**, *225*, 115611. [CrossRef]
40. Li, H.; Ji, C.-Y.; Zong, X.-N.; Zhang, Y.-Q. Body mass index growth curves for Chinese children and adolescents aged 0 to 18 years. *Zhonghua Er Ke Za Zhi.* **2009**, *47*, 493–498.
41. Lu, Q.; Strodl, E.; Liang, Y.; Huang, L.-H.; Hu, B.-J.; Chen, W.-Q. Joint Effects of Prenatal Folic Acid Supplement with Prenatal Multivitamin and Iron Supplement on Obesity in Preschoolers Born SGA: Sex Specific Difference. *Nutrients* **2023**, *15*, 380. [CrossRef]
42. Knol, M.J.; VanderWeele, T.J. Recommendations for presenting analyses of effect modification and interaction. *Int. J. Epidemiol.* **2012**, *41*, 514–520. [CrossRef]
43. Mao, G.; Nachman, R.M.; Sun, Q.; Zhang, X.; Koehler, K.; Chen, Z.; Hong, X.; Wang, G.; Caruso, D.; Zong, G.; et al. Individual and Joint Effects of Early-Life Ambient $PM_{2.5}$ Exposure and Maternal Prepregnancy Obesity on Childhood Overweight or Obesity. *Environ. Health Perspect.* **2017**, *125*, 067005. [CrossRef]
44. Bloemsma, L.D.; Dabelea, D.; Thomas, D.S.K.; Peel, J.L.; Adgate, J.L.; Allshouse, W.B.; Martenies, S.E.; Magzamen, S.; Starling, A.P. Prenatal exposure to ambient air pollution and traffic and indicators of adiposity in early childhood: The Healthy Start study. *Int. J. Obes.* **2022**, *46*, 494–501. [CrossRef]
45. Chiu, Y.-H.M.; Hsu, H.-H.L.; Wilson, A.; Coull, B.A.; Pendo, M.P.; Baccarelli, A.; Kloog, I.; Schwartz, J.; Wright, R.O.; Taveras, E.M.; et al. Prenatal particulate air pollution exposure and body composition in urban preschool children: Examining sensitive windows and sex-specific associations. *Environ. Res.* **2017**, *158*, 798–805. [CrossRef]
46. Qureshi, R.; Jadotte, Y.; Zha, P.; Porter, S.A.; Holly, C.; Salmond, S.; Watkins, E.A. The association between prenatal exposure to environmental tobacco smoke and childhood obesity: A systematic review. *JBI Database Syst. Rev. Implement. Rep.* **2018**, *16*, 1643–1662. [CrossRef]
47. Kuh, D.; Ben-Shlomo, Y.; Lynch, J.; Hallqvist, J.; Power, C. Life course epidemiology. *J. Epidemiol. Community Health* **2003**, *57*, 778–783. [CrossRef]
48. Wu, X.Y.; Han, L.H.; Zhang, J.H.; Luo, S.; Hu, J.W.; Sun, K. The influence of physical activity, sedentary behavior on health-related quality of life among the general population of children and adolescents: A systematic review. *PLoS ONE* **2017**, *12*, e0187668. [CrossRef]

49. Martin, A.; Booth, J.N.; Laird, Y.; Sproule, J.; Reilly, J.J.; Saunders, D.H. Physical activity, diet and other behavioural interventions for improving cognition and school achievement in children and adolescents with obesity or overweight. *Cochrane Database Syst. Rev.* **2018**, *3*, CD009728. [CrossRef]
50. Weihrauch-Blüher, S.; Wiegand, S. Risk Factors and Implications of Childhood Obesity. *Curr. Obes. Rep.* **2018**, *7*, 254–259. [CrossRef]
51. Cleland, V.; Crawford, D.; A Baur, L.; Hume, C.; Timperio, A.; Salmon, J. A prospective examination of children's time spent outdoors, objectively measured physical activity and overweight. *Int. J. Obes.* **2008**, *32*, 1685–1693. [CrossRef]
52. Burdette, H.L.; Whitaker, R.C.; Daniels, S.R. Parental report of outdoor playtime as a measure of physical activity in preschool-aged children. *Arch. Pediatr. Adolesc. Med.* **2004**, *158*, 353–357. [CrossRef]
53. Gray, C.; Gibbons, R.; Larouche, R.; Sandseter, E.B.H.; Bienenstock, A.; Brussoni, M.; Chabot, G.; Herrington, S.; Janssen, I.; Pickett, W.; et al. What Is the Relationship between Outdoor Time and Physical Activity, Sedentary Behaviour, and Physical Fitness in Children? A Systematic Review. *Int. J. Environ. Res. Public Health* **2015**, *12*, 6455–6474. [CrossRef]
54. Wittmeier, K.D.; Mollard, R.C.; Kriellaars, D.J. Physical Activity Intensity and Risk of Overweight and Adiposity in Children. *Obesity* **2008**, *16*, 415–420. [CrossRef]
55. Leppänen, M.H.; Nyström, C.D.; Henriksson, P.; Pomeroy, J.; Ruiz, J.R.; Ortega, F.B.; Cadenas-Sánchez, C.; Löf, M. Physical activity intensity, sedentary behavior, body composition and physical fitness in 4-year-old children: Results from the ministop trial. *Int. J. Obes.* **2016**, *40*, 1126–1133. [CrossRef]
56. Davison, K.K.; Birch, L.L. Childhood overweight: A contextual model and recommendations for future research. *Obes. Rev.* **2001**, *2*, 159–171. [CrossRef]
57. World Health Organization. Global Recommendations on Physical Activity for Health. 2010. Available online: http://www.ncbi.nlm.nih.gov/books/NBK305057/ (accessed on 24 February 2024).
58. Wang, G.; DiBari, J.; Bind, E.; Steffens, A.M.; Mukherjee, J.; Bartell, T.R.; Bellinger, D.C.; Hong, X.; Ji, Y.; Wang, M.-C.; et al. In utero exposure to mercury and childhood overweight or obesity: Counteracting effect of maternal folate status. *BMC Med.* **2019**, *17*, 216. [CrossRef]
59. Tsai, C.-C.; Tiao, M.-M.; Sheen, J.-M.; Huang, L.-T.; Tain, Y.-L.; Lin, I.-C.; Lin, Y.-J.; Lai, Y.-J.; Chen, C.-C.; Chang, K.-A.; et al. Obesity programmed by prenatal dexamethasone and postnatal high-fat diet leads to distinct alterations in nutrition sensory signals and circadian-clock genes in visceral adipose tissue. *Lipids Health Dis.* **2019**, *18*, 19. [CrossRef]
60. Claycombe, K.J.; Vomhof-DeKrey, E.E.; Garcia, R.; Johnson, W.T.; Uthus, E.; Roemmich, J.N. Decreased beige adipocyte number and mitochondrial respiration coincide with increased histone methyl transferase (G9a) and reduced FGF21 gene expression in Sprague–Dawley rats fed prenatal low protein and postnatal high-fat diets. *J. Nutr. Biochem.* **2016**, *31*, 113–121. [CrossRef]
61. Rahmalia, A.; Giorgis-Allemand, L.; Lepeule, J.; Philippat, C.; Galineau, J.; Hulin, A.; Charles, M.-A.; Slama, R. Pregnancy exposure to atmospheric pollutants and placental weight: An approach relying on a dispersion model. *Environ. Int.* **2012**, *48*, 47–55. [CrossRef]
62. Hoffman, D.J.; Powell, T.L.; Barrett, E.S.; Hardy, D.B. Developmental origins of metabolic diseases. *Physiol. Rev.* **2021**, *101*, 739–795. [CrossRef]
63. Harary, M.D.; Akinyemi, A.; Charron, M.J.; Fuloria, M. Fetal Growth and Intrauterine Epigenetic Programming of Obesity and Cardiometabolic Disease. *NeoReviews* **2022**, *23*, e363–e372. [CrossRef]
64. Lavigne, E.; Ashley-Martin, J.; Dodds, L.; Arbuckle, T.E.; Hystad, P.; Johnson, M.; Crouse, D.L.; Ettinger, A.S.; Shapiro, G.D.; Fisher, M.; et al. Air Pollution Exposure During Pregnancy and Fetal Markers of Metabolic function: The MIREC Study. *Am. J. Epidemiol.* **2016**, *183*, 842–851. [CrossRef]
65. Van den Hooven, E.H.; de Kluizenaar, Y.; Pierik, F.H.; Hofman, A.; van Ratingen, S.W.; Zandveld, P.Y.; Lindemans, J.; Russcher, H.; Steegers, E.A.; Miedema, H.M.; et al. Chronic air pollution exposure during pregnancy and maternal and fetal C-reactive protein levels: The Generation R Study. *Environ. Health Perspect.* **2012**, *120*, 746–751. [CrossRef]
66. Friedman, C.; Dabelea, D.; Thomas, D.S.K.; Peel, J.L.; Adgate, J.L.; Magzamen, S.; Martenies, S.E.; Allshouse, W.B.; Starling, A.P. Exposure to ambient air pollution during pregnancy and inflammatory biomarkers in maternal and umbilical cord blood: The Healthy Start study. *Environ. Res.* **2021**, *197*, 111165. [CrossRef]
67. Sen, S.; Simmons, R.A. Maternal antioxidant supplementation prevents adiposity in the offspring of Western diet-fed rats. *Diabetes* **2010**, *59*, 3058–3065. [CrossRef]
68. Saenen, N.D.; Vrijens, K.; Janssen, B.G.; Roels, H.A.; Neven, K.Y.; Berghe, W.V.; Gyselaers, W.; Vanpoucke, C.; Lefebvre, W.; De Boever, P.; et al. Lower Placental Leptin Promoter Methylation in Association with Fine Particulate Matter Air Pollution during Pregnancy and Placental Nitrosative Stress at Birth in the ENVIRONAGE Cohort. *Environ. Health Perspect.* **2017**, *125*, 262–268. [CrossRef]
69. Cai, J.; Zhao, Y.; Liu, P.; Xia, B.; Zhu, Q.; Wang, X.; Song, Q.; Kan, H.; Zhang, Y. Exposure to particulate air pollution during early pregnancy is associated with placental DNA methylation. *Sci. Total Environ.* **2017**, *607–608*, 1103–1108. [CrossRef]

toxics

MDPI

Article

Exploring the Burden of PM2.5-Related Deaths and Economic Health Losses in Beijing

Xiaoqi Wang [1], Bart Julien Dewancker [1,*], Dongwei Tian [2] and Shao Zhuang [3]

[1] Faculty of Environmental Engineering, The University of Kitakyushu, Kitakyushu 808-0135, Japan; qi1981@163.com
[2] School of Architecture and Urban Planning, Beijing University of Civil Engineering and Architecture, Beijing 100044, China; tiandongwei77@163.com
[3] School of Landscape Architecture, Beijing Forestry University, Beijing 100083, China; no81terry@bjfu.edu.cn
* Correspondence: bart@kitakyu-u.ac.jp

Abstract: Air pollution is one of the major global public health challenges. Using annual fine particulate matter (PM2.5) concentration data from 2016 to 2021, along with the global exposure mortality model (GEMM), we estimated the multi-year PM2.5-pollution-related deaths divided by different age groups and diseases. Then, using the VSL (value of statistical life) method, we assessed corresponding economic losses and values. The number of deaths attributed to PM2.5 in Beijing in 2021 fell by 33.74 percent from 2016, while health economic losses would increase by USD 4.4 billion as per capita disposable income increases year by year. In 2021, the average annual concentration of PM2.5 in half of Beijing's municipal administrative districts is less than China's secondary ambient air quality standard (35 $\mu g/m^3$), but it can still cause 48,969 deaths and corresponding health and economic losses of USD 16.31 billion, equivalent to 7.9 percent of Beijing's GDP. Therefore, it is suggested that more stringent local air quality standards should be designated to protect public health in Beijing.

Keywords: fine particulate matter; public health; mortality burden; economic value

1. Introduction

Air pollution is one of the major challenges facing global public health [1]. In 2022, according to the Global Burden of Disease (GBD), a study revealed that air pollution ranked fourth among various risk factors [2]. Fine particulate matter ($PM_{2.5}$) pollution is the main pollutant in urban atmosphere. $PM_{2.5}$ refers to dust or drifting dust with a diameter of 2.5 μm or less in ambient air. Atmospheric $PM_{2.5}$ pollution poses a grave public health risk, and the death toll is increasing. The Global Burden of Disease study indicated that $PM_{2.5}$ exposure led to approximately 6.67 million additional deaths worldwide and 1.42 million deaths in China in 2019 [3]. Therefore, addressing air pollution as a public health issue is one of the most urgent tasks facing the world [4], and quantifying and accurately assessing the death burden and economic loss related to $PM_{2.5}$ is one of the important tasks [5].

The impact of pollutant concentrations on public health has long been part of the focus of the WHO (World Health Organization). A precise and comprehensive evaluation of the health effects associated with pollutant concentrations remains a top priority for the WHO. Additionally, the accurate assessment of mortality rates and economic losses attributable to $PM_{2.5}$ pollution is of utmost importance. In the field of epidemiology, many models, such as the IER (integrated exposure–response) model [6], the NLP (non-linear programming) model [7], and the LL model (log–linear programming) [8], are used to estimate cause-specific mortality. However, these models have many uncertainties; for example, they do not evaluate the health hazards related to both indoor and outdoor PM2.5 pollution differently. Compared to other models, the GEMM model initiated by Burnett et al. (2018) [9] takes into account a wider range of health endpoints, considers indoor and outdoor sources of pollution, ADAPTS data, and specific conditions in different regions, and maintains high accuracy and relevance in applications in different regions of the world [10,11]. Therefore, this study utilized the GEMM model to assess the long-term health impacts of $PM_{2.5}$ pollution in 16 districts in Beijing. Recent research findings have shown the health impact assessment of $PM_{2.5}$ by using ground monitoring data combined with pollution exposure mortality models at national and urban agglomeration scales. Bell et al. (2007) conducted research about the influence of temporal and spatial differences within the chemical composition of $PM_{2.5}$ on health in the United States, and the results showed that the daily changes in the composition of $PM_{2.5}$ had an important impact on health [12]. Song et al. (2016) discussed the distribution features of $PM_{2.5}$ in China's air environment in 2013 and explored the health effects of $PM_{2.5}$ by taking four health endpoints of PM2.5 [13]. Yin et al. extracted the annual $PM_{2.5}$ concentrations of 16 districts in Beijing in 2012, estimated the external cost by using the statistical life value method (VSL) and the revised human capital method (AHC), and found that among all health effects, the economic losses caused by $PM_{2.5}$-related deaths took up more than four-fifths of the total external cost [14].

In response to the negative effects caused by air pollution in cities, the Chinese government and local governments have implemented and updated standards of air quality and conducted specific control measures since 2013, when the state council initiated the Air Pollution Prevention and Control Action Plan [15]. While some studies report improvements in air quality and public health outcomes, others highlight persistent challenges, such as enforcement issues, regional disparities, and the need for more stringent standards. Today, more and more evidence proves that low concentrations of $PM_{2.5}$ still cause health damage, and the goal of reducing $PM_{2.5}$ concentration is urgent. Therefore, there is an urgent need for an effective evaluation method of $PM_{2.5}$ pollution, which can offer essential information for regional policy goals, assess the public health impact of coordinating air pollution measures and reducing $PM_{2.5}$ emissions, and identify potential economic benefits, to further develop scientific and economic reduction strategy.

Previous regional studies in China [13–18] mostly used low-resolution $PM_{2.5}$ concentration values as exposure and mostly estimated $PM_{2.5}$-attributed death relying on the comprehensive exposure–response model, non-linear model, log–linear model, and other models, but there are many uncertainties in the above models. Compared with the IER model, the GEMM proposed by Burnett et al. (2018) may take a more refined approach and data in assessing exposure, allowing them to more accurately capture changes and impacts in exposure levels. The GEMM combines data and results from multiple studies to create a more comprehensive assessment framework with some flexibility to adapt and modify for different regions and research needs. This flexibility allows GEMM to adapt to different environments and study conditions to provide more accurate and applicable health risk assessment results. The current commonly used health assessment model is the classical global burden of disease integrated risk function (GBD-IER) [16], while the recently proposed global exposure mortality model (GEMM) is less commonly used. This study seeks to address these limitations by proposing an alternative approach that combines high-resolution $PM_{2.5}$ concentration data with a refined analysis of health outcomes, thereby offering a more accurate and comprehensive assessment of the health impacts of $PM_{2.5}$ pollution.

The terrain in Beijing is relatively flat, but the contradiction between air pollution control and economic development is prominent. As the capital of China, the complex urban heat island effect in Beijing makes the transport of air and pollutants more complicated. It is one of the cities with serious air pollution in China, and haze has become one of the highly concerned issues among Beijing residents. Although the annual average concentration of $PM_{2.5}$ in Beijing improved in recent years, there is still a significant gap compared to developed countries and regions [17]. At the same time, with the worsening of the aging population, the burden of deaths and economic losses related to $PM_{2.5}$ may further increase, posing a heavy burden on the medical service system [17,18].

This study leveraged advanced monitoring techniques to procure $PM_{2.5}$ concentration data of high spatial resolution, thereby ensuring detailed and granular insights into the air quality across various districts of Beijing. By harnessing the global exposure mortality model (GEMM), this study meticulously estimated the mortality burden that can be directly attributed to $PM_{2.5}$ pollution over a six-year period from 2016 to 2021. This model is renowned for its robustness and enhanced predictive accuracy, which is crucial for quantifying the public health effects of exposure to particulate matter. Further enriching the scope of the research, this study integrated the statistical value of life (VSL) approach—a method that assigns a monetary value to the prevention of fatalities, thereby providing a quantifiable economic perspective on health outcomes. By applying the VSL method, the research was able to compute the economic repercussions stemming from health detriments linked to $PM_{2.5}$ pollution. This economic valuation is particularly significant as it transcends the abstract and oftentimes imperceptible nature of air pollution's health effects, translating it into a concrete financial framework that can be readily comprehended and acted upon by policymakers and the public alike. The culmination of these methods yielded results that offer a comprehensive and scientifically rigorous foundation for potential policy reform. The findings underscore the critical interplay between air quality and public health and provide an evidentiary basis for the revision of local standards of air quality in Beijing. By considering both the health and economic benefits, this study presents a compelling case for the implementation of more stringent air quality regulations.

2. Materials and Methods

2.1. Data

This research encompassed an analysis of 16 districts in Beijing to comprehensively assess the repercussions of PM pollution on public health and economic well-being from 2016 to 2021. This study meticulously gathered key data required for this evaluation, emphasizing the significance of data accessibility in this context.

To determine the annual average $PM_{2.5}$ concentration in Beijing from 2016 to 2021, this study relied on the "China Long Time Series with high spatial resolution (1 km × 1 km)" dataset, known as ChinaHigh PMx. The $PM_{2.5}$ data were acquired from research from Donkelaar et al. [19]. This dataset, derived from a combination of various data sources, including land use, air emission, meteorological data, and satellite remote sensing technology, was instrumental in providing a detailed estimation of $PM_{2.5}$ levels [20]. Furthermore, the population data and death data were obtained from the "Beijing 7th National Population Census Main Data Bulletin," and the insufficient data years were obtained from the Beijing Municipal National Economic and Development Bulletin for 2016–2021 [21]. Additionally, the GDP of each region was obtained from the annual "Statistical Bulletin of National Economic and Social Development," enabling a comprehensive analysis of economic factors alongside pollution-related data.

We have conducted unified and standardized processing of the data, which included PM2.5 concentration, total resident population, and GDP in the 16 districts of Beijing. All data were unified from 2016 to 2021 to ensure the consistency of the study data. The research results were standardized; that is, the monetary units of the output results of the Beijing VSL model from 2016 to 2021 were unified into US dollars. $PM_{2.5}$ data were intercepted after spatial segmentation by ArcGIS Pro software. The smallest unit was the district-level administrative region, and there were no outliers or missing values.

2.2. Mortality Effect Assessment Method

The global exposure mortality model (GEMM) represents a cutting-edge epidemiological framework designed to quantify the health effects of exposure to various risk factors, with a strong focus on air pollution, specifically particulate matter (PM). The GEMM is built upon a rich bedrock of data compiled from a multitude of cohort studies conducted globally. These studies provide extensive empirical evidence on the relationships between exposure to different levels of air pollutants and the resulting mortality risks.

One of the key features of the GEMM is its non-linear exposure–response function, which allows for the estimation of mortality risk even at very low levels of pollution, a domain where many traditional models falter. This is particularly crucial as it enables health impact assessments across a broad spectrum of air pollution concentrations, encompassing both high- and low-exposure scenarios.

The model is adept at evaluating the mortality burden attributable to a variety of air pollutants, for instance, $PM_{2.5}$, ozone, nitrogen dioxide, etc. It takes into account factors such as age, location, and underlying health conditions, which are critical for accurate mortality estimations. The GEMM's versatility allows for its application in diverse geographical settings and can adapt to varying air quality standards, providing insights that are both locally relevant and globally comprehensive.

The GEMM is an approach to estimating mortality that differs from simpler linear models by providing a more nuanced understanding of the health risks of air pollution. This includes the ability to capture the drastic increase in risk at high pollution levels and the stabilizing of the risk curve at lower levels, which are consistent with the saturation effects observed in epidemiological studies. Quantitative estimates of attributable mortality are based on disease-specific hazard ratio models that incorporate risk information from multiple $PM_{2.5}$ sources (outdoor and indoor air pollution from the use of solid fuels and secondhand and active smoking), requiring assumptions about equivalent exposure and toxicity. It constructed a $PM_{2.5}$-mortality hazard ratio function based only on cohort studies of outdoor air pollution that cover the global exposure range. The GEMM modeled the shape of the association between $PM_{2.5}$ and non-accidental mortality using data from 41 cohorts from 16 countries in the global exposure mortality model (GEMM).

This study assessed the mortality effect of $PM_{2.5}$ based on the exposure–response model and combined it with the $PM_{2.5}$-attributable mortality burden assessment method proposed by Xiao et al. in the Global Burden of Disease study in 2015 [22]. The calculation formulas are as follows:

$$M_{ij} = \gamma_{0i} \times AF_{ij} \times POP_j \tag{1}$$

$$AF_{ij} = \frac{RR - 1}{RR} \tag{2}$$

where i represents the endpoints of different health effects, and j represents the grid. M_{ij} represents the excess deaths attributable to $PM_{2.5}$. γ_{0i} refers to the baseline mortality rates for different diseases. POP_j is the exposed population of each grid. AF_{ij} represents an attribution score. RR is the relative risk degree. This study was estimated by the GEMM.

The GEMM is an exposure–response model proposed by Burnett's team in 2018 to evaluate the health effects of $PM_{2.5}$ [9]. This model is the first exposure–response model to consider the Chinese population and cover the global PM concentration exposure range (2.4–84.0 μg/m). The calculation formulas are as follows:

$$GEMM(\Delta z_i) = \exp\{\beta T(\Delta z_i|\alpha, \mu, \nu)\} \tag{3}$$

$$T(\Delta z_i|\alpha, \mu, \nu) = \log(1 + \Delta z_i/\alpha)/\{1 + \exp[-(\Delta z_i - \mu)/\nu]\} \tag{4}$$

$$\Delta z_i = \max(0, z_j - z_{cf}) \tag{5}$$

In the formulas, z represents the average annual $PM_{2.5}$ concentration for each grid. z_{cf} refers to the counterfactual minimum $PM_{2.5}$ concentration, which assumes that at this concentration, $PM_{2.5}$ has no effect on health and takes a value of 2.4 μg/m. β represents the exposure–response model coefficient. $T(\Delta z_i|\alpha, \mu, \nu)$ is a complex transformation function for concentration, where the (α, μ, ν) parameter defines the quantitative relation between $PM_{2.5}$ and mortality. According to the research results of Burnet et al. [9], there are two models in the GEMM model that quantify the premature deaths due to $PM_{2.5}$, namely GEMM NCD+LRI and GEMM 5-COD. The former can comprehensively assess the health effects of all non-communicable diseases and respiratory infections induced by $PM_{2.5}$ pollution, as the latter can separately assess five related chronic diseases that are closely linked to $PM_{2.5}$ pollution. These include ischemic heart disease (IHD), stroke (STR), chronic pulmonary obstruction (COPD), lung cancer (LC), and lower respiratory tract infections (LRIs). The GEMM model was utilized to calculate the impacts of variations in $PM_{2.5}$ concentrations on the endpoint of population health effects. We selected the GEMM 5-COD model to study the health effects of 5 causes of death, including ischemic heart disease (IHD), stroke (STR), chronic pulmonary obstruction (COPD), lung cancer (LC), and lower respiratory tract infections (LRIs), caused by $PM_{2.5}$ pollution. Different health responses to atmospheric $PM_{2.5}$ in 12 variant age groups were quantified as well.

2.3. Health Economic Benefit Evaluation Method

The VSL (value of statistical life) is a methodological method used in the field of health economics and environmental economics to quantify the monetary value associated with reducing the risk of death. This concept is particularly utilized in cost-benefit analyses where it is essential to weigh the costs of implementing safety measures against the expected benefits of reducing risks to humans' health. The VSL model is not about the value of an individual's life per se but rather the value that a group or society places on marginal changes in the risk of death. For example, if individuals in a population are willing to pay a certain amount, collectively, for a reduction in mortality risk that results in one fewer death among them, this amount can be considered the VSL. To calculate VSL, data on individuals' risk preferences are gathered, often through labor market studies, where wage differentials are analyzed based on job risk levels. These data are then used to infer the amount of money people are willing to pay for small decreases in their probability of death, often termed the "willingness to pay" (WTP) to reduce risk. Essentially, if a population is willing to pay a certain aggregate amount for a measure that reduces the risk of death, that amount can be divided by the changes in the death toll to estimate the VSL.

Using the widely adopted statistical life value method and focusing on cities, this study further assesses the health economic losses attributable to $PM_{2.5}$ pollution [23,24]. It takes the research findings from Beijing in 2012 as the baseline statistical life value. Through the unit value transfer method, the statistical life value for Beijing from 2016 to 2021 is estimated [25].

$$VSL_{k,t} = VSL_{base} \times \left(\frac{G_{c,t}}{G_{base}}\right)^{\beta} \times (1 + \%\Delta P_c + \%\Delta G_c)^{\beta} \tag{6}$$

in which $VSL_{k,t}$ stands for the amended VSL value of city c in year t. The VSL for Beijing in the baseline year of 2012 is set at USD 132,000, approximately RMB 936,000 [14]. $G_{c,t}$ stands for the urban GDP per capita in year t, while G_{base} refers to the baseline per capita GDP, which is the 2012 per capita GDP of Beijing. The income elasticity coefficient is set at 0.8, following the recommendation of the Organisation for Economic Co-operation and Development (OECD) [26]. $\%\Delta P_c$ is the factor that accounts for the percentage change in the consumer price index (CPI), and $\%\Delta G_c$ is the per capita GDP from the baseline year to year t for city c. By multiplying the calculated result with the deaths linked to $PM_{2.5}$, the total health economic burden for a city in a given year can be determined as follows:

$$E = VSL_{c,t} \times M_{ij} \tag{7}$$

3. Results

3.1. Analysis of $PM_{2.5}$ Concentrations in Various Districts of Beijing

According to Figure 1 and Table 1, from 2016 to 2021, there is a clear downward trend in all areas of Beijing. Some regions start with higher values and then decline at different rates. For example, in 2016, Dongcheng District had the highest $PM_{2.5}$ concentration at 75.26 $\mu g/m^3$. By 2021, the maximum concentration becomes 38.90 $\mu g/m^3$ in the Daxing zone. The Dongcheng District decreased from 75.26 $\mu g/m^3$ in 2016 to 35.07 $\mu g/m^3$ in 2021, a decrease of 53.4%. The Huairou region decreased from 47.06 $\mu g/m^3$ in 2016 to 29.74 $\mu g/m^3$ in 2021, a 36.8% decrease, although the Huairou region consistently maintained low $PM_{2.5}$ aggregation levels. The $PM_{2.5}$ concentration in central areas (such as Dongcheng and Xicheng) decreased significantly from a high level, elaborating that the measures of urban air quality improvement have had a significant effect. Although the initial concentration in suburban areas (e.g., Huairou and Miyun) was low, it also showed a steady downward trend.

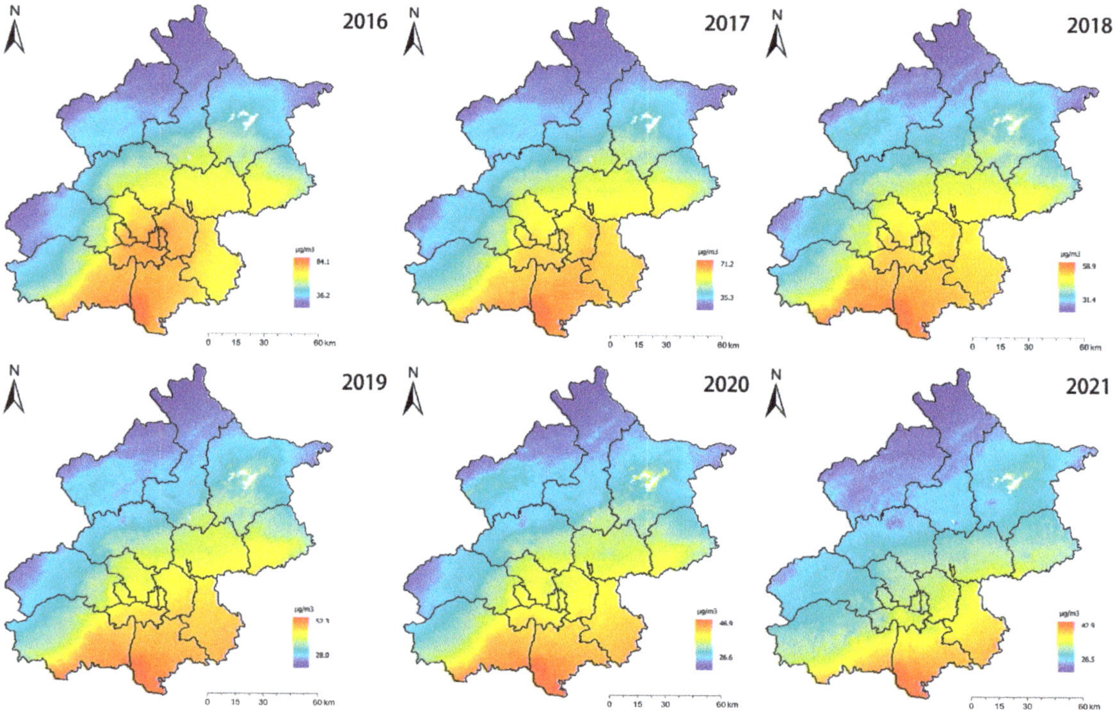

Figure 1. Spatial layout of $PM_{2.5}$ concentrations in 16 districts in Beijing from 2016 to 2021.

Table 1. $PM_{2.5}$ concentrations in 16 districts in Beijing from 2016 to 2021 ($\mu g/m^3$).

	2016	2017	2018	2019	2020	2021
Changping	58.17	50.26	43.76	37.32	34.33	31.83
Chaoyang	72.75	60.65	50.84	44.46	39.48	35.54
Daxing	73.97	64.34	53.75	47.79	42.83	38.90
Dongcheng	75.26	60.74	50.93	44.42	39.08	35.07
Fangshan	62.18	54.91	48.03	42.18	38.22	34.98
Fengtai	73.56	61.07	51.65	45.13	40.33	35.19
Haidian	68.64	57.52	48.98	41.92	38.22	33.80
Huairou	47.06	43.30	38.03	33.47	31.04	29.74
Mentougou	49.22	46.25	41.20	35.78	32.99	31.66
Miyun	50.74	46.19	40.64	36.35	32.98	31.54
Pinggu	61.18	53.64	45.38	40.96	36.44	33.72
Shijingshan	71.72	59.63	50.87	43.25	39.47	34.48
Shunyi	66.22	57.05	48.15	42.20	37.74	34.05
Tongzhou	69.04	61.57	51.20	46.08	41.19	37.73
Xicheng	75.75	60.45	50.97	44.11	38.94	35.09
Yanqing	45.17	42.89	38.22	33.38	31.41	29.57

From the perspective of space, over the years, the districts with high $PM_{2.5}$ aggregation levels mainly located in the central urban area of Beijing and some areas in the south, including Haidian District, Dongcheng District, Xicheng District, Fengtai District, along with parts of Fangshan District and Daxing District. The central region has implemented a series of policies and measures to reduce pollutant emissions and improve air quality, including promoting clean energy, limiting industrial emissions, and raising vehicle emission standards, which have played an important role in reducing $PM_{2.5}$ concentration. According to Table 1, Gu'an City, Hebei Province, also has a higher value of $PM_{2.5}$ concentration, and the aggregation level is similar to that of the central city. The government can promote public transport, encourage the use of low-emission vehicles, reduce vehicle exhaust emissions, and reduce the negative impact of traffic on air quality. Increase the use of clean energy (such as wind and solar energy), reduce the dependence on traditional high-polluting energy, and fundamentally reduce pollutant emissions.

3.2. Deaths and Health Related to $PM_{2.5}$ Pollution

Using $PM_{2.5}$ exposure levels and population data from Beijing, combined with the GEMM model, the numbers of premature deaths attributable to $PM_{2.5}$ from 2016 to 2021 were estimated. In 2016, Chaoyang District had the highest number of premature deaths at 13,590, which fell to 7833 by 2021, a reduction of 42.4%. Apart from Chaoyang, Haidian and Fengtai Districts also saw significant decreases in premature deaths, dropping from 12,346 to 6884 and from 8156 to 4547, respectively. A stable downward trend in premature deaths was observed across all districts, aligning with the decreasing trend in $PM_{2.5}$ concentrations. Urban areas such as Dongcheng, Xicheng, and Chaoyang experienced larger declines in premature deaths, possibly due to their denser populations and higher initial pollution levels. Suburban areas like Huairou, Miyun, and Yanqing, despite having lower initial death counts, also showed a downward trend, indicating overall improvements in air quality. The data from all districts highlight the diminishing negative effect of $PM_{2.5}$ pollution on health (Table 2). Reducing $PM_{2.5}$ exposure and translating into improved health outcomes, the first step is to reduce the concentration of $PM_{2.5}$ in the air by reducing the sources of $PM_{2.5}$ emissions, including industry, traffic, and other pollution sources. We will reduce traffic congestion and exhaust emissions by rationally planning urban layouts, increasing green coverage, and improving transportation systems.

There is a consistent decrease in the figures of premature deaths caused by $PM_{2.5}$ pollution across all age groups over the six-year period. The range of decrease across the age groups is relatively uniform, with the percentage change varying from approximately −32.24% for the 25–29 age group to −35.21% for the 80+ age group. The younger age groups (25–29 to 40–44) have shown a slightly lower percentage decrease in premature deaths compared to the older age groups. The middle age groups (45–49 to 60–64) also follow the decreasing trend but are in the middle range of the percentage decrease. The older age groups (65–69 to 80+) have the highest percentage decrease in premature deaths caused by $PM_{2.5}$ pollution (Figure 2). $PM_{2.5}$ pollution is associated with various diseases. There has been a notable decrease in the number of deaths from these conditions. Specifically, IHD-related deaths decreased from 16,648 to 11,297 over the analyzed period. This significant drop could be attributed to both enhanced medical treatments and interventions and a reduction in exposure to $PM_{2.5}$ pollution, which is a known one of the essential heart disease risk factors. Deaths from lung cancer (LC) attributed to $PM_{2.5}$ pollution fell from 9691 in 2016 to 6253 in 2021. This decline reflects the potential impact of public health initiatives aimed at reducing pollution and smoking alongside advancements in cancer treatment and early detection. Lower respiratory infection (LRI) deaths decreased from 8029 to 5366, underscoring the importance of cleaner air in preventing respiratory infections, particularly among vulnerable populations such as the elderly and children. Stroke-related deaths saw a reduction from 12,443 to 7701 (Figure 2).

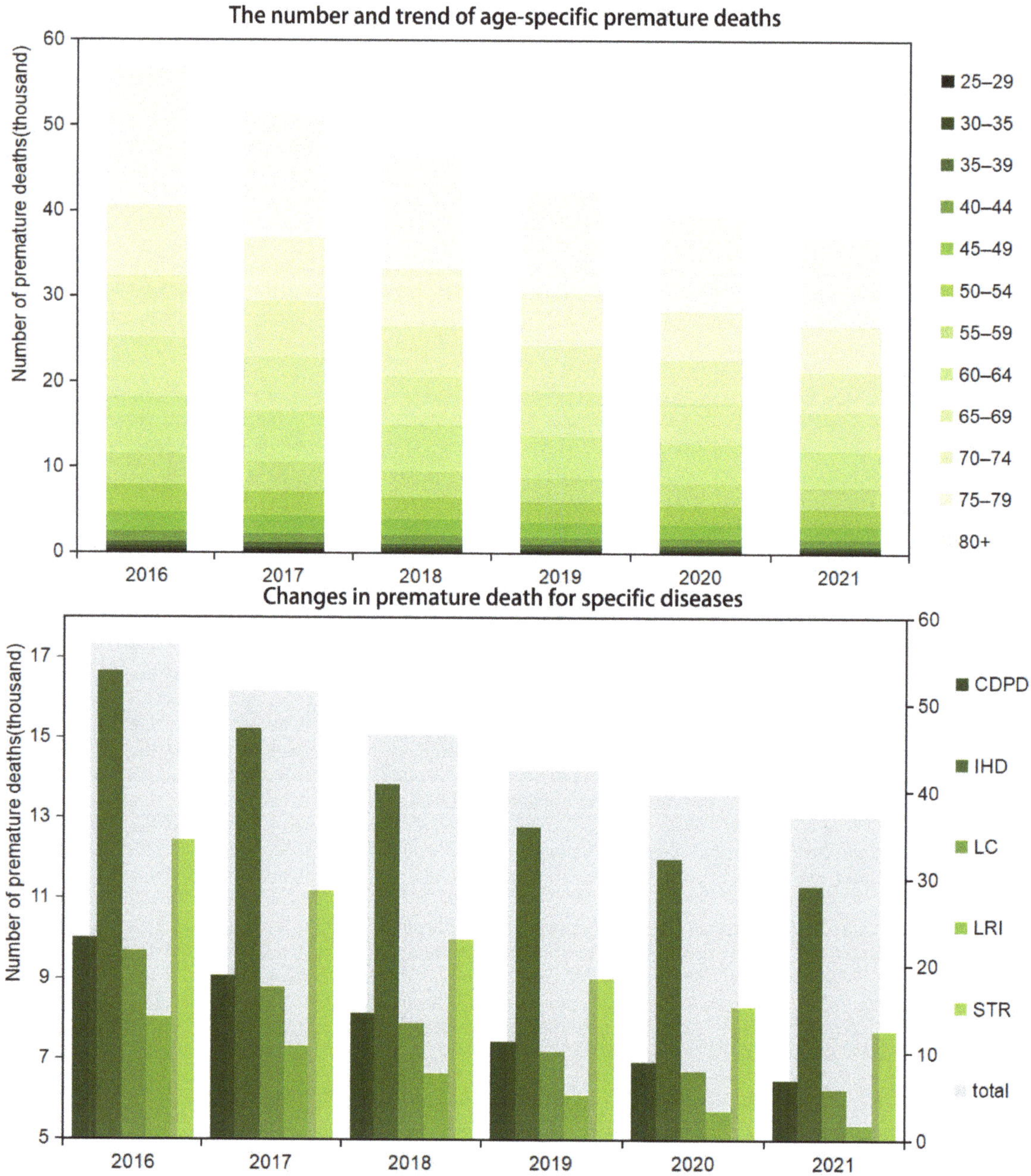

Figure 2. The trend of premature deaths attributed to $PM_{2.5}$ in Beijing from 2016 to 2021 (IHD, ischemic heart disease; LC, lung cancer; LRI, lower respiratory infection; STR, stroke; COPD, chronic obstructive pulmonary disease).

Table 2. Number of deaths related to $PM_{2.5}$ pollution in 16 districts of Beijing, 2016–2021.

	2016	2017	2018	2019	2020	2021
Changping	6281 (4805–7527)	5897 (4493–7100)	5561 (4225–6724)	5154 (3906–6258)	5044 (3818–6136)	4801 (3632–5850)
Chaoyang	13,590 (10,468–16,161)	11,980 (9175–14,337)	10,523 (8022–12,667)	9365 (7118–11,319)	8388 (6362–10,170)	7833 (5932–9522)
Daxing	5971 (4602–7097)	5750 (4411–6867)	5333 (4070–6408)	5194 (3954–6264)	5098 (3872–6168)	4799 (3639–5821)
Dongcheng	3065 (2364–3641)	2618 (2005–3133)	2259 (1722–2719)	1971 (1498–2382)	1711 (1298–2076)	1594 (1207–1938)
Fangshan	3508 (2688–4194)	3423 (2614–4110)	3264 (2485–3936)	3165 (2403–3830)	3125 (2369–3793)	2951 (2235–3589)
Fengtai	8156 (6284–9695)	7163 (5487–8570)	6298 (4803–7578)	5581 (4243–6742)	4974 (3774–6028)	4547 (3443–5529)
Haidian	12,346 (9492–14,711)	10,817 (8272–12,968)	9519 (7249–11,471)	8312 (6310–10,062)	7458 (5654–9051)	6884 (5210–8377)
Huairou	1087 (827–1312)	1059 (804–1281)	999 (757–1212)	935 (707–1138)	918 (694–1119)	892 (674–1088)
Mentougou	925 (704–1115)	924 (703–1115)	895 (679–1084)	852 (645–1036)	851 (644–1036)	834 (631–1017)
Miyun	1404 (1070–1691)	1342 (1020–1620)	1258 (954–1524)	1189 (901–1444)	1143 (865–1392)	1108 (838–1350)
Pinggu	1357 (1039–1623)	1277 (975–1535)	1176 (894–1421)	1108 (840–1342)	1055 (799–1282)	1003 (759–1221)
Shijingshan	2263 (1742–2693)	1982 (1517–2373)	1750 (1334–2106)	1530 (1162–1850)	1380 (1046–1673)	1260 (954–1533)
Shunyi	3626 (2784–4326)	3498 (2674–4195)	3300 (2512–3979)	3189 (2421–3859)	3127 (2370–3795)	2930 (2218–3565)
Tongzhou	4962 (3816–5912)	4922 (3771–5887)	4672 (3562–5623)	4637 (3527–5599)	4591 (3484–5560)	4349 (3296–5279)
Xicheng	4530 (3494–5380)	3889 (2978–4655)	3416 (2604–4111)	3006 (2284–3633)	2664 (2020–3231)	2487 (1883–3024)
Yanqing	838 (637–1013)	833 (633–1008)	789 (598–958)	732 (554–891)	726 (549–884)	697 (527–851)

3.3. *$PM_{2.5}$ Health and Economic Benefits*

According to Table 3, the overall trend across most districts indicates an increase in the VSL linked to $PM_{2.5}$ pollution over the six years, reflecting a growing economic cost of health impacts led by $PM_{2.5}$. Dongcheng District, Chaoyang District, Haidian District, and Shijingshan District show significant upward trends, with Dongcheng District and Chaoyang District experiencing the most substantial increases. Tongzhou District and Shunyi District show relatively stable or decreasing trends towards the end of the period, suggesting possible improvements in air quality, effective pollution control measures, or changes in the demographic or economic makeup affecting the valuation of health impacts.

In Figure 3, the overall trend indicates an increase in the economic losses due to $PM_{2.5}$ pollution, with the total rising from USD 11.91 billion in 2016 to a peak of USD 16.78 billion in 2020 before slightly decreasing to USD 16.31 billion in 2021. Notably, different districts exhibit varying patterns of change, with some districts showing a consistent increase, others experiencing fluctuations, and a few witnessing a decrease in the later years. Districts like Haidian and Chaoyang have shown a consistent increase in losses over the years. These areas are significant economic and educational hubs, implying higher population densities and potentially more vehicular and industrial emissions contributing to pollution levels, thereby increasing health and economic costs. Daxing presents a notable fluctuation, with a sharp increase from 2016 to 2019, followed by a significant decrease. This could be attributed to specific local industrial activities or infrastructural developments, such as the construction and subsequent operation of the Beijing Daxing International Airport, which might have initially increased pollution levels before mitigation measures were implemented. Shunyi district and Daxing district, after initial increases, show a decrease in losses in the later years. The Pandemic since 2020, which caused the closure of Daxing Airport, has resulted in a significant loss of GDP and, consequently, a reduction in the value of statistical life. From the perspective of urban areas, Haidian District and Chaoyang District account for most of the $PM_{2.5}$-related health economic losses in Beijing, and the growth rate and total amount of Haidian District are significantly higher than other districts. Chaoyang District grew at a steady rate between 2016 and 2021. Daxing District had a fast growth rate between 2016 and 2018, but it has decreased significantly since 2019. At the same time, the health and economic losses related to $PM_{2.5}$ in Xicheng District are also high but have always remained in a relatively stable state.

Table 3. The value of statistical life in 16 districts of Beijing from 2016 to 2021 ($\times 10^4$ USD).

	2016	2017	2018	2019	2020	2021
Changping	6.52	8.01	9.51	10.29	12.35	13.19
Chaoyang	18.44	23.79	29.74	32.93	40.56	44.36
Daxing	15.34	41.10	48.71	55.75	26.81	14.80
Dongcheng	41.07	54.98	49.33	59.13	81.11	91.76
Fangshan	9.27	12.02	12.81	11.52	12.04	11.19
Fengtai	9.26	11.99	15.17	18.00	23.04	24.69
Haidian	19.56	25.76	34.40	42.84	58.56	66.66
Huairou	10.47	12.30	14.23	14.20	17.29	20.04
Mentougou	8.24	9.02	10.11	12.71	15.40	19.23
Miyun	8.64	11.39	13.40	14.37	16.71	20.29
Pinggu	8.64	11.02	12.52	13.51	15.08	16.67
Shijingshan	11.50	14.64	18.88	21.57	32.42	43.77
Shunyi	20.17	23.70	25.87	25.35	24.34	22.64
Tongzhou	7.79	7.05	8.12	9.15	10.81	10.63
Xicheng	34.17	46.41	57.76	60.62	67.12	79.81
Yanqing	6.89	8.62	10.38	11.66	14.23	14.52

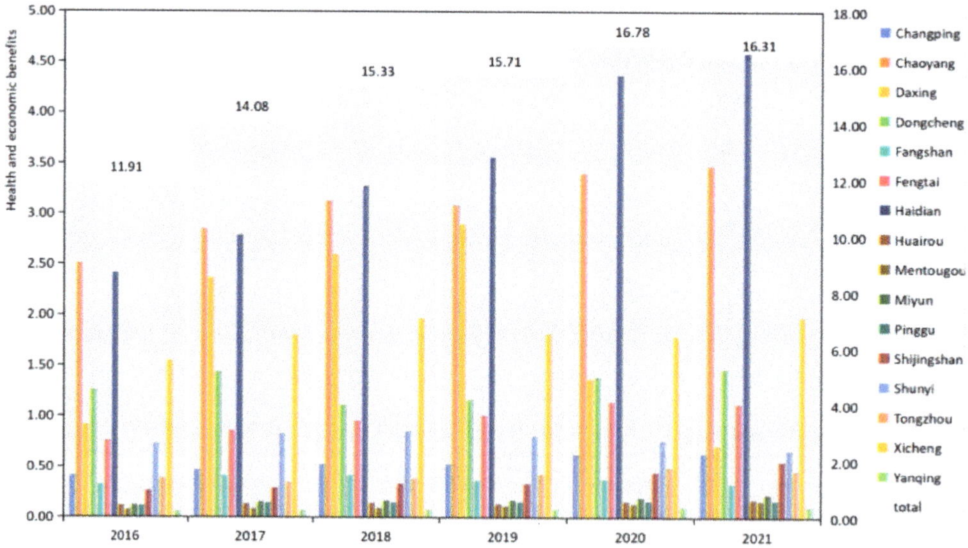

Figure 3. Health and economic losses caused by $PM_{2.5}$ pollution in 16 districts of Beijing from 2016 to 2021 (billion USD).

4. Discussion

4.1. The Attributable Disease Burden of $PM_{2.5}$ in Beijing Showed a Decreasing and Stable Trend

This study focuses on the atmospheric heavy pollution area of Beijing. By using $PM_{2.5}$ data with high-resolution, the international mainstream GEMM method was used to comprehensively evaluate the atmospheric $PM_{2.5}$-attributed deaths and time trends of five causes (COPD, IHD, LC, LRI, and STR), twelve age groups (25–29, 30–35, 35–39, 40–44, 45–49, 50–55, 55–59, 60–64, 65–69, 70–74, 75–79, and 80+), and the total numbers of deaths in Beijing from 2016 to 2021.

In 2012, the NAAQS (the Chinese National Ambient Air Quality Standard), initiated by the Ministry of Environmental Protection of China, listed $PM_{2.5}$ as one of the six pollutants monitored and assessed by AQI [27]. Subsequently, a series of relevant documents have also introduced practical prevention and control actions to improve the air quality in Beijing [28]. The results of this study show that the atmospheric $PM_{2.5}$ concentration in Beijing decreased significantly from 2016 to 2021, but it was still higher than all the national and international standards, including the national secondary standard, the national primary standard, and the WHO guideline standard. Although the attributable death burden of $PM_{2.5}$ in Beijing remains high, due to the improvement in air pollution in Beijing in recent years, the $PM_{2.5}$-attributable deaths of five diseases in 2021 have decreased to a certain extent compared with 2016.

4.2. Comparison with Other Studies concerning $PM_{2.5}$-Attributed Deaths and Economic Losses

Compared with previous studies on the disease burden of long-term exposure to $PM_{2.5}$, the advantage of this study is that it uses remote sensing $PM_{2.5}$ data with 1 km high spatial resolution and divides them by district level. At the same time of refinement, the spatial heterogeneity of $PM_{2.5}$ concentration and exposed population was also considered to a great extent. In terms of the total number of deaths, we updated the excess deaths and economic losses attributable to $PM_{2.5}$ in the Beijing area of China based on the innovative GEMM model, based on the calculation of different age groups and the number of deaths.

This study deepens the knowledge of the impacts of $PM_{2.5}$ pollution, consistently indicating that $PM_{2.5}$ pollution represents a severe public health issue, leading to a significant mortality burden [29–32]. $PM_{2.5}$ poses a serious health threat as their small size allows them to penetrate deep into the human respiratory system. Beyond its direct effects on human health, $PM_{2.5}$ pollution also has profound economic impacts, resulting in substantial economic losses. These losses stem not only from increased healthcare costs but also from indirect factors such as sick leave and decreased productivity. Estimating the economic and health losses is a complex process involving the assessment of the statistical value of life, measurement of pollution levels, the degree of population exposure, and the size of the affected population. The statistical value of life, which represents how much money people are willing to pay to reduce the risk of death, varies across different studies due to cultural, economic, and social values. Similarly, factors like pollution concentration, exposure levels, and population size can vary by region, time, and research methodology, leading to inconsistencies in the estimated economic health losses. All in all, $PM_{2.5}$ pollution not only poses a grave threat to human health but also causes significant economic losses. Addressing this challenge requires global cooperation and comprehensive strategies, including reducing emissions, raising public health awareness, and strengthening policy implementation to alleviate the health and economic burdens of $PM_{2.5}$ pollution. Furthermore, the methods for assessing economic health losses need further research and standardization to more accurately reflect the true impact of $PM_{2.5}$ pollution and provide a scientific basis for policymaking. For example, Maji et al. [33] estimated that the total economic loss related to pollution in China in 2016 was about USD 101.39 billion, accounting for 0.91% of GDP. For example, Maji et al. [33] estimated that China's total pollution-related economic loss in 2016 was about USD 101.39 billion, accounting for GDP. Among them, the $PM_{2.5}$-related death toll in Beijing was 18.58 thousand, and the economic loss was USD 4.75 billion. This is slightly lower than the number of related deaths (73.92 thousand) and economic losses

(USD 11.91 billion) in 2016 in this study. This is mainly because the statistical value of life in Beijing at the time assessed by the study was much lower than that estimated in this study. Han et al.'s findings suggest that economic losses attributable to long-term $PM_{2.5}$ exposure in the eastern region, where Beijing is located, were as high as USD 275.6 billion per year during 2015–2019 [34]. Meanwhile, Xie et al. showed that without effective control measures, it is estimated that by 2030, $PM_{2.5}$ pollution will lead to RMB 210 billion of health expenditure and RMB 10 trillion of health economic losses in China [31]. Previous studies have confirmed that the improvement in air quality in China in recent years has brought considerable health benefits [34–36]. Therefore, it is necessary to further take effective air pollution control measures, which will also bring considerable economic benefits. For example, the study by Xu et al. simulated the air quality benefits of the Air Pollution Prevention and Control Action Plan in Beijing in the middle of its implementation and found that the implementation of the policy could reduce external costs by USD 120 million in 2014–2016, which is significant [35].

4.3. Policy Implications

In recent years, new changes have taken place in China's air pollution situation. In order to meet the management needs of ambient air quality in the new era and coordinate environmental protection and economic development, it is necessary to revise the current ambient air quality standards in China [36]. It is worth noting that the formulation and implementation of local air quality standards is of great significance to improve the scientific and precise level of air pollution prevention and control. For example, the US state of California has formulated a series of air quality standards and pollution prevention and control policies based on local conditions, in particular strict control of important pollution sources such as motor vehicle emissions, and has made important progress in improving air quality, energy conservation, and emission reduction and ensuring people's health [37–39]. Beijing is one of the regions with the largest population density and the most active political and economic activities in China, and it is also a key area for air pollution prevention and control in China. Since the release of the "The Atmospheric Ten", the air quality in Beijing has been greatly improved. Taking Beijing as a pilot city, the formulation of China's local air standards for $PM_{2.5}$ will help promote the transformation and upgrading of local economic growth models, industrial structures, and technologies and promote the use of clean energy and green economic development to form a low-carbon policy guided by carbon neutrality goals [39–41].

Beijing has implemented stringent air pollution control measures over the years, including restrictions on coal-fired power plants, vehicle emission standards, and promotion of green energy, which could explain the overall trend of increasing losses peaking in 2020, as the cumulative effect of pollution on health becomes more pronounced before policies start to significantly mitigate these effects [42]. The economic development in certain districts can lead to increased construction, traffic, and industrial emissions, contributing to higher $PM_{2.5}$ levels and associated health costs [43]. Conversely, economic shifts towards less polluting industries or the relocation of heavy industries out of urban centers can reduce pollution levels [44]. Growing public awareness about the health impacts of $PM_{2.5}$ pollution, coupled with improvements in healthcare services, might influence the economic valuation of health losses as more people seek treatment and adopt preventive measures [29].

In order to further reduce the emission of air pollutants such as $PM_{2.5}$ and continuously improve air quality, it is recommended to adopt a series of regional pollution source control measures. In terms of industrial emissions, it is recommended to establish more stringent emission standards and encourage enterprises to adopt clean energy and efficient purification technologies. At the same time, the promotion of new energy vehicles and the improvement of public transport systems should be accelerated to effectively reduce traffic emissions. For the dust in the construction process, it is recommended to strictly manage and promote green construction standards. In addition, measures such as strengthening public environmental awareness education and expanding urban green areas will encourage the public to adopt a green lifestyle.

It is also crucial to further improve air quality monitoring and early warning systems, increase investment in environmental governance, implement differentiated policies, and improve public health services. It is recommended to encrypt air quality monitoring sites to improve the accuracy and timeliness of monitoring data and to release health warning information in a timely manner in combination with meteorological forecasting to reduce public exposure risks. It is recommended to increase investment in environmental technology research and development, support scientific and technological innovation in clean energy and pollution control, and invest in improving environmental infrastructure. According to the pollution characteristics and economic development level of different regions, it is suggested to formulate differentiated environmental protection policies and strengthen environmental governance cooperation among regions. Through strengthening health education and improving the level of medical services, public health services should be improved so as to provide more comprehensive health protection for the public. These recommendations are designed to continuously improve air quality and public health while also helping to mitigate economic losses and jointly build a greener and healthier future.

While this study underscores the importance of stringent local air quality standards and pollution control measures, implementing these policies faces several challenges. Enforcement mechanisms must be robust and adaptable to ensure compliance across diverse sectors. Engaging stakeholders, including industry, local communities, and policymakers, is essential for fostering a collaborative approach to air pollution mitigation. Moreover, the allocation of resources for monitoring, enforcement, and public awareness campaigns is critical for the success of these measures. Drawing on lessons from cities that have successfully improved air quality, such as Tokyo and London, can provide valuable insights into overcoming these challenges.

4.4. Limitations, Uncertainties, Feasibility, Cost-Effectiveness, and Unintended Consequences in Estimating $PM_{2.5}$-Attributed Deaths

This study presents a comprehensive analysis of $PM_{2.5}$ pollution in Beijing and its attributed mortality burden. However, it is crucial to acknowledge the inherent limitations and uncertainties associated with our data and methodology. The estimation of $PM_{2.5}$-attributed deaths relies on the global exposure mortality model (GEMM), which, while robust, is subject to uncertainties related to exposure assessment, population susceptibility, and the transferability of risk estimates across different populations. Additionally, spatial and temporal variations in $PM_{2.5}$ concentrations within Beijing may lead to underestimation or overestimation of exposure in certain districts. Future research should aim to refine exposure assessment methods and explore the heterogeneity of health impacts within urban populations.

The feasibility and cost-effectiveness of proposed pollution control measures are paramount for their successful implementation. Policies must balance environmental benefits with economic impacts, particularly on industries and employment. For instance, transitioning to cleaner energy sources requires significant investment and infrastructure development. Additionally, unintended consequences, such as the displacement of pollution to neighboring regions or increased financial burdens on low-income households, must be carefully considered. Mitigation strategies, including economic incentives for clean technologies and targeted support for affected communities, can help address these issues.

5. Conclusions

This study meticulously gathered data on the annual average concentrations of permanent residents, GDP, and $PM_{2.5}$ across 16 districts of Beijing from 2016 to 2021. Utilizing the GEMM method, we calculated the deaths caused by $PM_{2.5}$ pollution, which showed a fluctuating yet concerning trend with numbers like 9157 in 2016, peaking at 12,723 in 2020 and reducing slightly to 12,352 in 2021. These data provide a stark explanation of the impact of $PM_{2.5}$ pollution on people's health. Further, this study evaluated the corresponding health economic losses using the health economic benefit evaluation method, revealing staggering economic impacts ranging from USD 9232.27 million in 2016 to USD 12,735.42 million in 2021.

The $PM_{2.5}$-pollution-related economic losses fluctuated across 16 districts from 2016 to 2021, illuminating the intricate relationship between urban development, environmental policies, and public health measures. While there is growing public awareness of the impact of air pollution on population health and economic development, changes and differences at the district level point to the need for a more nuanced approach to pollution prevention and health risk management. Given the serious mortality burden and economic losses attributed to $PM_{2.5}$ exposure in Beijing, it becomes imperative to reevaluate and tighten the annual average standards for $PM_{2.5}$ air quality. The current situation demands a more scientific, precise, and localized approach to pollution prevention and control tailored to the evolving dynamics of atmospheric pollution. Establishing more rigorous and comprehensive local environmental air quality management standards is crucial for Beijing. Such measures should not only aim at meeting but surpassing the national standards, taking into account the specific challenges and needs of the city's diverse districts.

There is a close relationship and influence between air pollutants and building disciplines. Air pollutants will have an impact on building materials, the indoor environment, building energy efficiency, and other aspects, and have an impact on the indoor environment. In addition, air pollutants also have a certain impact on building energy conservation. The architectural discipline fully considers the harm and impact of air pollutants in the design and construction process, improves the comfort and health level of the indoor environment, and realizes the green, low-carbon, and sustainable development of buildings. Beijing's experience underscores the critical importance of sustained, comprehensive strategies that balance economic growth with environmental sustainability and public health. The path forward requires not just stringent standards but a collective effort to transform awareness into action, ensuring a healthier future for all residents.

Author Contributions: Conceptualization, B.J.D. and X.W.; methodology, B.J.D. and S.Z.; data curation, B.J.D. and X.W.; writing—review and editing, D.T., B.J.D. and S.Z. All authors have read and agreed to the published version of the manuscript.

Funding: This work was supported by the Beijing Key Laboratory of Urban Spatial Information Engineering (20230110), the Geological Disaster Monitoring Project of Mining Cave-In in Liuzhizhoushan Sports Park, Haizhou District, Lianyungang City.

Institutional Review Board Statement: Not applicable.

Informed Consent Statement: Informed consent was obtained from all subjects involved in the study.

Data Availability Statement: Data are contained within the article.

Acknowledgments: The authors are grateful to the editor and reviewers for their valuable comments and suggestions.

Conflicts of Interest: The authors declare no conflicts of interest.

References

1. Ioannis, M.; Elisavet, S.; Agathangelos, S.; Eugenia, B. Environmental and Health Impacts of Air Pollution: A Review. *Front. Public Health* **2020**, *8*, 505570.
2. Global Burden of Disease Collaborative Network. *Global Burden of Disease Study 2022*; Institute for Health Metrics and Evaluation (IHME): Seattle, WA, USA, 2022.
3. Ying, L.; Qing, G.; Wen, G.; Wu, D.; Xi, H.; Kai, Z. Meteorological factors related to winter severe PM2.5 pollution in China: In perspective of thresholds and relation of occurrence frequency with East Asian trough. *Atmos. Pollut. Res.* **2024**, *15*, 102002.
4. World Health Organization. *WHO Global Air Quality Guidelines: Particulate Matter (PM2.5 and PM10), Ozone, Nitrogen Dioxide, Sulfur Dioxide and Carbon Monoxide*; World Health Organization: Geneva, Switzerland, 2021.
5. Luo, G.; Zhang, L.; Hu, X.; Qiu, R. Quantifying public health benefits of PM2.5 reduction and spatial distribution analysis in China. *Sci. Total Environ.* **2020**, *719*, 137445. [CrossRef]

6. Tian, D.; Wang, J.; Xia, C.; Zhang, J.; Zhou, J.; Tian, Z.; Zhao, J.; Li, B.; Zhou, C. The relationship between green space accessibility by multiple travel modes and housing prices: A case study of Beijing. *Cities* **2024**, *145*, 104694. [CrossRef]
7. Turrini, E.; Carnevale, C.; Finzi, G.; Volta, M. A non-linear optimization programming model for air quality planning including co-benefits for GHG emissions. *Sci. Total Environ.* **2018**, *621*, 980–989. [CrossRef] [PubMed]
8. Ferreira, D.C.; Marques, R.C.; Nunes, A.M. Pay for performance in health care: A new best practice tariff-based tool using a log-linear piecewise frontier function and a dual–primal approach for unique solutions. *Oper. Res.* **2021**, *21*, 2101–2146.
9. Richard, B.; Hong, C.; Mieczysław, S.; Neal, F.; Bryan, H.; Arden, P.; Donkela, V. Global estimates of mortality associated with long-term exposure to outdoor fine particulate matter. *Proc. Natl. Acad. Sci. USA* **2018**, *115*, 9592–9597.
10. Maji, K.J. Substantial changes in PM2.5 pollution and corresponding premature deaths across China during 2015–2019: A model prospective. *Sci. Total Environ.* **2020**, *729*, 138838. [PubMed]
11. Bayat, R.; Ashrafi, K.; Motlagh, M.; Hassanvand, M.; Daroudi, R.; Fink, G.; Künzli, N. Health impact and related cost of ambient air pollution in Tehran. *Environ. Res.* **2019**, *176*, 108547. [CrossRef] [PubMed]
12. Bell, M.L. Spatial and temporal variation in PM2.5 chemical composition in the United States for health effects studies. *Environ. Health Perspect.* **2007**, *115*, 989–995. [CrossRef] [PubMed]
13. Song, Y.; Wang, X.; Maher, B.; Li, F.; Xu, C.; Liu, X.; Zhang, Z. The spatial-temporal characteristics and health impacts of ambient fine particulate matter in China. *J. Clean. Prod.* **2016**, *112*, 1312–1318. [CrossRef]
14. Tian, D.; Zhang, J.; Li, B.; Xia, C.; Zhu, Y.; Zhou, C.; Wang, Y.; Liu, X.; Yang, M. Spatial analysis of commuting carbon emissions in main urban area of Beijing: A GPS trajectory-based approach. *Ecol. Indic.* **2024**, *159*, 111610. [CrossRef]
15. Cai, S.; Wang, Y.; Zhao, B.; Wang, S.; Chang, X.; Hao, J. The impact of the "air pollution prevention and control action plan" on PM2.5 concentrations in Jing-Jin-Ji region during 2012–2020. *Sci. Total Environ.* **2017**, *580*, 197–209. [CrossRef] [PubMed]
16. Zhao, J.; Shao, Z.; Xia, C.; Kai, F.; Ran, C.; Jun, Z. Ecosystem services assessment based on land use simulation: A case study in the Heihe River Basin, China. *Ecol. Indic.* **2022**, *143*, 109402. [CrossRef]
17. Batterman, S.; Xu, L.; Chen, F.; Chen, F.; Zhong, X. Characteristics of PM2.5 concentrations across Beijing during 2013–2015. *Atmos. Environ.* **2016**, *145*, 104–114. [CrossRef] [PubMed]
18. Zíková, N.; Wang, Y.; Yang, F.; Li, X.; Tian, M.; Hopke, P. On the source contribution to Beijing PM2.5 concentrations. *Atmos. Environ.* **2016**, *134*, 84–95. [CrossRef]
19. Van, D.A.; Hammer, M.S.; Bindle, L.; Brauer, M. Monthly global estimates of fine particulate matter and their uncertainty. *Environ. Sci. Technol.* **2021**, *55*, 15287–15300.
20. Wei, J.; Huang, W.; Li, Z.; Xue, W.; Peng, Y.; Sun, L.; Cribb, M. Estimating 1-km-resolution $PM_{2.5}$ concentrations across China using the space-time random forest approach. *Remote Sens. Environ.* **2019**, *231*, 111221. [CrossRef]
21. National Bureau of Statistics of China. Beijing 7th National Census Bulletin. 2021. Available online: https://www.stats.gov.cn/english/PressRelease/202105/t20210510_1817185.html (accessed on 20 February 2024).
22. Xiao, Q.; Liang, F.; Ning, M.; Zhang, Q.; Bi, J.; He, K.; Lei, Y.; Liu, Y. The long-term trend of $PM_{2.5}$-related mortality in China: The effects of source data selection. *Chemosphere* **2021**, *263*, 127894. [CrossRef] [PubMed]
23. Tian, D.; Wen, Z.; Sun, Y. Analyzing the Spatial Interaction Characteristics of Urban Area Shared Bicycle Systems: A Case Study of Beijing's Central Area. *Buildings* **2023**, *13*, 2646. [CrossRef]
24. Huang, D.; Zhang, S. Health benefit evaluation for $PM_{2.5}$ pollution control in Beijing-Tianjin-Hebei region of China. *China Environ. Sci.* **2013**, *33*, 166–174.
25. Yin, H.; Pizzol, M.; Xu, L. External costs of PM2.5 pollution in Beijing, China: Uncertainty analysis of multiple health impacts and costs. *Environ. Pollut.* **2017**, *226*, 356–369. [CrossRef] [PubMed]
26. Lanzi, E. *The Economic Consequences of Outdoor Air Pollution 2016: The Economic Consequences of Outdoor Air Pollution*; OECD: Paris, France, 2016.
27. You, M. Addition of PM 2.5 into the national ambient air quality standards of China and the contribution to air pollution control: The case study of Wuhan, China. *Sci. World J.* **2014**, *2014*, 768405. [CrossRef] [PubMed]
28. Li, W.; Shao, L.; Wang, W.; Li, H.; Wang, X.; Li, Y.; Li, W.; Jones, T.; Zhang, D. Air quality improvement in response to intensified control strategies in Beijing during 2013–2019. *Sci. Total Environ.* **2020**, *744*, 140776. [CrossRef]
29. Wu, R.; Dai, H.; Geng, Y.; Xie, Y.; Masui, T.; Liu, Z.; Qian, Y. Economic impacts from PM2.5 pollution-related health effects: A case study in Shanghai. *Environ. Sci. Technol.* **2017**, *51*, 5035–5042. [CrossRef] [PubMed]
30. Xie, Y.; Dai, H.; Zhang, Y.; Wu, Y.; Hanaoka, T.; Masui, T. Comparison of health and economic impacts of PM2.5 and ozone pollution in China. *Environ. Int.* **2019**, *130*, 104881. [CrossRef] [PubMed]
31. Xie, Y.; Dai, H.; Dong, H.; Hanaoka, T.; Masui, T. Economic impacts from PM2.5 pollution-related health effects in China: A provincial-level analysis. *Environ. Sci. Technol.* **2016**, *50*, 4836–4843. [CrossRef]
32. Song, C.; He, J.; Wu, L.; Jin, T.; Chen, X.; Li, R.; Ren, P.; Zhang, L.; Mao, H. Health burden attributable to ambient PM2.5 in China. *Environ. Pollut.* **2017**, *223*, 575–586. [CrossRef] [PubMed]
33. Maji, K.J.; Ye, W.; Arora, M.; Nagendra, S.M. PM2.5-related health and economic loss assessment for 338 Chinese cities. *Environ. Int.* **2018**, *121*, 392–403. [CrossRef]
34. Han, C.; Xu, R.; Ye, T.; Xie, Y.; Zhao, Y.; Liu, H.; Yu, W.; Zhang, Y.; Li, S.; Zhang, Z.; et al. Mortality burden due to long-term exposure to ambient PM2.5 above the new WHO air quality guideline based on 296 cities in China. *Environ. Int.* **2022**, *166*, 107331. [CrossRef]

35. Xu, X.; Zhang, W.; Zhu, C.; Li, J.; Wang, J.; Li, P.; Zhao, P. Health risk and external costs assessment of PM2.5 in Beijing during the "Five-year Clean Air Action Plan". *Atmos. Pollut. Res.* **2021**, *12*, 101089. [CrossRef]
36. Wang, Z.; Tan, Y.; Guo, M.; Cheng, M.; Gu, Y.; Chen, S.; Wu, X.; Chai, F. Prospect of China's ambient air quality standards. *J. Environ. Sci.* **2023**, *123*, 255–269. [CrossRef] [PubMed]
37. Samuelsen, S.; Zhu, S.; Kinnon, M.M.; Yang, O.K.; Dabdub, D.; Brouwer, J. An episodic assessment of vehicle emission regulations on saving lives in California. *Environ. Sci.* **2020**, *55*, 547–552. [CrossRef] [PubMed]
38. Lurmann, F.; Avol, E.; Gilliland, F. Emissions reduction policies and recent trends in Southern California's ambient air quality. *J. Air Waste Manag.* **2015**, *65*, 324–335. [CrossRef] [PubMed]
39. Shi, X.; Zheng, Y.; Lei, Y.; Xue, W.; Yan, G.; Liu, X.; Cai, B.; Tong, D.; Wang, J. Air quality benefits of achieving carbon neutrality in China. *Sci. Total Environ.* **2021**, *795*, 148784. [CrossRef]
40. Tang, R.; Zhao, J.; Liu, Y.; Huang, X.; Zhang, Y.; Zhou, D.; Ding, A.; Nielsen, C.P.; Wang, H. Air quality and health co-benefits of China's carbon dioxide emissions peaking before 2030. *Nat. Commun.* **2022**, *13*, 1008. [CrossRef]
41. Cheng, J.; Tong, D.; Zhang, Q.; Liu, Y.; Lei, Y.; Yan, G.; Yan, L.; Yu, S.; Cui, R.Y.; Clarke, L.; et al. Pathways of China's PM2.5 air quality 2015–2060 in the context of carbon neutrality. *Natl. Sci. Rev.* **2021**, *8*, nwab078. [CrossRef] [PubMed]
42. Zhang, S.; Wu, Y.; Wu, X.; Li, M.; Ge, Y.; Liang, B.; Xu, Y.; Zhou, Y.; Liu, H.; Fu, L.; et al. Historic and future trends of vehicle emissions in Beijing, 1998–2020: A policy assessment for the most stringent vehicle emission control program in China. *Atmos. Environ.* **2014**, *89*, 216–229. [CrossRef]
43. Tian, X.; Dai, H.; Geng, Y.; Wilson, J.; Wu, R.; Xie, Y.; Hao, H. Economic impacts from PM2.5 pollution-related health effects in China's road transport sector: A provincial-level analysis. *Environ. Int.* **2018**, *115*, 220–229. [CrossRef]
44. Shen, J.; Wei, Y.; Yang, Z. The impact of environmental regulations on the location of pollution-intensive industries in China. *J. Clean. Prod.* **2017**, *148*, 785–794. [CrossRef]

toxics

MDPI

Article

The Possible Role of $PM_{2.5}$ Chronic Exposure on 5-Year Survival in Patients with Left Ventricular Dysfunction Following Coronary Artery Bypass Grafting

Tomasz Urbanowicz [1,*], Krzysztof Skotak [2], Anna Olasińska-Wiśniewska [1], Krzysztof J Filipiak [3,4], Aleksandra Płachta-Krasińska [5], Jakub Piecek [6], Beata Krasińska [4], Zbigniew Krasiński [7], Andrzej Tykarski [4] and Marek Jemielity [1]

[1] Cardiac Surgery and Transplantology Department, Poznan University of Medical Sciences, 61-701 Poznan, Poland
[2] Institute of Environmental Protection–National Research Institute, 02-170 Warsaw, Poland
[3] Institute of Clinical Science, Maria Sklodowska-Curie Medical Academy, 00-136 Warsaw, Poland
[4] Department of Hypertensiology, Angiology and Internal Medicine, Poznan University of Medical Sciences, 61-701 Poznan, Poland
[5] Department of Ophthalmology, Poznan University of Medical Sciences, 61-701 Poznan, Poland
[6] Student Research Group, Medical Faculty, Poznan University of Medical Sciences, 61-107 Poznan, Poland
[7] Department of Vascular, Endovascular Surgery, Angiology and Phlebology, Poznan University of Medical Science, 61-701 Poznań, Poland
* Correspondence: turbanowicz@ump.edu.pl

Abstract: Background: The survival benefit of surgical revascularization in multivessel coronary artery disease is well understood, though it can be modified by left ventricular dysfunction. Chronic exposure to air pollutants has gained more attention recently as a possible non-traditional morbidity and mortality cardiovascular risk factor. This study identified possible 5-year mortality risk factors related to postoperative left ventricular performance, including air pollutants. Patients: There were 283 patients (244 (86%) males) with a median age of 65 (60–70) years enrolled in the retrospective analysis. All patients were referred for off-pump coronary artery revascularization due to chronic coronary syndrome that presented as a multivessel coronary artery disease. They were divided into three groups depending on the postoperative course of left ventricular fraction (LVEF 50% or more (169 patients), LVEF between 41 and 49% (61 patients), and LVEF 40% or less (53 patients)). Results: The overall survival rate was 84% (237 patients) in a median follow-up time of 5.3 (4.8–6.1) years. The median (Q1–Q3) chronic air pollution exposures for the analyzed group were 19.3 (16.9–22.4) $\mu g/m^3$ for fine particles such as $PM_{2.5}$, 25.8 (22.5–29.4) $\mu g/m^3$ for coarse particles such as PM_{10}, and 12.2 (9.7–14.9) $\mu g/m^3$ for nitric dioxide (NO_2). The mortality in the first group (LVEF at least 50%) was 23 (13.6%), in the second group (LVEF 41–49%) was 9 (15%), and in the third group (LVEF 40% or less) was 14 (26%). The multivariable regression analysis for the five-year mortality risk in the first group revealed the predictive value of dyslipidemia (HR: 3.254, 95% CI: 1.008–10.511, $p = 0.049$). The multivariable regression analysis for five-year mortality risk in the second group revealed the predictive value of dyslipidemia (HR: 3.391, 95% CI: 1.001–11.874, $p = 0.050$) and $PM_{2.5}$ (HR: 1.327, 95% CI: 1.085–1.625, $p = 0.006$). In the third group (severely decreased LVEF), chronic $PM_{2.5}$ exposure was found to be significant (HR: 1.518, 95% CI: 1.50–2.195, $p = 0.026$) for 5-year mortality prediction. Conclusions: Traditional risk factors, such as dyslipidemia, are pivotal in the 5-year mortality risk following surgical revascularization. Chronic exposure to ambient air pollutants such as $PM_{2.5}$ may be an additional risk factor in patients with left ventricular dysfunction.

Keywords: OPCAB; CAD; air pollution; $PM_{2.5}$; LVEF

1. Introduction

Coronary artery atherosclerotic disease is characterized by an increased mortality risk. Non-traditional risk factors such as air pollution have gained more attention due to constant climate change [1,2]. Our previous analysis revealed the possible relationship between coronary artery disease progression, air pollution [3], and ambient temperature [4].

The current assessment of ischemic disease advancement involves anatomical and functional evaluation to optimize symptom reduction and address major adverse cardiovascular event threats [5]. The percutaneous and surgical interventions present satisfactory results and indicate a personalized approach [6]. In the meta-analysis at the 5-year follow-up by Formica et al. [7], higher incidences of all-cause mortality, myocardial infarction, and repeat revascularization were revealed among patients with multivessel coronary disease or left main disease treated with percutaneous interventions.

The two surgical techniques, off-pump and on-pump surgery, did not reveal significant long-term outcome differences in the randomized trial of Quin et al. [8]. Though still limited in overall application number, the off-pump surgical technique presents satisfactory results, especially in high-risk patients [8–10]. In the results of the recently published SYNTASES trial [7], 10-year mortality adjusted for significant confounders was significantly lower following on-pump surgical revascularization than with off-pump and percutaneous approaches.

Although the survival benefit of surgical revascularization in multivessel coronary artery disease is well understood, it can be modified by left ventricular dysfunction. Previous analysis pointed out the survival benefit of surgical over percutaneous therapies in multivessel disease in patients with left ventricular dysfunction [11]. Even asymptomatic mild left ventricular impaired function limits the prognosis and may progress to more advanced stages [12]. Heart dysfunction induces inflammatory activation related to mitochondrial dysfunction [13]. The presented phenomenon is characterized by impaired energy production, oxidative stress, and disrupted calcium homeostasis. Airborne fine particles are one of the strong external stimuli for inflammatory activation [14].

Accurately managing traditional coronary artery disease risk factors is essential for long-term results optimization. In their meta-analysis, Bond et al. [8] presented the relationship between ambient air pollution exposure and increased risk for all-cause cardiovascular morbidity and morbidity. Our previous studies revealed an increased risk for coronary disease progression related to air pollutants [15].

This study aimed to identify possible 5-year mortality risk factors, including air pollutants related to postoperative left ventricular performance. The mortality risk assessment was performed based on demographical and clinical characteristics, including non-traditional cardiovascular elements such as environmental factors.

2. Materials and Methods

There were 283 consecutive patients (244 (86%) males) with a median age of 65 (60–70) years enrolled in the retrospective analysis. All patients were referred for off-pump coronary artery revascularization due to chronic coronary syndrome, which presented as a multivessel disease. Co-morbidities that characterized the patients included arterial hypertension (222 (78%)), dyslipidemia (149 (53%)), and diabetes mellitus (111 (39%)). They were divided into three groups according to the current classification of heart failure based on the postoperative course of left ventricular ejection fraction (LVEF 50% or more (169 patients), an LVEF between 41–49% (61 patients), and an LVEF 40% or less (53 patients), as presented in Table 1.

Table 1. Groups' demographical and clinical characteristics.

Parameters	Group 1 LVEF ≥ 50% n = 169	Group 2 LVEF 41–49% n = 61	Group 3 LVEF ≤ 40% n = 53	*p* Group 1 vs. Group 2	*p* Group 1 vs. Group 3	*p* Group 2 vs. Group 3
Demographical						
Age (years) (median (Q1–Q3)	64 (60–72)	64 (58–69)	64 (59–68)	0.322	0.186	0.795
Sex (male (%))	142 (84)	52 (85)	49 (92)	0.627	0.124	0.324
BMI (median (Q1–Q3)	28.4 (26.6–30.9)	28.4 (26.3–31.0)	28.7 (26.6-31.5)	0.624	0.74	0.532
Co-morbidities						
Arterial hypertension (n, %)	128 (76)	49 (80)	45 (85)	0.349	0	0.302
Dyslipidemia (n, %)	89 (53)	30 (49)	30 (57)	0.724	0.457	0.639
Diabetes mellitus (n, %)	57 (34)	21 (34)	19 (36)	0.859	0.778	0.928
PAD (n, %)	18 (11)	5 (8)	4 (8)	0.61	0.512	0.883
CAD diagnosis:						
Left main disease (n, %)	51 (30)	19 (31)	14 (26)	0.873	0.73	0.68
Two-vessel disease (n, %)	49 (29)	18 (30)	14 26)	1	0.862	0.835
Three-vessel disease (n, %)	69 (41)	24 (39)	25 (47)	0.88	0.43	0.451

Abbreviations: BMI—body mass index, CAD—coronary artery disease, LVEF—left ventricular ejection fraction, n—number.

2.1. Air Pollution Exposure Methodology

Three health-relevant air pollutants were considered for our study: particulate matter with a diameter of 10 microns or less (PM_{10}), particulate matter with a diameter of 2.5 microns or less ($PM_{2.5}$), and nitrogen dioxide (NO_2).

The level of individual patients' exposure was assessed using spatial distributions of air concentration fields across Poland, as provided by the Chief Inspectorate of Environmental Protection. Maps of air pollutants PM_{10}, $PM_{2.5}$, and NO_2 were derived from the results of the National Air Quality Modelling (NAQM) system, elaborated by the Institute of Environmental Protection–National Research Institute in Poland (IEP-NRI), in line with the Environmental Protection Act in Poland (Art 66, paragraph 6). The NAQM base consists of two components: (1) high-resolution bottom-up emission inventory maps of air pollutants stored in the Central Emission Database [16] and (2) air concentration maps elaborated using the GEM-AQ model, which operates in the Copernicus Atmosphere Monitoring Service—Regional Production (CAMS2_40) [17].

2.2. Statistical Analysis

The normality of the distribution of variables was tested with the Shapiro–Wilk test. The t-test, Cochran–Cox test, Mann–Whitney tests, and Fisher's exact test were used where applicable to compare the variables between groups. Multivariable Cox regression was performed to analyze the predictors of long-term mortality. Demographic (age, sex, body mass index (BMI)), clinical (arterial hypertension, diabetes mellitus, hypercholesterolemia, peripheral artery disease, surgical details), laboratory (troponin, creatinine, uric acid), and air pollution ($PM_{2.5}$, PM_{10}, NO_2) data were evaluated. Statistical analysis was performed using Statistica 13 by TIBCO. $p < 0.05$ was considered statistically significant.

2.3. Bioethics Committee

Informed consent was obtained from all participants. This study was conducted in accordance with the Declaration of Helsinki and approved by the Institutional Review Board (or Ethics Committee) of Poznan University of Medical Sciences, Poznan, Poland (protocol code 55/20 from 16 January 2020), for studies involving humans.

3. Results

The overall survival rate was reported to be 84% (237 patients) in a median follow-up time of 5.3 (4.8–6.1) years. There were no perioperative deaths and no major adverse coronary events reported in the analyzed group. All patients were operated on through median sternotomy in the off-pump technique. The mean graft number was 2.3 (0.7), and the median hospitalization time was 12 (9–14) days, as presented in Table 2.

Table 2. Perioperative characteristics.

Parameters	Group 1 LVEF ≥ 50% n = 169	Group 2 LVEF 41–49% n = 61	Group 3 LVEF ≤ 40% n = 53	p Group 1 vs. Group 2	p Group 1 vs. Group 3	p Group 2 vs. Group 3
Preoperative laboratory results:						
WBC (×10^9/L) (median (Q1–Q3))	7.70 (6.47–8.93)	7.84 (6.41–8.83)	7.44 (6.59–8.51)	0.612	0.738	0.716
Hb (mmol/L) (median (Q1–Q3))	8.8 (8.2–9.3)	8.7 (8.2–9.15)	8.90 (8.40–9.30)	0.972	0.699	0.416
Plt (×10^9/L) (median (Q1–Q3))	219 (187–259)	225 (188–262)	222 (182–263)	0.896	0.961	0.863
Creatinine (µmol/L) (median (Q1–Q3))	98 (79–114)	93 (74–108)	95 (89–107)	0.578	0.685	0.893
CRP (mg/L) (median (Q1–Q3))	6 (5–8)	6 (3–8)	6 (5–8)	0.64	0.934	0.756
Preoperative echocardiography:						
LVED (mm) (median (Q1–Q3))	50 (44–55)	57 (53–60)	61 (57–64)	<0.001	<0.001	<0.001
LVEF (%) (median (Q1–Q3))	53 (50–57)	40 (38–43)	31 (27–34)	<0.001	<0.001	<0.001
Off-pump surgery:						
Skin-to-skin time (min) (median (Q1–Q3))	132 (119–167)	139 (121–170)	161 (120–182)	0.289	0.116	0.189
Number of grafts (n, mean (SD))	2.2 (0.8)	2.4 (0.7)	3.0 (0.8)	0.148	0.047	0.563
Troponin max (ng/mL) (median (Q1–Q3))	1.698 (0.789–4.334)	1.47 (0.603–3.416)	2.37 (0.942–4.125)	0.452	0.453	0.187
Overall hospitalization: (days) (mean (SD))	10 (2)	11 (3)	14 (3)	0.608	0.043	0.278
Complications:						
Bleeding (n, (%))	2 (1)	1 (2)	1 (2)	1	1	0.561
Wound infection (n, (%))	3 (2)	2 (3)	1 (2)	0.61	1	1

Abbreviations: CRP—C-reactive protein, Hb—hemoglobin, LVED—left ventricular end-diastolic diameter, LVEF—left ventricular ejection fraction, n—number, Plt—platelet count, Q—quartile, SD—standard deviation, WBC—white blood cells count.

Postoperative exposure to ambient air pollutants was calculated individually for each patient. The median (Q1–Q3) chronic air pollution exposures for the analyzed group were 19.3 (16.9–22.4) µg/m^3 for fine particles such as $PM_{2.5}$, 25.8 (22.5–29.4) µg/m^3 for coarse particles such as PM_{10}, and 12.2 (9.7–14.9) µg/m^3 for nitric dioxide (NO2). The mortality rates in groups were as follows: in the first group (LVEF at least 50%) 23 (13.6%), in the second group (LVEF 41–49%) 9 (15%), and in the third group (LVEF 40% or less) 14 (26%) patients died. The detailed follow-up information is presented in Table 3.

Table 3. Patients' characteristics in follow-up.

Parameters	Group 1 LVEF ≥ 50% n = 169	Group 2 LVEF 41–49% n = 61	Group 3 LVEF ≤ 40% n = 53	p Group 1 vs. Group 2	p Group 1 vs. Group 3	p Group 2 vs. Group 3
Mean follow-up time (years) (mean (SD)	5.3 (1.1)	5.5 (1.1)	5.4 (1.1)	0.919	0.814	0.818
Follow-up laboratory results:						
WBC (×10^9/L) (median (Q1–Q3))	8.32 (7.04–9.73)	8.6 (6.96–10.31)	8.91 (7.68–10.49)	0.797	0.152	0.535
Hb (mmol/L) (median (Q1–Q3))	7.0 (6.6–7.4)	6.8 (6.5–7.45)	6.9 (6.5–7.5)	0.915	0.767	0.709
Plt (×10^9/L) (median (Q1–Q3))	264 (211–322)	258 (220–303)	272 (222–354)	0.988	0.509	0.502
Creatinine (µmol/L) (median (Q1–Q3))	92 (79–104)	94 (75–105)	93 (81.5–100.6)	0.589	0.847	0.892
Uric acid (µmol/L) (median (Q1–Q3))	5.72 (4.85–6.99)	5.94 (5.01–6.63)	6.00 (4.98–7.64)	0.961	0.346	0.946
Hb1Ac (%) (median (Q1–Q3))	6.4 (6.0–6.9)	6.5 (6.1–7.1)	6.4 (6.0–7.0)	0.928	0.879	0.945
Lipidogram:						
Total cholesterol (mmol/L) (median (Q1–Q3))	4.0 (3.3–4.7)	3.7 (3.1–4.2)	3.8 (3.5–4.2)	0.131	0.212	0.441
LDL (mmol/L) (median (Q1–Q3))	2.2 (1.6–2.9)	1.7 (1.3–2.4)	2.1 (1.6–2.3)	0.034	0.145	0.123
HDL (mmol/L) (median (Q1–Q3))	1.2 (0.9–1.5)	1.0 (0.9–1.3)	1.1 (1.0–1.2)	0.11	0.48	0.423
TG (mmol/L) (median (Q1–Q3))	1.4 (1.1–1.8)	1.5 (1.0–1.9)	1.5 (1.0–1.5)	0.324	0.052	0.365
Follow-up echocardiography						
LVED (mm) (median) (Q1–Q3)	48 (42–52)	55 (51–58)	57 (53–61)	<0.001	<0.001	<0.001
LVEF (%) (median (Q1–Q3)	55 (50–60)	44 (41–47)	33 (30–37)	<0.001	<0.001	<0.001
Postoperative pharmacotherapy:						
B-blockers (n (%))	169 (100)	61 (100)	53 (100)	1	1	1
ACE-I (n (%))	151 (89)	56 (92)	21 (40)	1	<0.001	<0.001
ARNI (n (%))	14 (8)	3 (5)	32 (60)	0.768	<0.001	<0.001
Diuretics (n (%))	29 (17)	17 (28)	34 (64)	0.092	<0.001	<0.001
SGLT2 inhibitors (n (%))	2 (1)	3 (5)	15 (28)	0.09	<0.001	0.004

Table 3. *Cont.*

Parameters	Group 1 LVEF ≥ 50% n = 169	Group 2 LVEF 41–49% n = 61	Group 3 LVEF ≤ 40% n = 53	*p* Group 1 vs. Group 2	*p* Group 1 vs. Group 3	*p* Group 2 vs. Group 3
Statins (n (%))	164 (97)	61 (100)	53 (100)	0.566	1	1
MRA (n (%))	3 (18)	5 (8)	45 (85)	0.034	<0.001	<0.001
ASA (n (%))	169 (100)	61 (100)	53 (100)	1	1	1
Insulin (n (%))	31 (18)	6 (10)	10 (19)	0.218	0.838	0.187
Metformin (n (%))	26 (15)	15 (25)	43 (81)	0.12	<0.001	<0.001
Ambient air pollution						
$PM_{2.5}$ (μg/m^3) (median (Q1–Q3)	18.9 (16.9–22.4)	20.6 (17.8–23.0)	18.9 (15.4–21.8)	0.152	0.614	0.108
PM_{10} (μg/m^3) (median (Q1–Q3)	25.3 (22.4–29.6)	26.7 (23.9–29.7)	25.0 (21.2–28.3)	0.237	0.37	0.053
NO_2 (μg/m^3) (median (Q1–Q3)	12.2 (9.99–15.62)	13.0 (10.1–15.1)	11.2 (9.3–14.5)	0.709	0.217	0.145
Five-year overall mortality (n, %)	23 (14)	9 (15)	14 (26)	0.831	0.036	0.161

Abbreviations: ACE-I—angiotensin-converting enzyme—inhibitor, ARNI—angiotensin receptor neprilysin inhibitors, ASA—aspirin, BMI—body mass index, Hb—hemoglobin, Hb1Ac—glycemic hemoglobin, HDL—high-density lipoprotein, LDL—low-density lipoprotein, LVED—left ventricular end-diastolic diameter, LVEF—left ventricular ejection fraction, MRA—mineralocorticoid receptor antagonist, n—number, NO2—nitric dioxide, $PM_{2.5}$—air pollution particle matter 2.5 μm or less, PAD—peripheral artery disease, PM_{10}—air pollution particle matter 10 μm or less, Plt—platelets, SD—standard deviation, SGLT2—sodium–glucose cotransporter-2, TG—triglycerides, Q—quartile, WBC—white blood cell count.

3.1. Logistic Regression Analysis

The multivariable Cox regression analysis for predicting 5-year all-cause mortality risk factors was performed separately for each group. This study included ambient air pollutant exposure in places of habitation, including fine particles such as $PM_{2.5}$ and coarse particles such as PM_{10} and NO_2.

3.2. Group 1

The univariable and multivariable Cox analysis of 5-year mortality risk in the first group (LVEF 50% or less) revealed the predictive value of dyslipidemia (HR: 3.254, 95% CI: 1.008–10.511, $p = 0.049$), presented in Table 4.

Table 4. Univariable and multivariable analysis for 5-year mortality prediction in patients operated on due to multivessel artery disease presenting in postoperative course normal left ventricular ejection fraction (LVEF >50%).

Parameters	Univariable			Multivariable		
	HR	95% CI	*p*	HR	95% CI	*p*
Demographical:						
Age	0.976	0.828–1.151	0.775			
Sex (male)	0.755	0.135–2.606	0.49			
BMI	0.976	0.828–1.151	0.755			
Clinical:						
Arterial hypertension	2.411	0.465–12.512	0.295			
Diabetes mellitus	2.402	0.702–8.218	0.163			
Hypercholesterolemia	4.246	1.152–15.646	0.03	3.254	1.008–10.511	0.049
PAD	1.145	1.044–3.871	0.437			
Perioperative:						
Number of grafts (2)	1.478	0.288–7.574	0.64			
Number of grafts (3)	1.579	0.309–8.078	0.583			
Arterial revascularization	0.91	0.567–1.245	0.592			
Troponin max	0.903	0.770–1.059	0.21			
Postoperative:						
Creatinine	0.995	0.970–1.022	0.726			
Uric acid	0.889	0.616–1.282	0.528			

Table 4. *Cont.*

Parameters	Univariable			Multivariable		
	HR	95% CI	*p*	HR	95% CI	*p*
Air pollution exposure:						
$PM_{2.5}$	0.979	0.688–1.392	0.906			
PM_{10}	0.955	0.723–1.370	0.977			
NO_2	1.012	0.871–1.175	0.879			

Abbreviations: BMI—body mass index, HR—hazard ratio, NO2—nitric dioxide, $PM_{2.5}$—air pollution particle matter 2.5 μm or less, PAD—peripheral artery disease, PM_{10}—air pollution particle matter 10 μm or less.

3.3. Group 2

The multivariable stepwise regression analysis for 5-year mortality risk in the second group (LVEF 40–49%) revealed the predictive value of dyslipidemia (OR: 3.391, 95% CI: 1.001–11.874, $p = 0.050$) and $PM_{2.5}$ (OR: 1.327, 95% CI: 1.085–1.625, $p = 0.006$) as presented in Table 5.

Table 5. Univariable and multivariable analysis for 5-year mortality prediction in patients operated on due to multivessel artery disease presenting in postoperative course reduced left ventricular ejection fraction (LVEF 40–49%).

Parameter	Univariable			Multivariable		
	HR	95% CI	*p*	HR	95% CI	*p*
Demographical:						
Age	0.82	0.521–1.291	0.39			
Sex (male)	0.047	0.01–4.086	0.18			
BMI	1.194	0.743–1.919	0.463			
Clinical:						
Arterial hypertension	4.366	0.280–10.672	0.196			
Diabetes mellitus	1.934	0.124–30.031	0.638			
Hypercholesterolemia	6.767	0.859–83.861	0.156	3.391	1.001–11.874	0.05
PAD	1.04	0.103–5.764	0.241			
Perioperative:						
Number of grafts (2)	0.053	0.001–33.6700	0.226			
Number of grafts (3)	0.062	0.002–43.703	0.227			
Arterial revascularization	0.902	0.567– 1.674	0.997			
Troponin max	1.015	0.805–1.278	0.902			
Postoperative:						
Creatinine	0.997	0.943–1.054	0.913			
Uric acid	1.155	0.282–4.726	0.841			
Air pollution exposure:						
$PM_{2.5}$	2.084	0.849–5.114	0.109	1.327	1.085–1.625	0.006
PM_{10}	1.009	0.122–1.250	0.113			
NO_2	1.429	0.829–2.464	0.199			

Abbreviations: BMI—body mass index, HR—hazard ratio, NO2—nitric dioxide, $PM_{2.5}$—air pollution particle matter 2.5 μm or less, PAD—peripheral artery disease, PM_{10}—air pollution particle matter 10 μm or less.

3.4. Group 3

The multivariable analysis stepwise regression analysis for 5-year mortality risk in the third group (LVEF 40% or less) revealed the predictive value of chronic $PM_{2.5}$ exposure (OR: 1.518, 95% CI: 1.50–2.195, $p = 0.026$), as shown in Table 6.

Table 6. Univariable and multivariable analysis for 5-year mortality prediction in patients operated on due to multivessel artery disease presenting in postoperative course significantly reduced left ventricular ejection fraction (LVEF < 40%).

Parameter	Univariable			Multivariable		
	HR	95% CI	*p*	HR	95% CI	*p*
Demographical:						
Age	1.032	0.868–1.228	0.719			
Sex (male)	4.061	0.681–10.603	0.996			
BMI	1.035	0.784–1.367	0.807			
Clinical:						
Arterial hypertension	1.374	0.477–21.139	0.633			
Diabetes mellitus	1.856	0.228–15.096	0.563			
Hypercholesterolemia	2.397	0.327–24.812	0.142			
PAD	1.496	0.484–11.671	0.401			
Perioperative:						
Number of grafts (2)	1.478	0.961–1.029	0.743			
Number of grafts (3)	1.579	0.309–8.078	0.583			
Arterial revascularization	0.91	0.567–1.245	0.592			
Troponin max	1.062	0.998–1.158	0.092			
Postoperative:						
Creatinine	0.994	0.970–1.022	0.726			
Uric acid	0.889	0.616–1.282	0.528			
Air pollution exposure:						
$PM_{2.5}$	1.311	0.588–2.923	0.509	1.518	1.050–2.195	0.026
PM_{10}	1.322	0.547–3.193	0.535			
NO_2	0.644	0.306–1.355	0.247			

Abbreviations: BMI—body mass index, HR—hazard ratio, NO2—nitric dioxide, $PM_{2.5}$—air pollution particle matter 2.5 µm or less, PAD—peripheral artery disease, PM_{10}—air pollution particle matter 10 µm or less.

4. Discussion

Our analysis points out the significance of non-traditional mortality risk factors such as air pollution alongside dyslipidemia in coronary disease patients who underwent surgical revascularization. Eugene Braunwald has already presented the influence of environmental factors, including ambient pollution, on increased mortality risk [18].

We confirmed the prognostic value of dyslipidemia on patients' survival following coronary artery revascularization. According to epidemiological studies, lipid-lowering therapy may decrease mortality risk in the current population, as coronary heart disease is the single leading cause of over 40% of CVD deaths [19]. Atherosclerosis is an age-related disorder representing the complex mechanisms leading to lipid-rich lesion formation in the circulatory system. The intricate balance between endothelium-derived relaxing factors, such as nitric oxide and prostacyclins, and contracting factors, such as superoxide anion and endothelin-1, is disturbed in atherosclerotic lesion formation, especially in dyslipidemic patients [20]. The impaired endothelial hemostasis is a critical contributor to aging and chronic cardiometabolic disorders. The mechanism of plaque development relies on inflammatory activation and involves various types of cells, including macrophages, endothelial, vascular smooth muscle cells, and endothelial progenitor cells that are induced. Recent studies highlight another process that may play a significant role in the mentioned process and that is stimulated by dyslipidemia, named cellular senescence [21]. Prasad, in his review [22], pointed out the significance of modifiable risk factor controls, like arterial hypertension, dyslipidemia, diabetes mellitus, hypertension, obesity, and chronic renal disease for primary, secondary, and even tertiary preventive care. The low-density lipoprotein concentration is considered a primary target in cardiovascular patients [23]. Our previous analysis revealed the protective role of LDL lowering in perioperative myocardial injury in coronary revascularization [24]. The study by Lim et al. presented the association between exposure to elevated LDL and non-HDL levels and increased postoperative mortality [25]. Our analysis highlights the significance of dyslipidemia's presence, despite statin therapy, on 5-year survival in surgically treated patients with multivessel coronary disease.

The exploration of the possible role of air pollution in long-term survival, especially in patients presenting with decreased ejection fraction, is the novelty of our analysis. The environmental factors may be prognostic factors of worse outcomes in certain groups of patients following surgical coronary revascularization. The decreased ejection fraction following the surgical revascularization signifies the heart failure-related inflammatory activation. Regardless of the underlying etiology, heart dysfunction induces cytokines and chemokines that modulate the phenotype and function of all myocardial cells, inflammatory activation in macrophages, and microvascular dysfunction [26]. Systemic inflammatory markers, presented as possible late mortality risk predictors [27] related to left ventricular dysfunction, were reported to decrease in coordination with myocardial improvement [28]. In the CANTOS trial, the use of anti-inflammatory therapies, following lipid-lowering strategies, led to significantly lower MACE risks [29].

Air pollutants induce inflammatory activation [30]. Fine particulate matter below 2.5 μm in diameter ($PM_{2.5}$) mainly arises from fossil fuel combustion during power generation, transportation, and industrial processes and has been identified as the main hazardous constituent [31]. $PM_{2.5}$ can cross the alveolar–capillary barrier, reach other body organs, and activate tissue-resident immune cells, inducing oxidative stress, triggering inflammatory reactions, and stimulating the autonomic nervous system. In experimental studies, the properties of $PM_{2.5}$ in vascular cell penetration and its direct toxic effects were investigated [32]. $PM_{2.5}$ can alter mitochondrial DNA and gene expression at the cellular level, resulting in dysfunction that may lead to cell death [33]. The relationship between ambient $PM_{2.5}$ and increased serum cardiac biomarkers and inflammatory and oxidate stress indices is postulated [34,35]. Chronic exposure to $PM_{2.5}$ is currently regarded as a subclinical marker of atherosclerosis and CV-related increased mortality [36]. This is the main novelty of our analysis, namely, pointing out the significance of environmental factors influencing predisposed patients in whom the inflammatory processes have already been activated. Our results bring a new perspective to ambient pollution exposure in the cardiovascular population, suggesting that the presented effect can be more pronounced in predisposed patients.

Epidemiological studies have already presented the association between $PM_{2.5}$ exposure and increased mortality risk [37]. The unique characteristic of our analysis is the personalized approach. The exposure to ambient air pollutants was separately calculated for each patient, indicating its influence on human organisms. We focused on patient-calculated chronic exposure to ambient pollution, suggesting its role in overall mortality. However, previous studies highlighted the significance of acute and chronic $PM_{2.5}$ changes in increased mortality risk [38].

Study limitation: The study was a single-center analysis performed on patients presenting with chronic coronary syndrome who were diagnosed with multivessel coronary disease. However, all patients underwent off-pump surgical revascularization in a high-volume center well experienced in the mentioned technique. The second limitation is the fact that study results are based on all-cause mortality results.

5. Conclusions

The traditional risk factors, such as arterial hypertension, play a pivotal role in the 5-year mortality risk following surgical revascularization. Chronic exposure to ambient air pollutants such as $PM_{2.5}$ may be regarded as an additional risk factor in patients after surgical revascularization with left ventricular dysfunction.

Author Contributions: Conceptualization, T.U. and K.S.; methodology, T.U.; software, K.S.; validation, K.S., A.O.-W. and A.P.-K.; formal analysis, T.U.; investigation, J.P.; resources, T.U.; data curation, J.P.; writing—original draft preparation, T.U.; writing—review and editing, A.O.-W., K.J.F., B.K., Z.K.,

A.P.-K., A.T. and M.J.; visualization, K.S.; supervision, M.J.; project administration, T.U. All authors have read and agreed to the published version of the manuscript.

Funding: This research received no external funding.

Institutional Review Board Statement: The study was conducted in accordance with the Declaration of Helsinki and approved by the Poznan University of Medical Sciences Ethics Committee (protocol code 55/20 from 16 January 2020).

Informed Consent Statement: Informed consent was obtained from all subjects involved in the study.

Data Availability Statement: Data supporting the reported results can be obtained by contacting the e-mail address of the correspondence author after presenting the justifiable reasons. Data is not available as a supplemental material due to privacy restrictions.

Conflicts of Interest: The authors declare no conflicts of interest.

References

1. Rajagopalan, S.; Al-Kindi, S.G.; Brook, R.D. Air Pollution and Cardiovascular Disease: JACC State-of-the-Art Review. *J. Am. Coll. Cardiol.* **2018**, *72*, 2054–2070. [CrossRef]
2. Liu, J.; Varghese, B.M.; Hansen, A.; Zhang, Y.; Driscoll, T.; Morgan, G.; Dear, K.; Gourley, M.; Capon, A.; Bi, P. Heat exposure and cardiovascular health outcomes: A systematic review and meta-analysis. *Lancet Planet Health* **2022**, *6*, e484–e495. [CrossRef]
3. Urbanowicz, T.; Skotak, K.; Olasińska-Wiśniewska, A.; Filipiak, K.J.; Bratkowski, J.; Wyrwa, M.; Sikora, J.; Tyburski, P.; Krasińska, B.; Krasiński, Z.; et al. Long-Term Exposure to PM10 Air Pollution Exaggerates Progression of Coronary Artery Disease. *Atmosphere* **2024**, *15*, 216. [CrossRef]
4. Urbanowicz, T.K.; Skotak, K.; Lesiak, M.; Olasińska-Wiśniewska, A.; Filipiak, K.J.; Bratkowski, J.; Szczepański, K.; Grodecki, K.; Tykarski, A.; Jemielity, M. Coronary artery culprit lesions progression and ambient temperature exposure—Personalised analysis. *Postępy Kardiol. Interwencyjnej* **2024**, *20*, 139–147. [CrossRef]
5. Bharmal, M.; Kern, M.J.; Kumar, G.; Seto, A.H. Physiologic Lesion Assessment to Optimize Multivessel Disease. *Curr. Cardiol. Rep.* **2022**, *24*, 541–550. [CrossRef]
6. Granger, C.B.; Krychtiuk, K.A.; Gersh, B.J. Personalizing Choice of CABG vs. PCI for Multivessel Disease: Predictive Model Falls Short. *J. Am. Coll. Cardiol.* **2022**, *79*, 1474–1476. [CrossRef] [PubMed]
7. Formica, F.; Gallingani, A.; Tuttolomondo, D.; Hernandez-Vaquero, D.; Singh, G.; Pattuzzi, C.; Maestri, F.; Niccoli, G.; Ceccato, E.; Lorusso, R.; et al. Long-Term Outcomes Comparison between Surgical and Percutaneous Coronary Revascularization in Patients with Multivessel Coronary Disease or Left Main Disease: A Systematic Review and Study Level Meta-Analysis of Randomized Trials. *Curr. Probl. Cardiol.* **2023**, *48*, 101699. [CrossRef] [PubMed]
8. Quin, J.A.; Wagner, T.H.; Hattler, B.; Carr, B.M.; Collins, J.; Almassi, G.H.; Grover, F.L.; Shroyer, A.L. Ten-Year Outcomes of Off-Pump vs. *On-Pump Coronary Artery Bypass Grafting in the Department of Veterans Affairs: A Randomized Clinical Trial. JAMA Surg.* **2022**, *157*, 303–310.
9. Dominici, C.; Salsano, A.; Nenna, A.; Spadaccio, C.; Mariscalco, G.; Santini, F.; Chello, M. On-pump beating-heart coronary artery bypass grafting in high-risk patients: A systematic review and meta-analysis. *J. Card. Surg.* **2020**, *35*, 1958–1978. [CrossRef] [PubMed]
10. Farina, P.; Gaudino, M.; Angelini, G.D. Off-pump coronary artery bypass surgery: The long and winding road. *Int. J. Cardiol.* **2019**, *279*, 51–55. [CrossRef] [PubMed]
11. Aksut, B.; Starling, R.; Kapadia, S. Stable coronary artery disease and left ventricular dysfunction: The role of revascularization. *Catheter. Cardiovasc. Interv.* **2017**, *90*, 777–783. [CrossRef] [PubMed]
12. Kosmala, W.; Marwick, T.H. Asymptomatic Left Ventricular Diastolic Dysfunction: Predicting Progression to Symptomatic Heart Failure. *JACC Cardiovasc. Imaging* **2020**, *13*, 215–227. [CrossRef] [PubMed]
13. Zuo, B.; Fan, X.; Xu, D.; Zhao, L.; Zhang, B.; Li, X. Deciphering the mitochondria-inflammation axis: Insights and therapeutic strategies for heart failure. *Int. Immunopharmacol.* **2024**, *139*, 112697. [CrossRef] [PubMed]
14. Lanas, F.; Saavedra, N.; Saavedra, K.; Hevia, M.; Seron, P.; Salazar, L.A. Effect of intermediate-term firewood smoke air pollution on cardiometabolic risk factors and inflammatory markers. *Front. Cardiovasc. Med.* **2023**, *10*, 1252542. [CrossRef] [PubMed]
15. Urbanowicz, T.; Skotak, K.; Filipiak, K.J.; Olasińska-Wiśniewska, A.; Szczepański, K.; Wyrwa, M.; Sikora, J.; Tykarski, A.; Jemielity, M. Long-Term Exposure of Nitrogen Oxides Air Pollution (NO_2) Impact for Coronary Artery Lesion Progression-Pilot Study. *J. Pers. Med.* **2023**, *13*, 1376. [CrossRef]
16. Available online: https://www.kobize.pl/en/article/national-database-on-greenhouse-gases-and-other-substances-emissions/id/1232/general-information (accessed on 27 March 2024).
17. European Air Quality, Copernicus, Atmosphere Monitoring Service. Available online: https://www.regional-evaluation.atmosphere.copernicus.eu/ (accessed on 27 March 2024).
18. Braunwald, E. Air pollution: Challenges and opportunities for cardiology. *Eur. Heart J.* **2023**, *44*, 1679–1681. [CrossRef]

19. US Preventive Services Task Force; Mangione, C.M.; Barry, M.J.; Nicholson, W.K.; Cabana, M.; Chelmow, D.; Coker, T.R.; Davis, E.M.; Donahue, K.E.; Jaén, C.R.; et al. Statin Use for the Primary Prevention of Cardiovascular Disease in Adults: US Preventive Services Task Force Recommendation Statement. *JAMA* **2022**, *328*, 746–753. [CrossRef]
20. Wang, L.; Cheng, C.K.; Yi, M.; Lui, K.O.; Huang, Y. Targeting endothelial dysfunction and inflammation. *J. Mol. Cell Cardiol.* **2022**, *168*, 58–67. [CrossRef]
21. Xiang, Q.; Tian, F.; Xu, J.; Du, X.; Zhang, S.; Liu, L. New insight into dyslipidemia-induced cellular senescence in atherosclerosis. *Biol. Rev. Camb. Philos Soc.* **2022**, *97*, 1844–1867. [CrossRef]
22. Prasad, K. Current Status of Primary, Secondary, and Tertiary Prevention of Coronary Artery Disease. *Int. J. Angiol.* **2021**, *30*, 177–186. [CrossRef]
23. Writing Committee; Lloyd-Jones, D.M.; Morris, P.B.; Ballantyne, C.M.; Birtcher, K.K.; Covington, A.M.; DePalma, S.M.; Minissian, M.B.; Orringer, C.E.; Smith, S.C., Jr.; et al. 2022 ACC Expert Consensus Decision Pathway on the Role of Nonstatin Therapies for LDL-Cholesterol Lowering in the Management of Atherosclerotic Cardiovascular Disease Risk: A Report of the American College of Cardiology Solution Set Oversight Committee. *J. Am. Coll. Cardiol.* **2022**, *80*, 1366–1418.
24. Urbanowicz, T.K.; Olasińska-Wiśniewska, A.; Michalak, M.; Gąsecka, A.; Rodzki, M.; Perek, B.; Jemielity, M. Cardioprotective Effect of Low Level of LDL Cholesterol on Perioperative Myocardial Injury in Off-Pump Coronary Artery Bypass Grafting. *Medicina* **2021**, *57*, 875. [CrossRef]
25. Lim, K.; Wong, C.H.M.; Lee, A.L.Y.; Fujikawa, T.; Wong, R.H.L. Influence of cholesterol level on long-term survival and cardiac events after surgical coronary revascularization. *JTCVS Open* **2022**, *10*, 195–203. [CrossRef]
26. Hanna, A.; Frangogiannis, N.G. Inflammatory Cytokines and Chemokines as Therapeutic Targets in Heart Failure. *Cardiovasc. Drugs Ther.* **2020**, *34*, 849–863. [CrossRef]
27. Urbanowicz, T.; Michalak, M.; Al-Imam, A.; Olasińska-Wiśniewska, A.; Rodzki, M.; Witkowska, A.; Haneya, A.; Buczkowski, P.; Perek, B.; Jemielity, M. The Significance of Systemic Immune-Inflammatory Index for Mortality Prediction in Diabetic Patients Treated with Off-Pump Coronary Artery Bypass Surgery. *Diagnostics* **2022**, *12*, 634. [CrossRef]
28. Abu Khadija, H.; Gandelman, G.; Ayyad, O.; Poles, L.; Jonas, M.; Paz, O.; Goland, S.; Shimoni, S.; Meledin, V.; George, J.; et al. Comparative Analysis of the Kinetic Behavior of Systemic Inflammatory Markers in Patients with Depressed versus Preserved Left Ventricular Function Undergoing Transcatheter Aortic Valve Implantation. *J. Clin. Med.* **2021**, *10*, 4148. [CrossRef]
29. Ridker, P.M.; Everett, B.M.; Thuren, T.; MacFadyen, J.G.; Chang, W.H.; Ballantyne, C.; Fonseca, F.; Nicolau, J.; Koenig, W.; Anker, S.D.; et al. Antiinflammatory Therapy with Canakinumab for Atherosclerotic Disease. *N. Engl. J. Med.* **2017**, *377*, 1119–1131. [CrossRef]
30. Goossens, J.; Jonckheere, A.C.; Seys, S.F.; Dilissen, E.; Decaesteker, T.; Goossens, C.; Peers, K.; Vanbelle, V.; Stappers, J.; Aertgeerts, S.; et al. Activation of epithelial and inflammatory pathways in adolescent elite athletes exposed to intense exercise and air pollution. *Thorax* **2023**, *78*, 775–783. [CrossRef]
31. Marchini, T. Redox and inflammatory mechanisms linking air pollution particulate matter with cardiometabolic derangements. *Free Radic. Biol. Med.* **2023**, *209*, 320–341. [CrossRef]
32. Su, R.; Jin, X.; Li, H.; Huang, L.; Li, Z. The mechanisms of $PM_{2.5}$ and its main components penetrate into HUVEC cells and effects on cell organelles. *Chemosphere* **2020**, *241*, 125127. [CrossRef]
33. Xu, Z.; Xu, X.; Zhong, M.; Hotchkiss, I.P.; Lewandowski, R.P.; Wagner, J.G.; Bramble, L.A.; Yang, Y.; Wang, A.; Harkema, J.R.; et al. Ambient particulate air pollution induces oxidative stress and alterations of mitochondria and gene expression in brown and white adipose tissues. *Part. Fibre Toxicol.* **2011**, *8*, 20–34. [CrossRef]
34. Vieira, J.L.; Guimaraes, G.V.; de Andre, P.A.; Cruz, F.D.; Saldiva, P.H.; Bocchi, E.A. Respiratory Filter Reduces the Cardiovascular Effects Associated with Diesel Exhaust Exposure: A Randomized, Prospective, Double-Blind, Controlled Study of Heart Failure: The FILTER-HF Trial. *JACC Heart Fail.* **2016**, *4*, 55–64. [CrossRef]
35. Eze, U.U.; Eke, I.G.; Anakwue, R.C.; Oguejiofor, C.F.; Onyejekwe, O.B.; Udeani, I.J.; Onunze, C.J.; Obed, U.J.; Eze, A.A.; Anaga, A.O.; et al. Effects of Controlled Generator Fume Emissions on the Levels of Troponin I, C-Reactive Protein and Oxidative Stress Markers in Dogs: Exploring Air Pollution-Induced Cardiovascular Disease in a Low-Resource Country. *Cardiovasc. Toxicol.* **2021**, *21*, 1019–1032. [CrossRef]
36. Chaulin, A.M.; Sergeev, A.K. The Role of Fine Particles (PM 2.5) in the Genesis of Atherosclerosis and Myocardial Damage: Emphasis on Clinical and Epidemiological Data, and Pathophysiological Mechanisms. *Cardiol. Res.* **2022**, *13*, 268–282. [CrossRef]
37. Liu, Y.; Yan, M. Trends in all causes and cause specific mortality attributable to ambient particulate matter pollution in China from 1990 to 2019: A secondary data analysis study. *PLoS ONE* **2023**, *18*, e0291262. [CrossRef]
38. Krittanawong, C.; Qadeer, Y.K.; Hayes, R.B.; Wang, Z.; Thurston, G.D.; Virani, S.; Lavie, C.J. $PM_{2.5}$ and cardiovascular diseases: State-of-the-Art review. *Int. J. Cardiol. Cardiovasc. Risk Prev.* **2023**, *19*, 200217. [CrossRef]

toxics

MDPI

Article

$PM_{2.5}$ Exposure Induces Glomerular Hyperfiltration in Mice in a Gender-Dependent Manner

Hao Wang, Li Ma, Yuqiong Guo, Lingyu Ren, Guangke Li and Nan Sang *

Shanxi Key Laboratory of Coal-Based Emerging Pollutant Identification and Risk Control, Research Center of Environment and Health, College of Environment and Resource, Shanxi University, Taiyuan 030006, China; wh1034824679@163.com (H.W.); ml384000330@163.com (L.M.); 18635827695@163.com (Y.G.); renlingyu9619@163.com (L.R.); liguangke@sxu.edu.cn (G.L.)

* Correspondence: sangnan@sxu.edu.cn

Abstract: As one of the most common air pollutants, fine particulate matter ($PM_{2.5}$) increases the risk of diseases in various systems, including the urinary system. In the present study, we exposed male and female C57BL/6J mice to $PM_{2.5}$ for 8 weeks. Examination of renal function indices, including creatinine (CRE), blood urea nitrogen (BUN), uric acid (UA), and urinary microalbumin, indicated that the kidneys of female mice, not male mice, underwent early renal injury, exhibiting glomerular hyperfiltration. Meanwhile, pathological staining showed that the kidneys of female mice exhibited enlarged glomerulus that filled the entire Bowman's capsule in the female mice. Afterward, we explored the potential causes and mechanisms of glomerular hyperfiltration. Variations in mRNA levels of key genes involved in the renin–angiotensin system (RAS) and kallikrein–kinin system (KKS) demonstrated that $PM_{2.5}$ led to elevated glomerular capillary hydrostatic pressure in female mice by disturbing the balance between the RAS and KKS, which in turn increased the glomerular filtration rate (GFR). In addition, we found that $PM_{2.5}$ increased blood glucose levels in the females, which enhanced tubular reabsorption of glucose, attenuated macular dense sensory signaling, induced renal hypoxia, and affected adenosine triphosphate (ATP) synthesis, thus attenuating tubuloglomerular feedback (TGF)-induced afferent arteriolar constriction and leading to glomerular hyperfiltration. In conclusion, this study indicated that $PM_{2.5}$ induced glomerular hyperfiltration in female mice by affecting RAS/KKS imbalances, as well as the regulation of TGF; innovatively unveiled the association between $PM_{2.5}$ subchronic exposure and early kidney injury and its gender dependence; enriched the toxicological evidence of $PM_{2.5}$ and confirmed the importance of reducing ambient $PM_{2.5}$ concentrations.

Keywords: $PM_{2.5}$; renal hyperfiltration; renin–angiotensin system; kallikrein–kinin system; tubular reabsorption; tubuloglomerular feedback

1. Introduction

Ambient fine particulate matter ($PM_{2.5}$)—characterized by a small particle size (all abbreviations in Table 1); a large relative surface area; and a complex composition containing heavy metals, polycyclic aromatic hydrocarbons (PAHs), carbonaceous particles (CP), and other organic compounds— is a leading risk factor in global health, and the health problems it poses have aroused widespread public concern [1]. While some countries, such as China, have seen significant reductions in $PM_{2.5}$ levels in the past few years, very few countries and regions meet the World Health Organization's Air Quality Guidelines for $PM_{2.5}$ [2]. $PM_{2.5}$ can enter the lungs via the respiratory tract and further enter the bloodstream, leading to various adverse health effects. Epidemiological studies indicate that $PM_{2.5}$ exposure can increase global deaths and disability-adjusted life years (DALYs) [3], as well as the prevalence of anemia, acute respiratory infections, and diseases of other systems [4]. Toxicological studies have suggested that $PM_{2.5}$ not only causes respiratory, cardiovascular, and neurological diseases but also accumulates in distal organs, such as the liver and kidneys [5,6]. In recent years, kidney disease has become a hidden epidemic worldwide. Studies have demonstrated that air pollution, including $PM_{2.5}$, contributes to decreased kidney function and accelerates the development of renal diseases [7–9]. On the one hand, $PM_{2.5}$ exposure causes renal impairment by directly inducing oxidative stress, inflammation, cytotoxicity, and angiotensin mediators [2,10,11]. Inflammation is one of the most common mechanisms by which $PM_{2.5}$ produces nephrotoxicity. For example, $PM_{2.5}$ can cause kidney injury through NLRP3-mediated inflammatory activation of macrophages with the activation of the IL-6/STAT3 pathway [12,13]. In addition, $PM_{2.5}$ induces abnormal renal sodium excretion mediated by renal D1 receptors [14]. On the other hand, $PM_{2.5}$ can also indirectly aggravate kidney damage along with the increasing prevalence of obesity, diabetes, hypertension, and genetic factors [15,16]. For example, blood glucose abnormalities can cause changes in the Rho/Rock signaling pathway and the Notch3-mediated mTOR signaling pathway, resulting in kidney injury [17,18]. Currently, studies on the nephrotoxicity of $PM_{2.5}$ mainly focus on acute and long-term exposure, and studies on subacute and subchronic exposure are lacking. Furthermore, $PM_{2.5}$ exhibits strong seasonality and geography. As a typical coal-fired city in northern China, Taiyuan often experiences hazy weather conditions during the winter heating period; it is of great interest to explore the effects of airborne $PM_{2.5}$ in this region on renal function [19]. Furthermore, gender difference is an important factor in disease risk assessment, but few studies have reported on the gender differences in the effects of $PM_{2.5}$ on renal injury in adult mice.

Table 1. The list of abbreviations.

Full Name	Abbreviations
fine particulate matter	$PM_{2.5}$
polycyclic aromatic hydrocarbons	PAHs
carbonaceous particles	CP
disability-adjusted life years	DALYs
end-stage renal disease	ESRD
glomerular filtration rate	GFR
creatinine	CRE
blood urea nitrogen	BUN
and uric acid	UA
Estimated glomerular filtration rate	e-GFR
adenosine triphosphate	ATP
hematoxylin and eosin	H&E
Enzyme-Linked Immunosorbent Assay	ELISA
angiotensin II	Ang II
mean ± standard error	SEM
renin–angiotensin system	RAS
kallikrein–kinin system	KKS
angiotensin I	Ang I
angiotensin-converting enzyme	*Ace*
angiotensin II type 1 receptor	*At1r*
Human Kidney-2	HK-2
kallikrein 1	*Klk-1*
bradykinin 1 receptor	*B1r*
bradykinin 2 receptor	*B2r*
interleukin 6	*Il-6*
tumor necrosis factor-α	*Tnf-α*
sodium-dependent glucose transporters	*Sglts*
glucose transporters	*Gluts*
serum- and glucocorticoid-inducible kinase 1	*Sgk-1*
hepatocyte nuclear factor -1α	*Hnf-1α*
tubuloglomerular feedback	TGF
A1 adenosine receptor	*A1ar*
Hypoxia-inducible factor 1α	*Hif-1α*

The kidney is an important urinary organ with endocrine functions, responsible for filtering blood plasma, excreting metabolic waste, reabsorbing nutrients, and regulating blood pressure to ensure a stable internal environment and normal metabolism [20]. The functional unit of the kidney is the nephron, composed of the renal corpuscle and tubules. The renal corpuscle consists of the Bowman's capsule and glomerulus, which is formed by capillaries branching off from afferent arterioles, and the branches of each capillary eventually converge to form the efferent arteriole. The tubule consists of the proximal tubule, the loops of Henle, and the distal tubule [21]. Blood enters the kidney via the renal artery and then passes through the afferent arterioles to the glomerulus. Driven by the effective filtration pressure, all components of the blood, except for macromolecules such as proteins and blood cells, travel through the glomerular filtration membrane to enter the Bowman's capsule and are discharged into the tubules (the proximal tubule, loop of Henle, and distal tubule). After reabsorption, urine is formed (Figure 1) [22]. Kidney injury is often accompanied by changes in the glomerular filtration rate (GFR) as well as alterations in tubular reabsorption function [23,24]. Numerous studies have shown that $PM_{2.5}$ affects the body's metabolism, causing the development of hyperglycemia, hyperlipidemia, and hypertension, all of which influence the kidneys as the disease progresses.

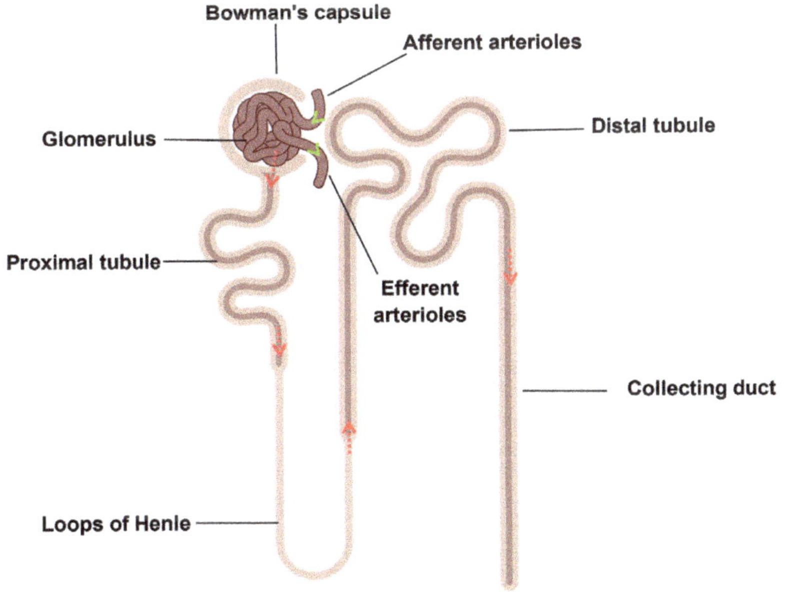

Figure 1. The composition and structure of the renal nephron (Red arrow represents the process of urine formation and green arrow represents the direction of blood flow. The elements were derived from Figdraw).

In this study, we exposed male and female C57BL/6J mice to $PM_{2.5}$ for 8 weeks to investigate its nephrotoxicity in different genders and the underlying mechanisms, thus enriching the toxicological evidence on $PM_{2.5}$ and aiding in the adoption of relevant regulations to reduce $PM_{2.5}$ pollution and improve human health.

2. Materials and Methods

2.1. Collection and Physicochemical Properties of $PM_{2.5}$

$PM_{2.5}$ was collected in Taiyuan, Shanxi province, China, using quartz filters (Φ90 mm, Munktell, Sweden) and a KC-1000 middle-volume air sampler (Laoshan Electronic Instrument, Qingdao, China) at a flow rate of 100 L/min (22 h/day) from November

2018 to March 2019. The extraction, storage, and physicochemical characterization of $PM_{2.5}$, as well as the preparation of $PM_{2.5}$ suspensions, were described in our previous studies [25–27]. There were 15 polycyclic aromatic hydrocarbons and 31 elements in $PM_{2.5}$, and their concentrations are listed in Table S1.

2.2. Animals and Exposure Experiments

Eight-week-old male and female C57BL/6J mice were provided by Beijing Vital River Laboratory Animal Technology Co., Ltd. (Beijing, China). After one week of acclimation, male and female mice were randomly divided into the $PM_{2.5}$-exposed and vehicle groups, 15 mice per group. Mice in the $PM_{2.5}$-exposed group were administrated $PM_{2.5}$ (3 mg/kg bw.) via nasal drip once every other day for 8 weeks, while mice in the vehicle control group were administered with an equal dose of the vehicle solution (blank quartz filters extraction). Urine was collected using metabolic cages in the eighth week of exposure. After exposure, blood was collected, the mice were sacrificed, and the kidneys were also collected and weighed, three of which from two groups were fixed using tissue fixation solution (n = 3).

2.3. Kidney Function Tests

Serum levels of creatinine (CRE), blood urea nitrogen (BUN), and uric acid (UA), as well as the levels of CRE and BUN in the urine, were determined using commercial kits (Nanjing Jiancheng Bioengineering Institute, Nanjing, Jiangsu, China). The estimated glomerular filtration rate (e-GFR) was calculated using the Cockcroft–Gault formula [28,29].

$$\mathrm{e} - GFR = \frac{(140 - \mathrm{age}) \times \mathrm{weight} \times 0.85(\mathrm{if\ female})}{72 \times \mathrm{serum\ creatinine}}$$

2.4. Measurements of ATP Content

Adenosine triphosphate (ATP) in the kidneys was determined using commercial kits (Beyotime Biotechnology, Shanghai, China).

2.5. Histological Analyses

Kidneys were fixed in 4% paraformaldehyde and then embedded in paraffin to prepare longitudinal kidney sections, which were stained with hematoxylin and eosin (H&E). The sections were observed using a microscope (OLYMPUS, Tokyo, Japan). Glomerulus analysis was performed to estimate the areas of the Bowman's capsule and glomerulus using the freehand selection tool in ImageJ software. Thirty glomerular cross-sectional areas were measured in each group. The Bowman's space was determined by subtracting the glomeruli area from the Bowman's capsule area.

2.6. Enzyme-Linked Immunosorbent Assay (ELISA)

The levels of microalbumin in the urine and the levels of angiotensin II (Ang II) in the serum were measured using commercial ELISA kits obtained from Animalunion Biotechnology (Shanghai, China).

2.7. Quantitative RT-PCR

The extraction, reverse transcription, and storage of total RNA from the kidneys of female mice were conducted as described previously [30]. The expression of genes was determined on a qTOWER 2.2 real-time PCR system (Analytic Jena AG, Jena, Germany) using TB Premix Ex Taq II kits (TaKaRa Bio, Shiga, Kyoto, Japan). The primers used are shown in Table 2.

Table 2. Primer sequences of the genes used in quantitative RT-PCR.

Gene	Primer Sequence (5′-3′)
Ace	*F: CTCCGCTCTTGATGCTGTC* *R: TTCTCCTCCGTGATGTTGGT*
At1r	*F: ATGTTTCTTGGTGGCTTGGTT* *R: CAGCAGCGTCTGATGATGAG*
Klk-1	*F: CAATGTGGGGGTATCCTGCTG* *R: GGGTATTCATATTTGACGGGTGT*
B1r	*F: TCCTTCTGCGTTCCGTCAA* *R: TTCAACTCCACCATCCTTACAA*
B2r	*F: AGGTGCTGAGGAACAACGA* *R: AGGAAGGTGCTGATCTGGAA*
Il-6	*F: TGATGGATGCTACCAAACTGGA* *R: TGTGACTCCAGCTTATCTCTTGG*
Tnf-α	*F: CCACGCTCTTCTGTCTACTGA* *R: GTTTGTGAGTGTGAGGGTCTG*
Sgk-1	*F: GGCACAAGGCAGAAGAAGTATT* *R: GGTCTGGAATGAGAAGTGAAGG*
Hnf-1α	*F: GACCTGACCGAGTTGCCTAAT* *R: CCGGCTCTTTCAGAATGGGT*
Sglt1	*F: CTCTTCGTCATCAGCGTCATC* *R: TCCTCCTCCTCCTTAGTCATCT*
Sglt2	*F: TCAGAACCAATAGAGGCACAGT* *R: CGGACAGGTAGAGGCGAATA*
Glut2	*F: GTCACACCAGCATACACAACA* *R: ACTTCGTCCAGCAATGATGAG*
A1ar	*F: ATCCTGGCTCTGCTTGCTATT* *R: GGCTTGTTCCACCTCACTCA*
Hif-1α	*F: ACCTTCATCGGAAACTCCAAAG* *R: CTCTTAGGCTGGGAAAAGTTAGG*
Gapdh	*F: AGAAGGTGGTGAAGCAGGCATC* *R: GATGGACTTCGGGAACGGACAG*
β-Actin	*F: GCTTCTTTGCAGCTCCTTCGT* *R: ATATCGTCATCCATGGCGAAC*

2.8. Data Analysis

Data are expressed as the mean ± standard error (SEM) and were analyzed using GraphPad Prism 8. Normal distribution was confirmed by the Shapiro–Wilk test ($p > 0.05$). Unpaired two-tailed t-tests were used to examine differences between the exposure group and the vehicle group. Differences were considered statistically significant when $p < 0.05$.

3. Results and Discussion

3.1. $PM_{2.5}$ Exposure Causes Early Renal Injury in Female Mice

CRE, BUN, and UA are metabolites excreted mainly through the kidneys and are all important indicators for assessing renal function and glomerular filtration [31,32]. Variation in GFR is a well-known phenomenon and the natural evolution of the glomerular damage observed during chronic degenerative diseases or after exposure to nephrotoxic substances. Similarly, changes in renal function and GFR induced by $PM_{2.5}$ exposure vary among existing studies [11,33–35]. In our study, the levels of serum CRE ($p = 0.0429$), BUN ($p = 0.0002$), and UA ($p = 0.0052$) were significantly lower in $PM_{2.5}$-exposed female mice than they were in the vehicle group, whereas the levels of CRE ($p = 0.0080$) and BUN ($p = 0.0161$) in the urine were significantly elevated (Figure 2A–E), which suggests increased glomerular filtration. A significant increase in glomerular filtration levels was calculated in female mice but not in male mice ($p = 0.0290$) (Figure 2F). This indicates that female mice were more susceptible to kidney damage caused by subchronic exposure to $PM_{2.5}$ than males.

Increased GFR implied that the kidney might be in a compensatory state, accompanied by increased glomerular capillary pressure, damaged endothelial cells, and increased capillary permeability, subsequently causing increased glomerular volume and proximal tubular load. Mehmet Kanbay et al. found that elevated GFR occurs in the early stages of kidney injury [36]. Urinary microalbumin is the most sensitive and reliable index for early diagnosis of renal function [37,38]. Importantly, the level of urinary microalbumin increased significantly in female mice exposed to $PM_{2.5}$ (p = 0.0026) (Figure 2G), proving that $PM_{2.5}$ exposure caused early kidney injury in female mice.

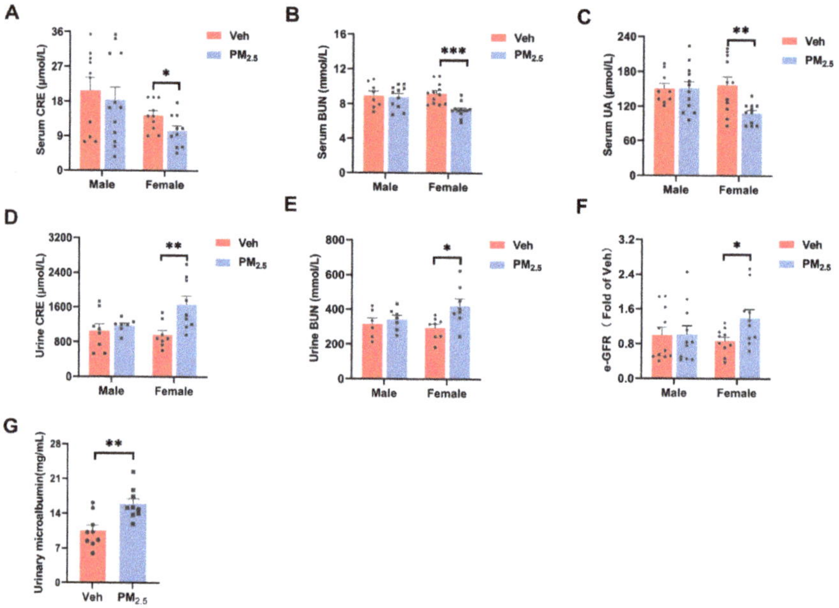

Figure 2. Effects of $PM_{2.5}$ on the renal function in mice. (**A–C**) Serum levels of CRE, BUN, and UA in mice. (**D**,**E**) Urine levels of CRE and BUN in mice. (**F**) Estimated glomerular filtration rate (e-GFR) of kidneys in mice. (**G**) Level of urinary microalbumin in female mice. The values are expressed as the mean ± SEM ($n \geq 6$). * $p < 0.05$, ** $p < 0.01$, *** $p < 0.001$. Veh, vehicle.

3.2. *$PM_{2.5}$ Exposure Alters Renal Pathomorphology in Female Mice*

Function influences structure and vice versa. Following eight-week exposure to $PM_{2.5}$, we found that female mice had a significantly decreased body weight (p = 0.0327), whereas the body weight of male mice did not exhibit any changes (Figure 3A). Furthermore, although both genders of mice showed no obvious alteration in kidney weight, the kidney/body weight ratio (%) of female mice showed a notable upward trend (p = 0.0129) (Figure 3B,C). Therefore, we supposed that the kidneys of female mice underwent compensatory enlargement following early injury. Similarly, Aurora Pérez-Gomez et al. discovered that the kidney activates hypertrophic molecular mechanisms that counteract the loss of renal function in the early stages [39]. Furthermore, early in the onset of diabetes, the kidneys enlarge due to glomerular enlargement [40].

According to previous studies, the enlargement of glomerular volume is one of the reasons for hyperfiltration. Glomerular hypertrophy has been implicated in the pathogenesis of several renal diseases, including diabetes mellitus, obesity-associated nephropathy, and focal segmental glomerulosclerosis [36,40–42]. The histological staining of kidney sections showed that $PM_{2.5}$-exposed female mice exhibited enlarged glomerulus that filled the entire Bowman's capsule, and the renal tubular cells were enlarged and tightly packed, whereas no changes were found in the kidneys of $PM_{2.5}$-exposed male mice (Figure 4A,B). It was statistically verified that the glomerular area was significantly elevated ($p = 0.0431$) and the Bowman's capsule area was unchanged in female mice after $PM_{2.5}$ exposure, resulting in a remarkable decrease in the Bowman's space area ($p < 0.0001$), whereas none of the males were changed (Figure 4C–E). Octavio Gamaliel Aztatzi-Aguilar et al. found that glomerular hypertrophy may be caused by glomerular inflammation, an imbalance of the RAS and KKS, and changes in blood pressure [11]. In addition, elevated blood glucose could also cause microvascular and podocyte damage, which in turn causes glomerular hypertrophy and kidney damage [43,44].

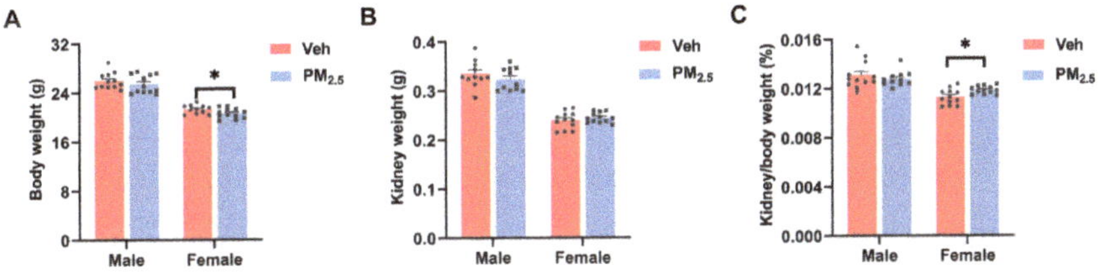

Figure 3. Effects of $PM_{2.5}$ exposure on (**A**) body weight, (**B**) kidney weight, and (**C**) kidney/body weight ratio. The values are expressed as the mean ± SEM ($n = 10$–12). * $p < 0.05$. Veh, vehicle.

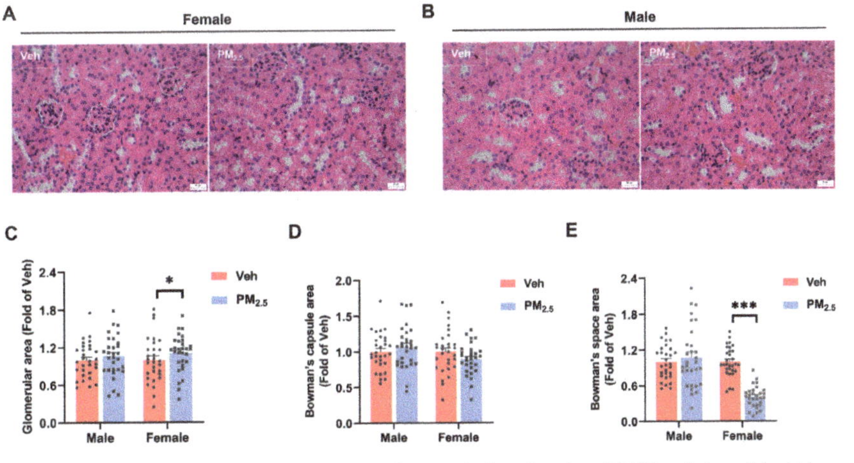

Figure 4. Effects of $PM_{2.5}$ exposure on renal pathomorphology in mice. (**A**) HE staining of the kidneys in female mice (magnification: 400×), and (**B**) HE staining of the kidneys in male mice (magnification: 400×). (**C**) Glomerular area. (**D**) Bowman's capsule area. (**E**) Bowman's space area. The values are expressed as the mean ± SEM ($n = 30$). * $p < 0.05$, *** $p < 0.001$. Veh, vehicle.

3.3. *$PM_{2.5}$ Exposure Causes Early Kidney Damage by Inducing the Imbalance of the Renin–Angiotensin System (RAS) and the Kallikrein–Kinin System (KKS)*

In addition to increased glomerular volume, an increase in glomerular capillary pressure can also result in glomerular hyperfiltration. The RAS and KKS play a crucial role in maintaining renal hemodynamics and transport function, as well as sodium and water reabsorption in distal renal units [34,35]. Increased activity and overexpression of relevant genes in the RAS and its imbalance with the KKS are among the most widely associated mechanisms of kidney disease. $PM_{2.5}$ exposure leads to elevated inflammation and altered endocrine signaling in the lung, which in turn trigger an imbalance between the renal RAS and KKS, affects glomerular filtration, and causes kidney damage [10,11,45,46]. In our past studies, we found that $PM_{2.5}$ exposure causes lung inflammation in mice [47]. Vasodilatation of the afferent arterioles and/or vasoconstriction of the efferent arterioles can increase the hydrostatic pressure in the glomerular capillaries, leading to glomerular hyperfiltration [36]. In the RAS, renin acts on plasma angiotensinogen, producing inactive angiotensin I (Ang I). Ang I is hydrolyzed by Ace to active Ang II, which can cause vasoconstriction of small arteries and increase blood pressure. In the KKS, Klk-1 converts kininogen to bradykinin, the latter binds to bradykinin receptors, exerting vasodilation and blood pressure-lowering effects. At the same time, Ace acts on bradykinin to convert it into inactive fragments [45,48]. These two systems are interdependent and function in regulating blood pressure and renal function (Figure 5A) [49–51].

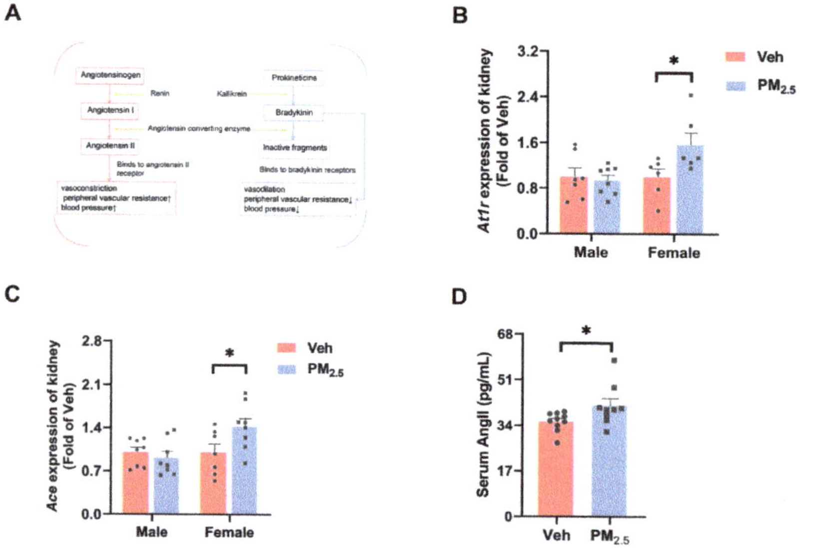

Figure 5. Effects of $PM_{2.5}$ exposure on the RAS in the kidney of mice. (**A**) Interactions of the RAS and KKS. (**B**,**C**) mRNA expression of RAS-related genes. (**D**) Serum levels of angiotensin II (Ang II) in female mice. The values are expressed as the mean ± SEM ($n \geq 6$). * $p < 0.05$. Veh, vehicle.

Octavio Gamaliel Aztatzi-Aguilar et al. found that acute and subchronic exposure to $PM_{2.5}$ induces the activation of the RAS and KKS [52]. However, the gender dependence of the expression of this endocrine signaling for indirect renal effects remains unclear. Consequently, we first determined the mRNA expression of angiotensin-converting enzyme (*Ace*) and angiotensin II type 1 receptor (*At1r*) in the RAS (Figure 5B,C). These genes are engaged in the endocrine pathway and angiotensin production. The results showed that the expression of *At1r* and *Ace* increased by 57.3% ($p = 0.0438$) and 42.5% ($p = 0.0452$), respectively, in $PM_{2.5}$-exposed female mice compared with those in vehicle female mice, whereas no changes were observed in male mice. Consistent with our findings, the expression of Ace and At1r was increased in human kidney-2 (HK-2) cells exposed to $PM_{2.5}$ and the kidneys of acutely exposed male rats [11,53]. Following this observation, we examined Ang II in the serum of female mice and found that elevated expression of Ace did increase Ang II in the serum ($p = 0.0406$) (Figure 5D), which can bind to *At1r* and cause vasoconstriction of the efferent arterioles, thus contributing to glomerular hyperfiltration [54]. On the other hand, Ang II can result in a high GFR by weakening the structural integrity of the slit diaphragm and affecting glomerular permeability [55,56].

Moreover, we examined the mRNA expression of kallikrein 1 (*Klk-1*), bradykinin 1 receptor (*B1r*), and bradykinin 2 receptor (*B2r*) in the KKS (Figure 6A–C), which are important mediators of vasodilation and inflammatory responses. Under pathological conditions, *B1r* expression increases in inflamed tissues [45]. The results demonstrated that the mRNA level of *Klk-1* in female mice was reduced by 37.8% ($p = 0.0294$) after $PM_{2.5}$ exposure, and the mRNA levels of *B1r* and *B2r* were not dramatically altered. In male mice, all of them underwent non-significant changes. At the same time, we examined the mRNA expression of interleukin 6 (*Il-6*) and tumor necrosis factor-α (*Tnf-α*) (Figure S1A,B), which exhibited few alterations in these two genes, suggesting that $PM_{2.5}$ exposure did not cause inflammation in the kidneys. Decreased *Klk-1* expression with increased *Ace* expression results in decreased bradykinin production and increased consumption, which further leads to elevated glomerular capillary blood pressure. Similarly, O. G. Aztatzi-Aguilar et al. found that $PM_{2.5}$ exposure induces early renal injury in rats by inducing an imbalance between the RAS and the KKS [45]. Kallikrein–kinin inhibits apoptosis, inflammation, hypertrophy, and fibrosis but promotes angiogenesis and neuroregeneration in the heart, kidney, brain, and blood vessels. It is worth noting that decreased kallikrein expression can reduce this unique ability of kallikrein–kinin to repair renal tubular injury [43].

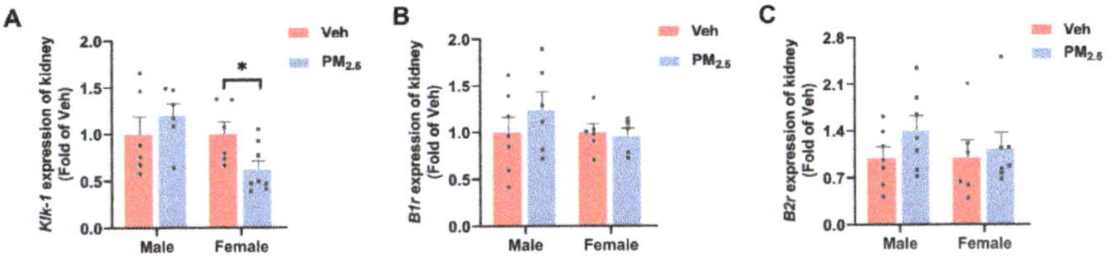

Figure 6. Effects of $PM_{2.5}$ exposure on the KKS and inflammation in the kidneys of female mice. (**A–C**) mRNA expression of *Klk-1*, *B1r*, and *B2r*. The values are expressed as the mean ± SEM ($n \geq 6$). * $p < 0.05$. Veh, vehicle.

In summary, $PM_{2.5}$ exposure may increase the glomerular capillary hydrostatic pressure by causing an imbalance of the RAS and KKS, which in turn leads to mild glomerular damage.

3.4. $PM_{2.5}$ Exposure Causes Early Kidney Damage by Impacting TGF

Tubuloglomerular feedback (TGF) is one of the essential mechanisms in the self-regulation of renal blood flow and GFR, and it is highly dependent on ATP and adenosine. When macula densa cells sense an increase in sodium chloride concentration in the renal tubular fluid, it stimulates the hydrolysis of ATP to adenosine, which is then released extracellularly and acts on the A1 adenosine receptor (*A1ar*) in the afferent arterioles, activating TGF and leading to the constriction of the afferent arterioles and a lower glomerular filtration rate [57,58].

3.4.1. $PM_{2.5}$ Exposure Influences TGF by Enhancing Renal Tubule Reabsorption of Glucose

Epidemiological studies have shown that for each 1 $\mu g/m^3$ increase in $PM_{2.5}$, the odds of impaired fasting blood glucose increase by 10.20% in non-diabetic adolescents [59]. Toxicological studies have demonstrated that $PM_{2.5}$ specifically affects insulin sensitivity and hepatic lipid metabolism in female mice [60]. In our work, there was a significant increase in blood glucose in female mice ($p = 0.0240$) but not in male mice (Figure 7A). Research has indicated that during the initial phases of diabetic nephropathy, there is an increase in the GFR [40]. Elevated blood glucose can increase renal blood flow and intraglomerular pressure through osmotic pressure, which increases the amount of glucose filtered through the glomerulus, thereby increasing glucose load, exposure, and reabsorption in the renal tubules.

The process of glucose reabsorption in the renal tubules is mainly dependent on sodium-dependent glucose transporters (*Sglts*) and glucose transporters (*Gluts*). Under hyperglycemia, serum- and glucocorticoid-inducible kinase 1 (*Sgk-1*) and hepatocyte nuclear factor-1α (*Hnf-1α*) can upregulate the expression of *Sglt1* and *Sglt2*, respectively, thereby increasing glucose reabsorption [61,62]. In our study, we found significantly upregulated expression of *Hnf-1α* ($p = 0.0376$), *Sgk-1* ($p = 0.0414$), *Sglt2* ($p = 0.0167$), and *Glut2* ($p = 0.0368$) in female mice following $PM_{2.5}$ exposure, whereas no significant change was found in the expression of *Sglt1* (Figure 7B–F), but *Sglt2* plays a greater role than *Sglt1* during reabsorption [63]. These results indicated that glucose reabsorption was elevated in the renal tubules of $PM_{2.5}$-exposed female mice. When the glomeruli are exposed to high concentrations of blood glucose, the glucose content in glomerular filtrate increases, which causes increased reabsorption of glucose from the proximal tubule, accompanied by increased reabsorption of sodium chloride in the proximal tubules, leading to a decrease in the concentration of sodium chloride in the distal tubule, as perceived by the macula densa cells; in this case, TGF was attenuated, thus leading to glomerular hyperfiltration [64,65]. SGLT2 inhibitors inhibit sodium and glucose reabsorption, leading to increased sodium in the macula densa, TGF activation, decreased glomerular hyperperfusion, high blood pressure, hyperfiltration, and recovery of renal function [66].

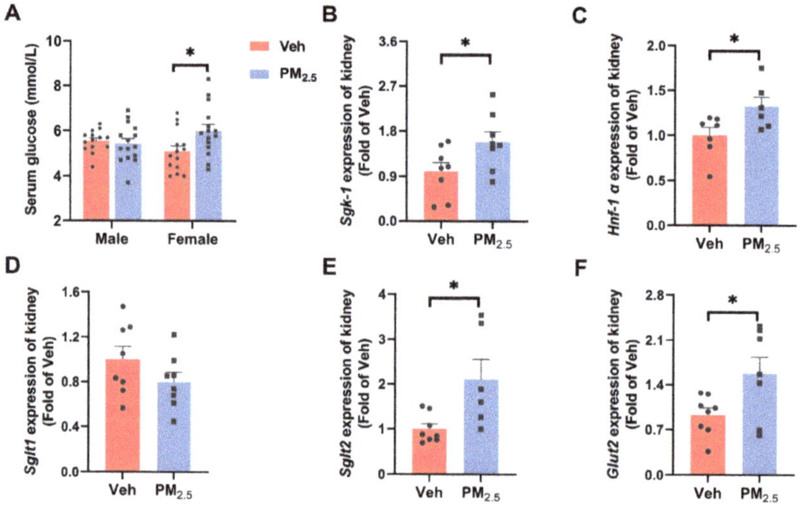

Figure 7. Effects of $PM_{2.5}$ exposure on renal tubular reabsorption of glucose in female mice. (**A**) Blood glucose levels in mice. (**B–F**) mRNA expression of reabsorption-related genes. The values are expressed as the mean ± SEM ($n \geq 6$). * $p < 0.05$. Veh, vehicle.

3.4.2. $PM_{2.5}$ Exposure Influences TGF by Inducing Renal Hypoxia and Decreased ATP Synthesis

As explained above, the concentration of sodium chloride in the macula densa was reduced, leading to an elevation in renin release, which further increased the production of Ang II and enhanced the vasoconstrictor effects [67]. Vasoconstriction, as well as enhanced tubular reabsorption, consumes large amounts of oxygen and ATP, resulting in renal hypoxic/ischemic injury [68]. Alberto Valdés et al. proved that exposure of renal proximal tubular cells to high glucose and hypoxic conditions decreases the synthesis of ATP [69]. Kiefer W Kious et al. indicated that chronic intermittent hypoxia leads to a higher glomerular filtration rate in rats [70]. Hypoxia-inducible factor 1α (*Hif-1α*) is a key mediator that adapts cells to hypoxia [71]. In this study, the mRNA level of *Hif-1α* in the kidneys of female mice was elevated (p = 0.0224) (Figure 8A), indicating that the kidney might be hypoxic. Renal hypoxia can cause mitochondrial dysfunction and affect ATP synthesis. Furthermore, we verified that $PM_{2.5}$ exposure significantly reduced the ATP content in the kidney of female mice (p = 0.0123) (Figure 8B), which could affect TGF and cause glomerular hyperfiltration. Notably, the mRNA levels of renal A1ar increased significantly in female mice after $PM_{2.5}$ exposure (p = 0.0019) (Figure 8C). This may be a compensatory increase in the inhibition of TGF action. Therefore, we concluded that $PM_{2.5}$ could cause mild kidney damage by affecting TGF, mainly because of enhanced renal tubule reabsorption of glucose and renal hypoxia.

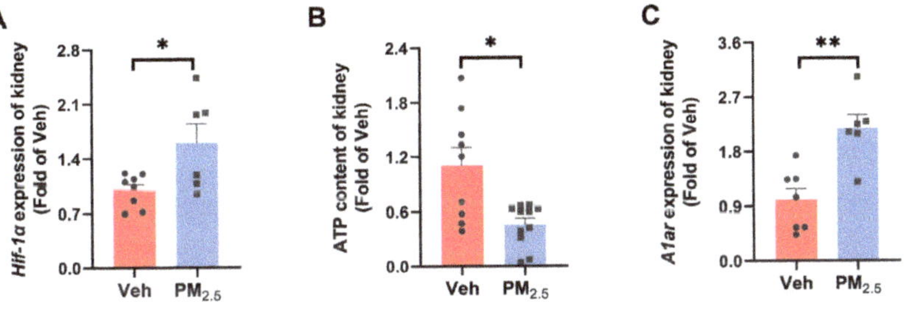

Figure 8. Effects of $PM_{2.5}$ exposure on renal hypoxia and ATP synthesis in female mice. (**A**) mRNA expression of Hif-1α. (**B**) ATP levels. (**C**) mRNA expression of A1ar. The values are expressed as the mean ± SEM ($n \geq 6$). * $p < 0.05$, ** $p < 0.01$. Veh, vehicle.

4. Conclusions

In the current study, we proved that eight weeks of $PM_{2.5}$ exposure induced early renal injury in female mice, manifested as glomerular hyperfiltration. The underlying reason for this was, on the one hand, that $PM_{2.5}$ induced an imbalance of the RAS and KKS in female mice. On the other hand, $PM_{2.5}$ caused elevated blood glucose in female mice, which in turn enhanced the reabsorption of glucose by the renal tubules, affected TGF, and resulted in renal hypoxia and decreased ATP (Figure 9). Our study provides valuable experimental evidence for the nephrotoxicity of $PM_{2.5}$ and elucidates the possible mechanisms underlying the renal effects of subchronic exposure to $PM_{2.5}$. However, as a typical outdoor air pollutant, exposure to $PM_{2.5}$ via oropharyngeal aspiration does not fully and accurately reflect its effects on the kidneys in the real environment. Therefore, it is of interest to explore the renal effects of $PM_{2.5}$ exposure in real environments. Additionally, due to the heterogeneity of $PM_{2.5}$, there is a need for a deeper exploration of the effects of specific components of $PM_{2.5}$ on kidney damage and their contribution to gender differences.

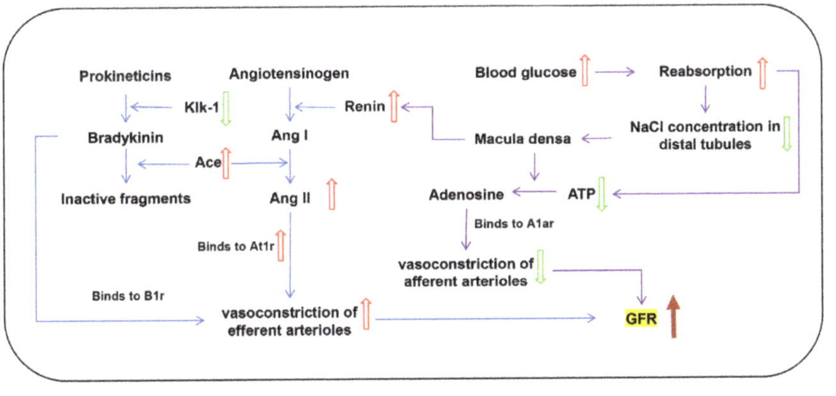

Figure 9. Diagram of the mechanism underlying renal injury in female mice caused by $PM_{2.5}$ exposure. (Red and dark red arrows represent ascending. Green arrows represent descending).

Supplementary Materials: The following are available online at https://www.mdpi.com/article/10.3390/toxics12120878/s1, Figure S1. Effects of $PM_{2.5}$ exposure inflammation in the kidney of mice. (A,B) The mRNA expression of inflammatory factor, Il-6 and Tnf-α. The values are expressed as the mean ± SEM (n ≥ 6). Veh, vehicle, Table S1. The contents of elements and polycyclic aromatic hydrocarbons in $PM_{2.5}$ samples.

Author Contributions: H.W., Conceptualization, Methodology, Validation, and Writing—original draft; L.M., Software and Formal analysis; Y.G., Methodology and Validation; L.R., Software; G.L.,

Investigation; N.S., Conceptualization, Writing—review and editing, and Supervision. All authors have read and agreed to the published version of the manuscript.

Funding: This research was funded by the National Science Foundation of China (No. 22036005), Special Fund for Scientific and Technological Innovation Talent Team of Shanxi Province (No. 202204051002024).

Institutional Review Board Statement: The animal study protocol was approved by the Committee of Scientific Research at Shanxi University (SXULL2020011, 8 April 2020).

Informed Consent Statement: Not applicable.

Data Availability Statement: Data are contained within the article.

Conflicts of Interest: The authors declare no conflicts of interest.

References

1. Yan, R.; Ma, D.; Liu, Y.; Wang, R.; Fan, L.; Yan, Q.; Chen, C.; Wang, W.; Ren, Z.; Ku, T.; et al. Developmental Toxicity of Fine Particulate Matter: Multifaceted Exploration from Epidemiological and Laboratory Perspectives. *Toxics* **2024**, *12*, 274. [CrossRef] [PubMed]
2. Jiang, Y.; Peng, Y.; Yang, X.; Yu, J.; Yu, F.; Yuan, J.; Zha, Y. $PM_{2.5}$ Exposure Aggravates Kidney Damage by Facilitating the Lipid Metabolism Disorder in Diabetic Mice. *PeerJ* **2023**, *11*, e15856. [CrossRef] [PubMed]
3. Sang, S.; Chu, C.; Zhang, T.; Chen, H.; Yang, X. The Global Burden of Disease Attributable to Ambient Fine Particulate Matter in 204 Countries and Territories, 1990–2019: A Systematic Analysis of the Global Burden of Disease Study 2019. Ecotoxicol. *Environ. Saf.* **2022**, *238*, 113588. [CrossRef] [PubMed]
4. Chaudhary, E.; George, F.; Saji, A.; Dey, S.; Ghosh, S.; Thomas, T.; Kurpad, A.V.; Sharma, S.; Singh, N.; Agarwal, S.; et al. Cumulative Effect of $PM_{2.5}$ Components Is Larger than the Effect of $PM_{2.5}$ Mass on Child Health in India. *Nat. Commun.* **2023**, *14*, 6955. [CrossRef] [PubMed]
5. Bandyopadhyay, A. Neurological Disorders from Ambient (Urban) Air Pollution Emphasizing UFPM and $PM_{2.5}$. Curr. *Pollut. Rep.* **2016**, *2*, 203–211. [CrossRef]
6. Yan, R.; Ji, S.; Ku, T.; Sang, N. Cross-Omics Analyses Reveal the Effects of Ambient $PM_{2.5}$ Exposure on Hepatic Metabolism in Female Mice. *Toxics* **2024**, *12*, 587. [CrossRef]
7. Lin, S.-Y.; Ju, S.-W.; Lin, C.L.; Hsu, W.-H.; Lin, C.-C.; Ting, I.-W.; Kao, C.-H. Air Pollutants and Subsequent Risk of Chronic Kidney Disease and End-Stage Renal Disease: A Population-Based Cohort Study. *Environ. Pollut.* **2020**, *261*, 114154. [CrossRef]
8. An, Y.; Liu, Z.-H. Air Pollution and Kidney Diseases: $PM_{2.5}$ as an Emerging Culprit. *Contrib. Nephrol.* **2021**, *199*, 274–284. [CrossRef]
9. Seltenrich, N. $PM_{2.5}$ and Kidney Function: Long-Term Exposures May Lead to Modest Declines. *Environ. Health Perspect.* **2016**, *124*, A168. [CrossRef]
10. Xu, W.; Wang, S.; Jiang, L.; Sun, X.; Wang, N.; Liu, X.; Yao, X.; Qiu, T.; Zhang, C.; Li, J.; et al. The Influence of $PM_{2.5}$ Exposure on Kidney Diseases. *Hum. Exp. Toxicol.* **2022**, *41*, 9603271211069982. [CrossRef]
11. Aztatzi-Aguilar, O.G.; Pardo-Osorio, G.A.; Uribe-Ramírez, M.; Narváez-Morales, J.; De Vizcaya-Ruiz, A.; Barbier, O.C. Acute Kidney Damage by $PM_{2.5}$ Exposure in a Rat Model. *Environ. Toxicol. Pharmacol.* **2021**, *83*, 103587. [CrossRef] [PubMed]
12. Lin, C.-H.; Wan, C.; Liu, W.-S.; Wang, H.-H. $PM_{2.5}$ Induces Early Epithelial Mesenchymal Transition in Human Proximal Tubular Epithelial Cells through Activation of IL-6/STAT3 Pathway. *Int. J. Mol. Sci.* **2021**, *22*, 12734. [CrossRef] [PubMed]
13. Pei, H.; Dai, X.; He, Z.; Tang, Z.; Zhu, Y.; Du, R. $PM_{2.5}$ Exposure Promotes the Progression of Acute Kidney Injury by Activating NLRP3-Mediated Macrophage Inflammatory Response. *Ecotoxicol. Environ. Saf.* **2024**, *278*, 116454. [CrossRef] [PubMed]
14. Lu, X.; Chen, K.; Zeng, J.; Ren, H.; Zeng, C. Abstract 281: Long-Term Exposure of $PM_{2.5}$ Causes Hypertension by Impaired Renal D1 Receptor Mediated Sodium Excretion via Up-Regulation of GRK4 Expression in SD Rats. *Hypertension* **2014**, *64*, A281. [CrossRef]
15. Lash, L.H. Environmental and Genetic Factors Influencing Kidney Toxicity. *Semin. Nephrol.* **2019**, *39*, 132–140. [CrossRef]
16. Kelly, D.M.; Anders, H.-J.; Bello, A.K.; Choukroun, G.; Coppo, R.; Dreyer, G.; Eckardt, K.-U.; Johnson, D.W.; Jha, V.; Harris, D.C.H.; et al. International Society of Nephrology Global Kidney Health Atlas: Structures, Organization, and Services for the Management of Kidney Failure in Western Europe. *Kidney Int. Suppl.* **2021**, *11*, e106–e118. [CrossRef]
17. Harnois, T.; Brishoual, S.; Vincent-Tassin, E.; Paris, I.; Bourmeyster, N.; Hadjadj, S. O46 Les Fluctuations Du Glucose Induisent Une Activation de La Fibrose Rénale Par Des Voies de Signalisation P38-MAP Kinase et Rho/Rock. *Diabetes Metab.* **2012**, *38*, A12. [CrossRef]
18. Cui, Y.; Fang, J.; Guo, H.; Cui, H.; Deng, J.; Yu, S.; Gou, L.; Wang, F.; Ma, X.; Ren, Z.; et al. Notch3-Mediated mTOR Signaling Pathway Is Involved in High Glucose-Induced Autophagy in Bovine Kidney Epithelial Cells. *Molecules* **2022**, *27*, 3121. [CrossRef]
19. Ji, S.; Guo, Y.; Yan, W.; Wei, F.; Ding, J.; Hong, W.; Wu, X.; Ku, T.; Yue, H.; Sang, N. $PM_{2.5}$ Exposure Contributes to Anxiety and Depression-like Behaviors via Phenyl-Containing Compounds Interfering with Dopamine Receptor. *Proc. Natl. Acad. Sci. USA* **2024**, *121*, e2319595121. [CrossRef] [PubMed]

20. Takasato, M.; Er, P.X.; Chiu, H.S.; Maier, B.; Baillie, G.J.; Ferguson, C.; Parton, R.G.; Wolvetang, E.J.; Roost, M.S.; Chuva de Sousa Lopes, S.M.; et al. Kidney Organoids from Human iPS Cells Contain Multiple Lineages and Model Human Nephrogenesis. *Nature* **2015**, *526*, 564–568. [CrossRef]
21. Gupta, N.; Morizane, R. Kidney Development to Kidney Organoids and Back Again. *Semin. Cell Dev. Biol.* **2022**, *127*, 68–76. [CrossRef] [PubMed]
22. Tekguc, M.; Gaal, R.C.V.; Uzel, S.G.M.; Gupta, N.; Riella, L.V.; Lewis, J.A.; Morizane, R. Kidney Organoids: A Pioneering Model for Kidney Diseases. *Transl. Res.* **2022**, *250*, 1–17. [CrossRef] [PubMed]
23. Xin, Y.; Liu, Y.; Liu, L.; Wang, X.; Wang, D.; Song, Y.; Shen, L.; Liu, Y.; Liu, Y.; Peng, Y.; et al. Dynamic Changes in the Real-Time Glomerular Filtration Rate and Kidney Injury Markers in Different Acute Kidney Injury Models. *J. Transl. Med.* **2024**, *22*, 857. [CrossRef]
24. Sancho-Martínez, S.M.; Blanco-Gozalo, V.; Quiros, Y.; Prieto-García, L.; Montero-Gómez, M.J.; Docherty, N.G.; Martínez-Salgado, C.; Morales, A.I.; López-Novoa, J.M.; López-Hernández, F.J. Impaired Tubular Reabsorption Is the Main Mechanism Explaining Increases in Urinary NGAL Excretion Following Acute Kidney Injury in Rats. *Toxicol. Sci.* **2020**, *175*, 75–86. [CrossRef] [PubMed]
25. Ku, T.; Li, B.; Gao, R.; Zhang, Y.; Yan, W.; Ji, X.; Li, G.; Sang, N. NF-κB-Regulated microRNA-574-5p Underlies Synaptic and Cognitive Impairment in Response to Atmospheric $PM_{2.5}$ Aspiration. *Part. Fibre Toxicol.* **2017**, *14*, 34. [CrossRef] [PubMed]
26. Xing, Q.; Wu, M.; Chen, R.; Liang, G.; Duan, H.; Li, S.; Wang, Y.; Wang, L.; An, C.; Qin, G.; et al. Comparative Studies on Regional Variations in $PM_{2.5}$ in the Induction of Myocardial Hypertrophy in Mice. *Sci. Total. Environ.* **2021**, *775*, 145179. [CrossRef] [PubMed]
27. Hou, Y.; Yan, W.; Guo, L.; Li, G.; Sang, N. Prenatal $PM_{2.5}$ Exposure Impairs Spatial Learning and Memory in Male Mice Offspring: From Transcriptional Regulation to Neuronal Morphogenesis. *Part. Fibre Toxicol.* **2023**, *20*, 13. [CrossRef] [PubMed]
28. Rivera-Caravaca, J.M.; Ruiz-Nodar, J.M.; Tello-Montoliu, A.; Esteve-Pastor, M.A.; Quintana-Giner, M.; Véliz-Martínez, A.; Orenes-Piñero, E.; Romero-Aniorte, A.I.; Vicente-Ibarra, N.; Pernias-Escrig, V.; et al. Disparities in the Estimation of Glomerular Filtration Rate According to Cockcroft-Gault, Modification of Diet in Renal Disease-4, and Chronic Kidney Disease Epidemiology Collaboration Equations and Relation With Outcomes in Patients With Acute Coronary Syndrome. *J. Am. Heart Assoc.* **2018**, *7*, e008725. [CrossRef]
29. Kumar, B.V.; Mohan, T. Retrospective Comparison of Estimated GFR Using 2006 MDRD, 2009 CKD-EPI and Cockcroft-Gault with 24 Hour Urine Creatinine Clearance. *J. Clin Diagn. Res.* **2017**, *11*, BC09–BC12. [CrossRef]
30. Guo, Y.; Ji, S.; Rong, S.; Hong, W.; Ding, J.; Yan, W.; Qin, G.; Li, G.; Sang, N. Screening Organic Components and Toxicogenic Structures from Regional Fine Particulate Matters Responsible for Myocardial Fibrosis in Male Mice. *Environ. Sci. Technol.* **2024**, *58*, 11268–11279. [CrossRef] [PubMed]
31. Shekoufeh, A.; Hassanali, A.; Nazanin, S.J.; Mohammad Aref, B.; Jamileh, S.; Amirashkan, M.; Hossein, K.J. Effect of High Doses of Salep Aqueous Extract on Serum Levels of Urea Nitrogen, Creatinine, Uric Acid, and Kidney Histopathological Changes in Adult Male Wistar Rats. *Arch. Razi. Inst.* **2023**, *78*, 1451–1461. [CrossRef] [PubMed]
32. Mirsharif, E.S.; Heidary, F.; Vaez Mahdavi, M.R.; Gharebaghi, R.; Pourfarzam, S.; Ghazanfari, T. Sulfur Mustard-Induced Changes in Blood Urea Nitrogen, Uric Acid and Creatinine Levels of Civilian Victims, and Their Correlation with Spirometric Values. *Iran. J. Public. Health* **2018**, *47*, 1725–1733. [PubMed]
33. Paoin, K.; Ueda, K.; Vathesatogkit, P.; Ingviya, T.; Buya, S.; Dejchanchaiwong, R.; Phosri, A.; Seposo, X.T.; Kitiyakara, C.; Thongmung, N.; et al. Long-Term Air Pollution Exposure and Decreased Kidney Function: A Longitudinal Cohort Study in Bangkok Metropolitan Region, Thailand from 2002 to 2012. *Chemosphere* **2022**, *287*, 132117. [CrossRef] [PubMed]
34. Wu, Y.-H.; Wu, C.-D.; Chung, M.-C.; Chen, C.-H.; Wu, L.-Y.; Chung, C.-J.; Hsu, H.-T. Long-Term Exposure to Fine Particulate Matter and the Deterioration of Estimated Glomerular Filtration Rate: A Cohort Study in Patients With Pre-End-Stage Renal Disease. *Front. Public Health* **2022**, *10*, 858655. [CrossRef]
35. Nolin, T.D.; Himmelfarb, J. Mechanisms of Drug-Induced Nephrotoxicity. In *Adverse Drug Reactions*, 1st ed.; Springer: Berlin/Heidelberg, Germany, 2010; pp. 111–130. [CrossRef]
36. Kanbay, M.; Copur, S.; Bakir, C.N.; Covic, A.; Ortiz, A.; Tuttle, K.R. Glomerular Hyperfiltration as a Therapeutic Target for CKD. *Nephrol Dial Transpl.* **2024**, *39*, 1228–1238. [CrossRef]
37. Oz-Sig, O.; Kara, O.; Erdogan, H. Microalbuminuria and Serum Cystatin C in Prediction of Early-Renal Insufficiency in Children with Obesity. *Indian. J. Pediatr.* **2020**, *87*, 1009–1013. [CrossRef]
38. Chiarelli, F.; Verrotti, A.; Morgese, G. Glomerular Hyperfiltration Increases the Risk of Developing Microalbuminuria in Diabetic Children. *Pediatr. Nephrol.* **1995**, *9*, 154–158. [CrossRef] [PubMed]
39. Pérez-Gomez, A.; Diaz-Tocados, J.M.; Coral, J.D.D.; Enriquez, M.C.; García-Carrasco, A.; Bardaji, A.M.; Revilla, J.M.V. #5799 Compensatory Hypertrophy of The Kidney Contributes to Loss of Klotho Kidney Through Pakt Signaling. *Nephrol. Dial. Transplant.* **2023**, *38*, gfad063d_5799. [CrossRef]
40. Yang, Y.; Xu, G. Update on Pathogenesis of Glomerular Hyperfiltration in Early Diabetic Kidney Disease. *Front. Endocrinol.* **2022**, *13*, 872918. [CrossRef]
41. Kataoka, H.; Mochizuki, T.; Nitta, K. Large Renal Corpuscle: Clinical Significance of Evaluation of the Largest Renal Corpuscle in Kidney Biopsy Specimens. *Contrib. Nephrol.* **2018**, *195*, 20–30. [CrossRef]
42. Toyota, E.; Ogasawara, Y.; Fujimoto, K.; Kajita, T.; Shigeto, F.; Asano, T.; Watanabe, N.; Kajiya, F. Global Heterogeneity of Glomerular Volume Distribution in Early Diabetic Nephropathy. *Kidney Int.* **2004**, *66*, 855–861. [CrossRef] [PubMed]

43. Stackhouse, S.; Miller, P.L.; Park, S.K.; Meyer, T.W. Reversal of Glomerular Hyperfiltration and Renal Hypertrophy by Blood Glucose Normalization in Diabetic Rats. *Diabetes* **1990**, *39*, 989–995. [CrossRef] [PubMed]
44. Daehn, I.S. Glomerular Endothelial Cell Stress and Cross-Talk With Podocytes in Early [Corrected] Diabetic Kidney Disease. *Front. Med.* **2018**, *5*, 76. [CrossRef]
45. Aztatzi-Aguilar, O.G.; Uribe-Ramírez, M.; Narváez-Morales, J.; De Vizcaya-Ruiz, A.; Barbier, O. Early Kidney Damage Induced by Subchronic Exposure to $PM_{2.5}$ in Rats. *Part. Fibre Toxicol.* **2016**, *13*, 68. [CrossRef] [PubMed]
46. Lin, C.-I.; Tsai, C.-H.; Sun, Y.-L.; Hsieh, W.-Y.; Lin, Y.-C.; Chen, C.-Y.; Lin, C.-S. Instillation of Particulate Matter 2.5 Induced Acute Lung Injury and Attenuated the Injury Recovery in ACE2 Knockout Mice. *Int. J. Biol. Sci.* **2018**, *14*, 253–265. [CrossRef] [PubMed]
47. Ji, X.; Yue, H.; Ku, T.; Zhang, Y.; Yun, Y.; Li, G.; Sang, N. Histone Modification in the Lung Injury and Recovery of Mice in Response to $PM_{2.5}$ Exposure. *Chemosphere* **2019**, *220*, 127–136. [CrossRef]
48. da Costa, P.L.N.; Wynne, D.; Fifis, T.; Nguyen, L.; Perini, M.; Christophi, C. The Kallikrein-Kinin System Modulates the Progression of Colorectal Liver Metastases in a Mouse Model. *BMC Cancer* **2018**, *18*, 382. [CrossRef]
49. Koumallos, N.; Sigala, E.; Milas, T.; Baikoussis, N.G.; Aragiannis, D.; Sideris, S.; Tsioufis, K. Angiotensin Regulation of Vascular Homeostasis: Exploring the Role of ROS and RAS Blockers. *Int. J. Mol. Sci.* **2023**, *24*, 12111. [CrossRef]
50. Regoli, D.; Gobeil, F. Critical Insights into the Beneficial and Protective Actions of the Kallikrein-Kinin System. *Vascul. Pharmacol.* **2015**, *64*, 1–10. [CrossRef]
51. Hornig, B.; Kohler, C.; Drexler, H. Role of Bradykinin in Mediating Vascular Effects of Angiotensin-Converting Enzyme Inhibitors in Humans. *Circulation* **1997**, *95*, 1115–1118. [CrossRef]
52. Aztatzi-Aguilar, O.G.; Uribe-Ramírez, M.; Arias-Montaño, J.A.; Barbier, O.; De Vizcaya-Ruiz, A. Acute and Subchronic Exposure to Air Particulate Matter Induces Expression of Angiotensin and Bradykinin-Related Genes in the Lungs and Heart: Angiotensin-II Type-I Receptor as a Molecular Target of Particulate Matter Exposure. *Part. Fibre Toxicol.* **2015**, *12*, 17. [CrossRef] [PubMed]
53. Kang, E.; Yim, H.E.; Nam, Y.J.; Jeong, S.H.; Kim, J.-A.; Lee, J.-H.; Son, M.H.; Yoo, K.H. Exposure to Airborne Particulate Matter Induces Renal Tubular Cell Injury in Vitro: The Role of Vitamin D Signaling and Renin-Angiotensin System. *Heliyon* **2022**, *8*, e10184. [CrossRef] [PubMed]
54. Pahlitzsch, T.; Liu, Z.Z.; Al-Masri, A.; Braun, D.; Dietze, S.; Persson, P.B.; Schunck, W.-H.; Blum, M.; Kupsch, E.; Ludwig, M.; et al. Hypoxia-Reoxygenation Enhances Murine Afferent Arteriolar Vasoconstriction by Angiotensin II. *Am. J. Physiol. Renal. Physiol.* **2018**, *314*, F430–F438. [CrossRef] [PubMed]
55. Königshausen, E.; Zierhut, U.M.; Ruetze, M.; Potthoff, S.A.; Stegbauer, J.; Woznowski, M.; Quack, I.; Rump, L.C.; Sellin, L. Angiotensin II Increases Glomerular Permeability by β-Arrestin Mediated Nephrin Endocytosis. *Sci. Rep.* **2016**, *6*, 39513. [CrossRef] [PubMed]
56. Axelsson, J.; Rippe, A.; Oberg, C.M.; Rippe, B. Rapid, Dynamic Changes in Glomerular Permeability to Macromolecules during Systemic Angiotensin II (ANG II) Infusion in Rats. *Am. J. Physiol. Renal. Physiol.* **2012**, *303*, F790–F799. [CrossRef] [PubMed]
57. Castrop, H. Mediators of Tubuloglomerular Feedback Regulation of Glomerular Filtration: ATP and Adenosine. *Acta Physiol.* **2007**, *189*, 3–14. [CrossRef]
58. Osswald, H.; Mühlbauer, B.; Vallon, V. Adenosine and Tubuloglomerular Feedback. *Blood Purif.* **2008**, *15*, 243–252. [CrossRef]
59. Yu, W.; Sulistyoningrum, D.C.; Gasevic, D.; Xu, R.; Julia, M.; Murni, I.K.; Chen, Z.; Lu, P.; Guo, Y.; Li, S. Long-Term Exposure to $PM_{2.5}$ and Fasting Plasma Glucose in Non-Diabetic Adolescents in Yogyakarta, Indonesia. *Environ. Pollut.* **2020**, *257*, 113423. [CrossRef]
60. Li, R.; Sun, Q.; Lam, S.M.; Chen, R.; Zhu, J.; Gu, W.; Zhang, L.; Tian, H.; Zhang, K.; Chen, L.-C.; et al. Sex-Dependent Effects of Ambient $PM_{2.5}$ Pollution on Insulin Sensitivity and Hepatic Lipid Metabolism in Mice. *Part. Fibre Toxicol.* **2020**, *17*, 14. [CrossRef]
61. Lang, F.; Görlach, A.; Vallon, V. Targeting SGK1 in Diabetes. *Expert Opin. Ther. Targets* **2009**, *13*, 1303–1311. [CrossRef]
62. Freitas, H.S.; Anhê, G.F.; Melo, K.F.S.; Okamoto, M.M.; Oliveira-Souza, M.; Bordin, S.; Machado, U.F. Na(+) -Glucose Transporter-2 Messenger Ribonucleic Acid Expression in Kidney of Diabetic Rats Correlates with Glycemic Levels: Involvement of Hepatocyte Nuclear Factor-1alpha Expression and Activity. *Endocrinology* **2008**, *149*, 717–724. [CrossRef]
63. Santer, R.; Calado, J. Familial Renal Glucosuria and SGLT2: From a Mendelian Trait to a Therapeutic Target. *Clin. J. Am. Soc. Nephrol.* **2010**, *5*, 133–141. [CrossRef] [PubMed]
64. Persson, P.; Hansell, P.; Palm, F. Tubular Reabsorption and Diabetes-Induced Glomerular Hyperfiltration. *Acta Physiol.* **2010**, *200*, 3–10. [CrossRef]
65. Vallon, V.; Thomson, S.C. The Tubular Hypothesis of Nephron Filtration and Diabetic Kidney Disease. *Nat. Rev. Nephrol* **2020**, *16*, 317–336. [CrossRef] [PubMed]
66. Gonzalez, D.E.; Foresto, R.D.; Ribeiro, A.B. SGLT-2 Inhibitors in Diabetes: A Focus on Renoprotection. *Rev. Assoc. Med. Bras.* **2020**, *66* (Suppl. 1), s17–s24. [CrossRef] [PubMed]
67. Schnermann, J. Juxtaglomerular Cell Complex in the Regulation of Renal Salt Excretion. *Am. J. Physiol.* **1998**, *274*, R263–R279. [CrossRef]
68. Vallon, V. The Proximal Tubule in the Pathophysiology of the Diabetic Kidney. *Am. J. Physiol. Regul. Integr. Comp. Physiol.* **2011**, *300*, R1009–R1022. [CrossRef] [PubMed]
69. Valdés, A.; Castro-Puyana, M.; García-Pastor, C.; Lucio-Cazaña, F.J.; Marina, M.L. Time-Series Proteomic Study of the Response of HK-2 Cells to Hyperglycemic, Hypoxic Diabetic-like Milieu. *PLoS ONE* **2020**, *15*, e0235118. [CrossRef]

70. Kious, K.W.; Savage, K.A.; Twohey, S.C.E.; Highum, A.F.; Philipose, A.; Díaz, H.S.; Del Rio, R.; Lang, J.A.; Clayton, S.C.; Marcus, N.J. Chronic Intermittent Hypoxia Promotes Glomerular Hyperfiltration and Potentiates Hypoxia-Evoked Decreases in Renal Perfusion and PO_2. *Front. Physiol.* **2023**, *14*, 1235289. [CrossRef]
71. Packer, M. Mechanisms Leading to Differential Hypoxia-Inducible Factor Signaling in the Diabetic Kidney: Modulation by SGLT2 Inhibitors and Hypoxia Mimetics. *Am. J. Kidney Dis.* **2021**, *77*, 280–286. [CrossRef]

MDPI AG
Grosspeteranlage 5
4052 Basel
Switzerland
Tel.: +41 61 683 77 34

Toxics Editorial Office
E-mail: toxics@mdpi.com
www.mdpi.com/journal/toxics

www.ingramcontent.com/pod-product-compliance
Lightning Source LLC
Chambersburg PA
CBHW061559210926
51850CB00009B/2158
9783725856770